MAMMOGRAPHY – RECENT ADVANCES

Edited by **Nachiko Uchiyama**
and **Marcelo Zanchetta do Nascimento**

Mammography – Recent Advances
Edited by Nachiko Uchiyama and Marcelo Zanchetta do Nascimento

Published by InTech
Janeza Trdine 9, 51000 Rijeka, Croatia

Publishing Process Manager Bojan Rafaj

Technical Editor Teodora Smiljanic

Cover Designer InTech Design Team

Additional hard copies can be obtained from orders@intechopen.com

Mammography – Recent Advances,
Edited by Nachiko Uchiyama and Marcelo Zanchetta do Nascimento
p. cm.
ISBN 978-953-51-0285-4

For EU product safety concerns:
IN TECH d.o.o., Prolaz Marije Krucifikse Kozulić 3, 51000 Rijeka, Croatia,
info@intechopen.com or visit our website at intechopen.com.

Meet the editors

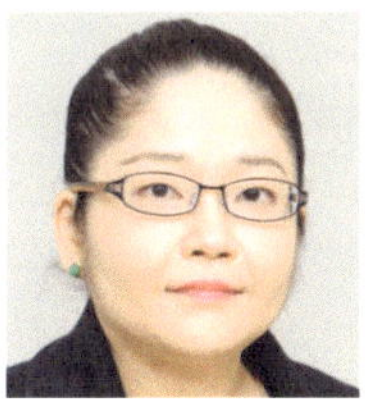

Nachiko Uchiyama M.D. graduated from Nippon Medical School, Tokyo, Japan in 1992 and was trained as trainee at Nippon Medical School from 1992 to 1994 and as resident and chief resident at Department of Diagnostic Radiology, National Cancer Center, Tokyo, Japan from 1994 to 1999. After residency, she worked as Assistant Professor at Department of Radiology, Nippon Medical School from 1999 to 2003. From 2003 to 2007, she worked as Staff and since 2007, has been working as Head of Staff at National Cancer Center, Tokyo, Japan. Board certifications are Radiological Society of North America, Japan Radiological Society, Japan Association of Breast Cancer Screening, Japanese Association for Cancer Detection and Diagnosis, The Japanese Society of Nuclear Medicine, and Certified Radiation Protection Supervisor, 1st Grade.

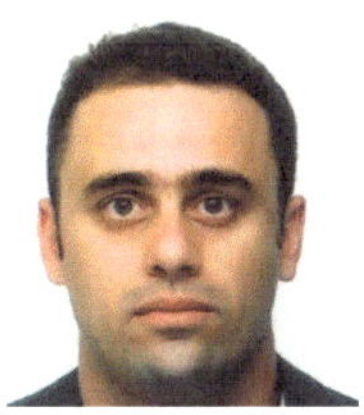

Marcelo Z. do Nascimento was born in Sao Jose do Rio Preto Brazil, in 1976. He received the high-level technologist degree from the University Center of Rio Preto, Sao Paulo, in 1996. He received his M.Sc. and Ph.D. in Electrical engineering from University of Sao Paulo, Sao Carlos, Brazil, in 2002 and 2005, respectively. Since 2006, he has been an Associate Professor of Center of Mathematical, Computation and Cognition, Federal University of ABC. His research interests include medical image processing, mammography, computer vision, and pattern recognition.

Contents

Preface

In this volume, the topics are constructed from a variety of contents: the bases of mammography systems, optimization of screening mammography with reference to evidence-based research, new technologies of image acquisition and its surrounding systems, and case reports with reference to up-to-date multimodality images of breast cancer.

Mammography has been lagged in the transition to digital imaging systems because of the necessity of high resolution for diagnosis. However, in the past ten years, technical improvement has resolved the difficulties and boosted new diagnostic systems. We hope that the reader will learn the essentials of mammography and will be forward-looking for the new technologies.

We want to express our sincere gratitude and appreciation to all the co-authors who have contributed their work to this volume.

Nachiko Uchiyama M.D.
National Cancer Center, Tokyo,
Japan

Dr. Marcelo Zanchetta do Nascimento
Universidad Federal do ABC, Santo André,
Brazil

Part 1

Optimization of Screening Mammography

1

Choice, Trust and Risk - The Policy Context and Mammography Screening

Karen Willis
University of Tasmania
Australia

1. Introduction

Mammography screening is now a well-established measure aimed at reducing mortality from breast cancer. However, while it is well established it is not without contention. Mammography screening has been the subject of fierce scientific debate about the evidence gathered using large scientific trials. There continues to be debate about the magnitude of benefit, issues of over-diagnosis, and the age at which screening should begin. These debates spill over into the policy arena where governments must decide which health measures to promote (and to fund). It is remarkable that policies about mammography screening differ between and within countries. This is particularly the case for policies establishing the age at which women should commence screening and the recommended interval between screening. Any policy decision about frequency of screening and lowering the age limit has resource implications and these must be weighed against the potential for benefit.

This chapter presents an international overview of the differing policy contexts in countries with mammography screening programs. It then explores the intersections between scientific knowledge, policy making and individual decision making with particular reference to the age at which screening should begin. Using research conducted with women in three different policy settings (two in Australian states and one in a Swedish county), it explores the differing ideas that form a crucial part of women's decisions to participate in screening. While most research focuses on women who don't participate in screening (there is a vast literature about the 'underutilisation' of mammography screening), we can learn much about health behaviour by talking with women who have chosen to be screened. This is particularly the case where screening is contentious.

The research at each of the sites comprised qualitative interviews with women aged 40-49 years who had participated in screening. Interestingly, the risk of breast cancer is not the main reason that women choose to be screened. For women in rural Uppsala, Sweden, trust in authorities was the dominant discourse; for women in rural Victoria, discourses of rights and choice predominated; and for women in rural Tasmania, trust in technology was a key reason for participating in screening. Women in rural areas also utilise services that are delivered in their local area because they highly value regional health services. These ideas are necessarily bound up in sociological concepts of choice, trust and risk. An understanding of these differing ways that women in different policy settings view the 'invitation to be screened' is an essential part of exploring what information women should receive about screening, and how they will respond to the provision of screening services.

2. The intersections between scientific and policy knowledge

In western developed countries, policies to reduce the mortality (and morbidity) from cancer have become a national health priority. Breast cancer is a major cause of mortality for women in many such countries, and the quest to reduce breast cancer mortality has seen early detection emerge as the leading policy strategy. The scientific evidence supporting early detection in the form of mammography screening is viewed as being strong – however, it is also contentious. The translation of scientific knowledge into public health policy is never a simple process, but this is all the more difficult when there is general agreement around the principle of early detection, but disagreement about factors such as the age at which screening should commence and screening intervals. The 'story' of the evidence surrounding mammography screening is quite well known. However, as is illustrated in the following re-cap of this story, scientific evidence alone doesn't provide all the required knowledge for successful policy implementation.

Randomised controlled trials are studies where the efficacy of an intervention is judged following random allocation of study participants into a study group that receives the intervention and a control group that does not receive the intervention. At the end of a specified period of time the results are compared. Evidence from such trials is regarded as 'the most scientifically rigorous method of hypothesis testing available in epidemiology' (Last, 1995: 140). Eight randomised controlled trials of mammography screening were conducted in the United States, the United Kingdom, Sweden, and Canada. The earliest of the trials was the Health Insurance Plan (HIP) of New York which was conducted in the 1960s (Shapiro et al., 1982). This was followed by Swedish trials commencing in the late 1970s and early 1980s: Malmö (Andersson et al., 1988), Two County (Tabár et al., 1985) and Stockholm (Frisell et al., 1991). At approximately the same time, a randomised controlled trial arm of the broader United Kingdom screening research commenced in Edinburgh (Roberts et al., 1990). Trials have been also been conducted in Canada (Miller et al., 1992a; 1992b), and Gothenberg in Sweden (Bjurstam et al., 1997). A trial in the United Kingdom from 1991 to 1997 aimed to identify the evidence of benefit for women below the age of 50 found a reduction of 17%, but this was not statistically significant (Baines, 2011). Proponents of screening mammography cite evidence from these trials that mass mammography screening as a population-based strategy reduces mortality from breast cancer by approximately 30% for women aged 50–74 years.

These findings have formed the scientific justification for breast cancer screening programs. The Australian policy setting can be used to illustrate the use of scientific policy and the broader political concerns that contribute to government decisions to establish a screening program. In the lead up to the introduction of the Australian screening program, the Screening Evaluation Coordination Unit (SECU) at the Australian Institute of Health conducted a review of the overseas evidence and reported to the Australian government on the feasibility of establishing a national breast cancer screening program (Australian Health Ministers' Advisory Council, Breast Cancer Screening Evaluation Screening Committee, 1990). In examining the scientific evidence, the SECU unit focused on the HIP and the Two

County trials as providing evidence of benefit. It also took into account other non-randomised trials that also showed a benefit from screening and included a discussion of the Malmö and United Kingdom (Edinburgh) trials which had not achieved statistical significance but had reported the potential for benefit from mass screening. Based on all the evidence considered, the SECU predicted that with a 70% participation rate in the targeted age group, the reduction in mortality from breast cancer would be around 16% (noting that this figure included non-participants and those outside the targeted age group) (Australian Health Ministers' Advisory Council, Breast Cancer Screening Evaluation Screening Committee, 1990: 26). The Australian policy documents reflect this claim by stating that an organised national screening program will result in a *significant* reduction in breast cancer mortality (National Advisory Committee for the Early Detection of Breast Cancer, 1992).

This review of scientific evidence was accompanied by feasibility research aimed at understanding issues associated with policy implementation. Feasibility studies, often in the form of pilot screening programs, were conducted in the five most populous Australian States. These pilot programs were aimed at applying the Australian context to the application of the selected scientific knowledge. Issues examined included strategies for encouraging women to participate in screening, psycho-social issues in implementation, analysis of the costs of screening, and technical aspects of service delivery.

Within the broader policy context in Australia, funding concerns also contributed to the need for a nationally organised program. The national universal health insurance program, Medicare, covered payments for diagnostic mammography for the relatively small number of symptomatic women (women with breast lumps or other potential signs of breast disease). However there was the perception that, increasingly, asymptomatic women were seeking to have mammograms. This blurring of the distinction between diagnostic and screening mammography (a population-wide program for well women) had the potential for a 'blow-out' of costs due to increased *de facto* screening mammography. Duckett (a former senior health bureaucrat and, from 1994 to 1996, secretary of the then Australian Department of Human Services and Health) points to the two aims of the mammography program: 'In addition to the health enhancement objective of promoting early detection of cancer and thus reducing breast cancer mortality, this program had the objective of moderating the previous rapid growth in expenditure on mammography' (1999: 81). Therefore, the decision to implement the screening policy seemed to bring together advocates arguing for the efficacy of reducing mortality from breast cancer, those establishing the feasibility of the programmatic aspects, as well as health bureaucrats concerned with expenditure.

Population based screening, however, is not without its critics. Since the incidence of the disease is much lower than in a diagnostic population, such screening programs require large numbers of well people to participate, in order to demonstrate effectiveness. For most people who participate in the mammography screening program, there will be no benefit, in terms of reduced morbidity or mortality. In a radio interview, one health bureaucrat encapsulated this aspect of screening programs by stating: 'It is a community action rather than an individual action and we can never, ever say to women that as individuals they individually will benefit' (Australian Broadcasting Corporation, 1998). In fact, at an individual level, for some women the outcome will be worse. The possibility of having a 'false negative' test result may mean that women are falsely reassured about the absence of breast cancer, a 'false positive' test result may subject women to a series of further tests, and the uncertainty resulting from indicators of benign breast disease may mean that treatment which is unwarranted will be recommended. Foster points out that, as a secondary prevention program, 'breast cancer screening cannot prevent breast cancer, nor can it promise a cure; it is rather an attempt to gain better control over the disease' (Foster, 1995: 116).

In addition to the criticism of the potential harm of screening as a population based strategy, there has been criticism calling into question the epidemiological evidence of benefit (for example, Schmidt, 1990). From the commencement of the promising reports about the possibilities of mammography, Dr Petr Skrabanek, a senior lecturer in community medicine at Trinity College in Ireland, maintained that the reduction in mortality was a substantial over-estimate of the evidence (Skrabanek, 1985). Dr Maureen Roberts (1989), who established the Edinburgh mammography program, argued that screening had not delivered the promised benefits in an article in the *British Medical Journal* published shortly after her death from breast cancer. More recently, following the Canadian study results, critics have focused on the lack of mortality benefit, the potential harm for women from the program in terms of over-diagnosis, and issues associated with screening asymptomatic, well women who have no breast problems. They claim that 'although politically attractive, the benefits of mass population screening, even in older women, are too small and the harm and cost generated too great to justify widespread implementation of screening mammography as a publicly funded health measure' (Wright & Mueller, 1995: 31). Further, in 1999, there was extensive media coverage in Sweden raising questions about the evidence from the trials, together with claims that the programs that have been implemented have not delivered the promised mortality benefits (Atterstam, 1999; Sjönell & Ståhle, 1999a; Gøtsche & Olsen, 2000). These critical voices, however, are not part of a vigorous and public debate about the efficacy of screening programs, rather emerging publicly only occasionally and generally dismissed by the central proponents of screening as 'ill informed', even endangering women's lives. As noted by Atterstam, the space for a critical point of view is minimal (1999: 1).

Ongoing debate has existed about the scientific evidence for screening women aged between 40 and 49 years. More recently, studies have attempted to ascertain the magnitude of benefit, but these results are contested. Commentary, dispute and refutation of claims from the Canadian trials that, in 1992, resulted in a questioning of benefit of population-based mammography screening continues ferociously almost 20 years later (Baines, 2011). The level of dispute also reveals the entrenched positions that various experts and commentators occupy in their reading of the scientific results from the trials. A recent review by Fletcher (2011) problematizes the changed landscape of screening, arguing that while it had its place as a secondary prevention measure, it is an 'imperfect tool' and that with progress in primary prevention and treatment, the need for screening should decrease. Such a message may be difficult to reconcile with the 'early detection is your best protection' message that forms part of the dominant discourse about breast cancer screening. That policies rest on dominant beliefs and often imperfect and uncertain science is evident when policies for breast cancer screening are explored.

3. Policy implementation and policy settings – an international overview

In arguing that policy is an ongoing process, rather than a finite event, Considine says, 'policy is the continuing work done by groups of policy actors who use available public institutions to articulate and express the things they value' (1994: 4). Understanding policy choices relating to mammography screening involves more than identifying who benefits and who loses. It is about understanding the dominant ways of thinking about an issue, the cultural dimensions of the issue, and whether policy players have their voices heard, or are excluded from the debate. Health policy is a broad area. In intervening in health at a policy level, governments are called on to undertake a variety of tasks relating to health financing for medical and hospital systems, as well as undertaking measures to redress health inequalities. Increasingly, governments are required to ensure provision for expensive high technologies in health and put in place programs to protect health. Texts analysing the politics of health and health policy portray the health system as complex, resource intensive and a site of much political contestation in the formal political arena (see, for example, Palmer & Short, 2010).

Palmer and Short claim that health policy is distinctive in three significant ways: first, the role of the dominant profession - the medical profession - in shaping policy direction is unprecedented in comparison to other policy areas; second, consumers are confronted with a complex arena of services where it is difficult to distinguish between 'good' and bad' services; and, third, the nature of health care means that decision making is often associated with life and death issues and, therefore, is psychologically stressful. This leads 'the community to see health care and its providers as being "different" (2010: 25). Accompanying this latter perception is the implicit assumption that consumers can trust health care providers, that governments will provide effective and efficient health care and that health care policies and innovations will have a sound basis in scientific research. This is particularly the case with policies involving technologies. However, the relationship between health care provision and research evidence is not clear cut (Davis & Howden-Chapmen, 1996).

As can be seen from the outline of evidence in the previous section, consensus about the evidence is widespread but not universal. Leaving aside the question of whether screening should be implemented at all, the lack of universal consensus is particularly important when governments and health authorities are deciding who they should be screening (i.e., the age at which screening should begin) and what the screening interval should be. These decisions are made combining a range of factors: resource implications and who should pay (it is more costly to extend the target group and to screen at shorter intervals); political implications (whether professional or consumer groups are demanding availability and access to services; where decision making fits within an election cycle); implementation implications including the structure of governance for health services and health workforce availability; geographical considerations; and how to access the target population groups - in particular whether active strategies for recruitment can be used or whether women are encouraged to self select into the screening program.

In addition to the issues identified above governance of a population based health program will affect the claims that can be made about its effectiveness in meeting targets. In many jurisdictions in western countries, two tiers of government are involved in policy direction and implementation. The roles that different levels of governments play in screening programs are diverse, with many devolving responsibility from a national government to state or county governments (BreastScreen Australia Evaluation, 2009). Thus, while the screening policy is decided at the national level, operational responsibility for the programs is devolved to levels of government such as states, territories, provinces or counties. This is particularly important to note in countries like Australia and Sweden where populations in various jurisdictions are low and may be dispersed. With different operational procedures, guidelines and recruitment strategies existing within countries, there is a risk of variation in population coverage, thus diminishing the capacity of the program to demonstrate overall population level benefits. In some countries, private providers coexist alongside the state services that are provided. Again, this has implications for determining policy parameters (such as eligibility and recruitment) as well as the determination of effectiveness.

In order to explore the differences in policy settings a desk top search was undertaken. It draws on two main sources - the international review of selected policy settings carried out by Australian policy makers (BreastScreen Australia Evaluation, 2009) (based primarily on stakeholder interviews) and the information provided by participating countries to the International Cancer Screening Network (2010) where English was available. In addition to the information provided, reports or publications of specific network members were downloaded, and further searching was undertaken where information was unclear (either by corresponding with member countries, further searching on participating country health websites, or through the academic literature). What emerges is a picture of considerable complexity. While generally established as government public health initiatives, there is a combination of public and private providers. The private sector plays a role in screening in a number of countries, with sole responsibility for parts of countries such as England and New Zealand. Objectives for participation are generally set at a national level (generally 70% of the total population, but 80% in England) with regions or specific services having operational responsibility. This brief description of the selected policy settings, with particular emphasis on the age at which screening is recommended or available, and where the information is available, the strategies for recruitment, highlights the differences in approach that exist both within and between different countries

Australia

Australia has a national government that determines policy but operational responsibility for service delivery is devolved to State/Territory governments. Screening is free of charge for women attending through the national program. In most (but not all) States/Territories, women aged 50-69 years are invited to attend screening at 2 year intervals. Invitations are based on the electoral roll (elections are compulsory in Australia); where access to the electoral roll is not possible, women are encouraged to attend for screening through advertising. In 2004-05, the participation rate for women in the 50-69 years target group was 56.2% (with variation between Australian states) (Australian Institute of Health and Welfare, 2008). Women aged 40-49 years can attend for screening, but whether, having attended, they will be invited back at 2 year intervals varies between individual states.

Canada

The Public Health Agency oversees the Canadian Breast Cancer Screening Initiative (Public Health Agency of Canada, 2008), but has less of a leadership role than other countries where national governments establish programs and devolve operational responsibility. Responsibility for mammography programs is devolved to the 12 Provinces/Territories, all of whom provide screening for women aged 50-69 years every two years. It is estimated that approximately 60% of women aged 50-69 years age group have had at least one mammogram (Hanson et al., 2009). All but three Provinces/Territories allow women to access the program from age 40 years. All programs allow women aged over 70 years to be screened. A range of strategies are used to invite women to participate - letters of invitation, media campaigns and referral from medical doctors. Policy documents indicate a reliance on doctors referring those women outside of the eligible age groups. In five of the Provinces/Territories, women aged 40-49 years are reinvited for screening on an annual basis; the remainder do not reinvite women in this age group.

England

England has a nationally coordinated screening program, but screening services are devolved to individual screening units in National Health Service (NHS) regions. Women aged 50-70 years are invited to attend and in 2004-05 overall 75% of women invited to screening attended (NHS, 2006). The invitations are based on general practice registers. Women are screened at three year intervals. Women aged over 70 years are able to continue to participate in the program if they wish to do so. From 2012, following the 'Age Trial' (Moss et al., 2006), that investigated the age at which screening should commence, women will be invited to attend screening from age 47 years.

Finland

Finland has a unitary government that provides an organised screening program based on a national population register. The target age group is 50-69 years and women are invited to attend screening when they turn age 50 years of age. In Finland there has been debate about the age range for mammography screening. Initially women aged 50-59 years received regular invitations to screening, and women aged 60-69 received 'irregular' invitations (depending on the municipality); from 2007 all women aged 50-69 have been invited to the free screening program. Participation in screening by the target population is very high, with 87.9% of women invited to screening in the past three years having participated (Palencia et al, 2010).

Ireland

In Northern Ireland women aged 50-70 years are invited to attend the screening program every three years. In the Republic of Ireland, women aged 50-69 years are invited every two years. Both programs are free. The register of eligible women is compiled using government and private health sources in addition to individual women registering. There is approximately a 73-75% acceptance of screening invitations in both Northern Ireland and the Republic of Ireland (Kinnear et al, 2010). Screening is provided via mobile and fixed site services.

Italy

With guidelines set at the national level, Italian mammography programs invite women aged 50-69 years to screening. The mammography programs are devolved to the 21 geographical regions and there are a total of 130 screening programs - 64 in the North, 39 in the Centre and 27 in the South and Islands. Some programs include women aged over 70 years. Since the commencement of screening programs some facilities include women aged 45-49 years as the national government has provided free biennial mammography for women in this age group. There are large differences in population participation between the regions, partially attributed to the fact that some programs in the Central and Southern regions have only recently been established, and due to dispersed populations some regions struggle to provide a biennial service to all women in the target age groups (Georgi et al., 2009).

Netherlands

Mammography is provided for all women aged 50-75 years of age. Women outside this age group may still access mammography, but the out-of-pocket expenses to do so will depend on their health insurance arrangements (all citizens are required to have health insurance). Approximately 84% of women invited to screening attend (Palencia et al, 2010).

New Zealand

Women aged 45-69 years are eligible to participate in screening in New Zealand, although the publicity materials emphasise that the greatest benefit is for women aged 50-69 years. For the two years up to December 2006, 60% of women aged 50-64 years had participated in screening, below the target of 70% and with high variation in participation between population groups (Thomson, Crengle & Lawrenson, 2009). Service delivery is devolved to eight regionally based lead providers, with funding responsibility the role of the central government. The private sector plays a key role in providing services. Women register for screening by phone or online. In some areas women are identified through general practice registers and are invited to screening.

Norway

Women aged 50-69 years are invited to be screened every two years. There are 26 stationary and 4 mobile screening units. The Central Population Registry of Norway is used to identify eligible women. Invitations are mailed to each eligible woman, suggesting a time for an appointment. Approximately 77% of all women invited participate do so (Kalager, et al, 2010).

Sweden

Sweden's central government has established mammography screening with delivery of mammography programs devolved to the 20 counties. While the two year screening interval is consistently applied, counties vary in whether women aged 40-49 years can access the program. The majority of counties invite women aged between 40-74 years to screening; six provinces invite women aged 50-69 years, and in a few cases the age range is slightly different again. Eligibility is based on the national population register. Screening is low cost, with women making a small co-payment for the service. The participation rate for women invited to screening is approximately 80% (Palencia et al, 2010).

United States of America

Guidelines for mammography screening in the Unites States of America emphasise the importance of clinical breast examination as well as mammography screening. While the Food and Drug Administration sets standards for mammography facilities, arrangements for screening are indicative of the health system more generally - where insurance coverage dictates recruitment and participation, and there is no organised national program beyond the setting of quality standards and guidelines for women. The United States Preventive TaskForce (2009) recommends mammography screening for women each two years commencing at age 50 years. Like the Australian policy context, the Taskforce emphasises that the decision to be screened between ages 40-49 years is an individual woman's decision and should be made taking account of personal beliefs about the benefits and harms. Various other stakeholders disagree with this advice and recommend screening from age 40 years. Women participate in screening through their health maintenance or health insurance organisations (although most states mandate that insurance companies reimburse all or part of the cost of mammography for their members). Uninsured and low income women aged over 40 years who qualify for Medicare health insurance are able to access a screening mammogram each year (with eligibility for a baseline mammogram between 35-39 years) (National Cancer Institute, 2010).

The selected international cases highlight the differences in policy in different health care settings. What is surprising is the level of scientific contention around the evidence particularly in relation to the magnitude of benefit for aged under 50 years. This plays out in differences within policy settings about women's participation in mammography screening. This is illustrated more clearly in the following section which reports on interview studies with women in three different policy settings who chose to participate in mammography screening.

4. Women's choice to be screened – different policy settings, different choices?

As previously stated, the age at which screening begins is a key site of policy difference, with the links between scientific evidence and policy knowledge unclear. The rest of this chapter focuses on this issue and explores the perspective of those women in different policy settings who have participated in screening programs while aged between 40-49 years. The aim is to highlight how embedded the policy context is in shaping what appears to be individual behaviour. Three policy settings have been chosen because their policy context differs for women aged 40-49 years. These three settings are two states in Australia and one county in Sweden. The first site is Tasmania. This island state is geographically isolated from the rest of Australia. It is a decentralised state. Of a total population of approximately 476,000 people, approximately 60% live outside the capital city of Hobart. The second site is the state of Victoria. Less decentralised than Tasmania, it has a population of 5.1 million people with 3.7 million people living in the capital city of Melbourne, but an extensive regional and rural hinterland that comprises 1.4 million people. The third site is Uppsala, Sweden. With a total population of approximately 336,000 people, Uppsala is also quite decentralised, with 40% of the population residing outside its major municipality.

The key difference between policy settings in Australia is whether they re-invite women in the 40-49 year age group once women have chosen to attend. As stated earlier, the Australian policy on screening targets women aged 50-69 years but allows women aged 40-49 years to make an individual decision about whether to participate in screening. Tasmania has a policy of reinviting women once they have attended once. In the more populous state of Victoria, women are not reinvited - rather they must make the decision themselves as to whether they continue to participate in screening while they are in the 40-49 year age group. Another key difference between these two states, relates to jurisdictional issues. Health providers in Tasmania are unable to access the electoral roll to call women to screening once they turn 50 years of age, relying on public information campaigns to encourage women to participate, whereas Victoria recruits women using the electoral roll. In both Tasmania and Victoria, mammogram facilities are provided both at fixed sites and through mobile services to rural areas. By contrast, the Swedish county of Uppsala actively invites women to screening at age 40 years, with a recruitment letter giving an appointment date and time for individual women to attend.

Of particular interest in this study was the decision making that rural women participated in when they decided to have a mammogram when aged 40-49 years. Rurality has been linked with poorer health outcomes and a key concern to policy makers in decentralised countries is how to best serve small populations in rural areas (Palmer and Short, 2010: 274). In each of the three policy settings examined, an emphasis has been placed on encouraging rural women's access either through mobile services (Tasmania and Victoria) or by locating mammography at smaller regional centres (Uppsala). Exploratory research in Tasmania found that screening rates in the 40-49 year age group were substantially above those estimated by BreastScreen Australia and in the Victorian setting were significantly lower. This indicates that perhaps some other factors related to rurality and the provision of services might be important in understanding women's decisions about mammography.

In order to examine women's decision making about mammography screening in these three different contexts, a qualitative study was designed. Using an interpretive methodological approach and a purposive sampling strategy, semi-structured interviews were conducted with women who had participated in mammography screening between the ages of 40-49 years. The interview schedule was in four sections. First, demographic information was obtained. Women were then asked about their ideas about health generally - the importance of health, and whether they took steps to maintain health. They were then asked about their screening history, their reasons for choosing to be screened, their ideas about mammography screening and their knowledge of contemporary debates about the age at which screening should commence. Finally, they were presented with some statements about mammography screening and asked whether they agreed or disagreed with them. These Likert questions were derived from the exploratory study originally carried out with women in the Tasmanian site (Willis and Baxter, 2003). While all questions (apart from the Likert scale questions) were open-ended enabling participants to reveal as much or as little as they wished, the schedule was designed to elicit responses from the broad ideas about health to specific information about their screening experiences. Where answers were unclear, additional probing questions were asked.

The interviews were audiotaped and transcribed verbatim. Analysis commenced with transcription of the first interview, ensuring that interviews were flexible enough to capture the important issues at each site. This was particularly important for those interviews carried out in Uppsala (see below). In both the Australian settings, the Chief Investigator interviewed all participants. In the Swedish study, the process differed a little because of the reliance on a Swedish interviewer (five interviews were conducted in English) and translation into English. This required attention to the ways that words and phrases are given meaning in the Swedish cultural context and how they could be best understood in English.

Interviews were analysed using a thematic analytical approach that incorporated both inductive and deductive elements. As the interview schedule had specific questions (outlined above), themes relating to reasons for attending were initially deductively derived from the data, but the contextual information presented by participants then allowed inductive exploration of these themes. Following transcription, each transcript was read, re-

Gorski, B., Tulinius, H., Thorlacius, S., Eerola, H., Nevanlinna, H., Syrjakoski, K., Kallioniemi, O. P., Thompson, D., Evans, C., Peto, J., Lalloo, F., Evans, D. G. & Easton, D. F. (2003). Average risks of breast and ovarian cancer associated with BRCA1 or BRCA2 mutations detected in case Series unselected for family history: a combined analysis of 22 studies, *Am J Hum Genet* 72: 1117–1130.

Autier, P., Boniol, M., Gavin, A. & Vatten, L. J. (2011). Breast cancer mortality in neighbouring European countries with different levels of screening but similar access to treatment: trend analysis of WHO mortality database, *BMJ* 343: d4411.

Bare, M., Sentis, M., Galceran, J., Ameijide, A., Andreu, X., Ganau, S., Tortajada, L., Planas, J. & of Sabadell Cerdanyola Research Group on Interval Cancers, B. C. S. P. B. (2008). Interval breast cancers in a community screening programme: frequency, radiological classification and prognostic factors, *Eur J Cancer Prev* 17: 414–421.

Barlow, W. E., White, E., Ballard-Barbash, R., Vacek, P. M., Titus-Ernstoff, L., Carney, P. A., Tice, J. A., Buist, D. S., Geller, B. M., Rosenberg, R., Yankaskas, B. C. & Kerlikowske, K. (2006). Prospective breast cancer risk prediction model for women undergoing screening mammography, *J Natl Cancer Inst* 98: 1204–1214.

Becker, G. S. (1964). *Human capital*, Columbia University Press, New York.

Berry, D. A., Cronin, K. A., Plevritis, S. K., Fryback, D. G., Clarke, L., Zelen, M., Mandelblatt, J. S., Yakovlev, A. Y., Habbema, J. D., Feuer, E. J., Intervention, C. & Collaborators, S. M. N. C. (2005). Effect of screening and adjuvant therapy on mortality from breast cancer, *N Engl J Med* 353: 1784–1792.

Berwick, D. (2005). *Translating new technologies into improved patient outcomes*, Saving women's lives. Strategies for improving breast cancer detection and diagnosis, National Academies Press (US), Washington (DC).

Berwick, D. M. (2003). Disseminating innovations in health care, *JAMA* 289: 1969–1975.

Black, W. C. (2000). Overdiagnosis: An underrecognized cause of confusion and harm in cancer screening, *J Natl Cancer Inst* 92: 1280–1282.

Carles, M., Vilaprinyo, E., Cots, F., Gregori, A., Pla, R., Roman, R., Sala, M., Macia, F., Castells, X. & Rue, M. (2011). Cost-effectiveness of early detection of breast cancer in Catalonia (Spain), *BMC Cancer* 11: 192.

Chen, J., Pee, D., Ayyagari, R., Graubard, B., Schairer, C., Byrne, C., Benichou, J. & Gail, M. H. (2006). Projecting absolute invasive breast cancer risk in white women with a model that includes mammographic density, *J Natl Cancer Inst* 98: 1215–1226.

Claus, E. B., Risch, N. & Thompson, W. D. (1991). Genetic analysis of breast cancer in the cancer and steroid hormone study, *Am J Hum Genet* 48: 232–242.

Costantino, J. P., Gail, M. H., Pee, D., Anderson, S., Redmond, C. K., Benichou, J. & Wieand, H. S. (1999). Validation studies for models projecting the risk of invasive and total breast cancer incidence, *J Natl Cancer Inst* 91: 1541–1548.

Cronin, K. A., Feuer, E. J., Clarke, L. D. & Plevritis, S. K. (2006). Impact of adjuvant therapy and mammography on U.S. mortality from 1975 to 2000: comparison of mortality results from the CISNET breast cancer base case analysis, *J Natl Cancer Inst Monogr* (36): 112–121.

Cummings, S. R., Tice, J. A., Bauer, S., Browner, W. S., Cuzick, J., Ziv, E., Vogel, V., Shepherd, J., Vachon, C., Smith-Bindman, R. & Kerlikowske, K. (2009). Prevention of breast cancer in postmenopausal women: approaches to estimating and reducing risk, *J Natl Cancer Inst* 101: 384–398.

Cutler, D. M. (2007). The lifetime costs and benefits of medical technology, *Technical Report 13478*, NBER Working Papers, National Bureau of Economic Research, Inc.

Domingo, L., Sala, M., Servitja, S., Corominas, J. M., Ferrer, F., Martinez, J., Macia, F., Quintana, M. J., Albanell, J. & Castells, X. (2010). Phenotypic characterization and risk factors for interval breast cancers in a population-based breast cancer screening program in Barcelona, Spain, *Cancer Causes Control* 21: 1155–1164.

Drummond, M. F., O'Brien, B. J., Stoddart, G. L. & Torrance, G. W. (1997). *Methods for the Evaluation of Health Care Programmes (2nd Edition)*, Oxford University Press, Oxford.

Duffy, S. W., Tabar, L., Olsen, A. H., Vitak, B., Allgood, P. C., Chen, T. H., Yen, A. M. & Smith, R. A. (2010). Absolute numbers of lives saved and overdiagnosis in breast cancer screening, from a randomized trial and from the Breast Screening Programme in England, *J Med Screen* 17: 25–30.

Ferlay, J., Autier, P., Boniol, M., Heanue, M., Colombet, M. & Boyle, P. (2007). Estimates of the cancer incidence and mortality in Europe in 2006, *Ann Oncol* 18: 581–592.

Feuer, E. J. (2006). Modeling the impact of adjuvant therapy and screening mammography on U.S. breast cancer mortality between 1975 and 2000: introduction to the problem, *J Natl Cancer Inst Monogr* (36): 2–6.

Finkler, S. A. (1982). The distinction between cost and charges, *Ann Intern Med* 96: 102–109.

Gail, M. H., Brinton, L. A., Byar, D. P., Corle, D. K., Green, S. B., Schairer, C. & Mulvihill, J. J. (1989). Projecting individualized probabilities of developing breast cancer for white females who are being examined annually, *J Natl Cancer Inst* 81: 1879–1886.

Gail, M. & Rimer, B. (1998). Risk-based recommendations for mammographic screening for women in their forties, *J Clin Oncol* 16: 3105–3114.

González-Páramo, J. M. (1994). *El sector público español: una aproximación a la panorámica actual. In: Gasto social y crecimiento económico en el estado de bienestar. Hacienda Pública Española Monografía n. 2*, Instituto de Estudios Fiscales, Madrid.

Gotzsche, P. C., Hartling, O. J., Nielsen, M., Brodersen, J. & Jorgensen, K. J. (2009). Breast screening: the facts–or maybe not, *BMJ* 338: b86.

Jorgensen, K. J. & Gotzsche, P. C. (2009). Overdiagnosis in publicly organised mammography screening programmes: systematic review of incidence trends, *BMJ* 339: b2587.

Jorgensen, K. J., Klahn, A. & Gotzsche, P. C. (2007). Are benefits and harms in mammography screening given equal attention in scientific articles? A cross-sectional study, *BMC Med* 5: 12.

Lee, S. J. & Zelen, M. (1998). Scheduling periodic examinations for the early detection of disease: Applications to breast cancer, *Journal of the American Statistical Association* 93: 1271–1281.

Lee, S. J. & Zelen, M. (2003). Modelling the early detection of breast cancer, *Ann Oncol* 14: 1199–1202.

Lee, S. J. & Zelen, M. (2008). Mortality modeling of early detection programs, *Biometrics* 64: 386–395.

Lee, S. & Zelen, M. (2006). A stochastic model for predicting the mortality of breast cancer, *J Natl Cancer Inst Monogr* pp. 79–86.

Lopez-Bastida, J., Serrano-Aguilar, P. & Duque-Gonzalez, B. (2003). Socioeconomic costs of cardiovascular disease and cancer in the Canary Islands (Spain) in 1998, *Gac Sanit* 17: 210–217.

Lowery, J. T., Byers, T., Hokanson, J. E., Kittelson, J., Lewin, J., Risendal, B., Singh, M. & Mouchawar, J. (2011). Complementary approaches to assessing risk factors for interval breast cancer, *Cancer Causes Control* 22: 23–31.

Mahnken, J. D., Chan, W., Freeman, D. H., J. & Freeman, J. L. (2008). Reducing the effects of lead-time bias, length bias and over-detection in evaluating screening mammography: a censored bivariate data approach, *Stat Methods Med Res* 17: 643–663.

Mandelblatt, J. S., Cronin, K. A., Bailey, S., Berry, D. A., de Koning, H. J., Draisma, G., Huang, H., Lee, S. J., Munsell, M., Plevritis, S. K., Ravdin, P., Schechter, C. B., Sigal, B., Stoto, M. A., Stout, N. K., van Ravesteyn, N. T., Venier, J., Zelen, M., Feuer, E. J., of the Cancer Intervention, B. C. W. G. & Network, S. M. (2009). Effects of mammography screening under different screening schedules: model estimates of potential benefits and harms, *Ann Intern Med* 151: 738–747.

Mandelblatt, J. S., Stout, N. & Trentham-Dietz, A. (2011). To screen or not to screen women in their 40s for breast cancer: is personalized risk-based screening the answer?, *Ann Intern Med* 155: 58–60.

Martinez-Alonso, M., Vilaprinyo, E., Marcos-Gragera, R. & Rue, M. (2010). Breast cancer incidence and overdiagnosis in Catalonia (Spain), *Breast Cancer Res* 12: R58.

Meltzer, D. (1997). Accounting for future costs in medical cost-effectiveness analysis, *J Health Econ* 16: 33–64.

Oliva, J. (1999). La valoración de los costes indirectos en economía de la salud, *Technical Report 9917*, Universidad Complutense de Madrid.

Oliva, J., Lobo, F., López-Bastida, J., Duque, B. & Osuna, R. (2004). Costes no sanitarios ocasionados por las enfermedades isquémicas del corazón en España, *Cuadernos Económicos de ICE* pp. 263–298.

Oostenbrink, J. B., Koopmanschap, M. A. & Rutten, F. F. (2002). Standardisation of costs: the dutch manual for costing in economic evaluations, *Pharmacoeconomics* 20: 443–454.

Ortún, V., Meneu, R. & Peiró, S. (2004). *El impacto de los servicios sanitarios sobre la salud*, Más recursos para la salud?, Masson-Salvat, Barcelona.

Parmigiani, G., Berry, D. & Aguilar, O. (1998). Determining carrier probabilities for breast cancer-susceptibility genes BRCA1 and BRCA2, *Am J Hum Genet* 62: 145–158.

Pauw, A. D., Stoppa-Lyonnet, D., Andrieu, N. & Asselain, B. (2009). Estimation of individual breast cancer risk: relevance and limits of risk estimation models, *Bull Cancer* 96: 979–988.

Pinto, J. L. (2001). *Cuánto vale la pena gastarse para ganar un año de vida ajustado por calidad? Un estudio empírico*, El valor monetario de la salud, Springer-Verlag, Barcelona.

Puig-Junoy, J. & Pinto, J. L. (2001). El coste de oportunidad del tiempo remunerado en la producción de salud, *Technical Report 39*, CRES-Universitat Pompeu Fabra.

Rauner, M., Gutjahr, W. J., Heidenberger, K., Wagner, J. & Paisa, J. (2010). Dynamic policy modeling for chronic diseases: metaheuristic-based identification of Pareto-optimal screening strategies, *Operations Research* 58: 1269–1286.

Roman, R., Sala, M., De La Vega, M., Natal, C., Galceran, J., Gonzalez-Roman, I., Baroja, A., Zubizarreta, R., Ascunce, N., Salas, D. & Castells, X. (2011b). Effect of false-positives and women's characteristics on long-term adherence to breast cancer screening, *Breast Cancer Res Treat* .

Roman, R., Sala, M., Salas, D., Ascunce, N., Zubizarreta, R., Castells, X. & Cumulative False Positive Risk Group. (2011a). Effect of protocol-related variables and women's

characteristics on the cumulative false-positive risk in breast cancer screening, *Ann Oncol* .
Rue, M., Carles, M., Vilaprinyo, E., Martinez-Alonso, M., Espinas, J. A., Pla, R. & Brugulat, P. (2008). Dissemination of periodic mammography and patterns of use, by birth cohort, in Catalonia (Spain), *BMC Cancer* 8: 336.
Rue, M., Vilaprinyo, E., Lee, S., Martinez-Alonso, M., Carles, M., Marcos-Gragera, R., Pla, R. & Espinas, J. A. (2009). Effectiveness of early detection on breast cancer mortality reduction in Catalonia (Spain), *BMC Cancer* 9: 326.
Sacristan, J. A., Oliva, J., Del Llano, J., Prieto, L. & Pinto, J. L. (2002). What is an efficient health technology in Spain?, *Gac Sanit* 16: 334–343.
Sala-i-Martin, X. (1992). Transfers, *Technical Report 4186*, NBER Working Papers, National Bureau of Economic Research, Inc.
Schousboe, J. T., Kerlikowske, K., Loh, A. & Cummings, S. R. (2011). Personalizing mammography by breast density and other risk factors for breast cancer: analysis of health benefits and cost-effectiveness, *Ann Intern Med* 155: 10–20.
Stout, N. K., Rosenberg, M. A., Trentham-Dietz, A., Smith, M. A., Robinson, S. M. & Fryback, D. G. (2006). Retrospective cost-effectiveness analysis of screening mammography, *J Natl Cancer Inst* 98: 774–782.
Tabar, L., Yen, M. F., Vitak, B., Chen, H. H., Smith, R. A. & Duffy, S. W. (2003). Mammography service screening and mortality in breast cancer patients: 20-year follow-up before and after introduction of screening, *Lancet* 361: 1405–1410.
Tice, J. A., Cummings, S. R., Smith-Bindman, R., Ichikawa, L., Barlow, W. E. & Kerlikowske, K. (2008). Using clinical factors and mammographic breast density to estimate breast cancer risk: development and validation of a new predictive model, *Ann Intern Med* 148: 337–347.
Tyrer, J., Duffy, S. W. & Cuzick, J. (2004). A breast cancer prediction model incorporating familial and personal risk factors, *Stat Med* 23: 1111–1130.
USPSTF (2009). Screening for breast cancer: U.S. Preventive Services Task Force recommendation statement, *Ann Intern Med* 151: 716–26, W–236.
Vilaprinyo, E., Gispert, R., Martinez-Alonso, M., Carles, M., Pla, R., Espinas, J. A. & Rue, M. (2008). Competing risks to breast cancer mortality in Catalonia, *BMC Cancer* 8: 331.
Vilaprinyo, E., Rue, M., Marcos-Gragera, R. & Martinez-Alonso, M. (2009). Estimation of age- and stage-specific Catalan breast cancer survival functions using US and Catalan survival data, *BMC Cancer* 9: 98.
Weinstein, M. C. (1990). Principles of cost-effective resource allocation in health care organizations, *Int J Technol Assess Health Care* 6: 93–103.
Xu, J. L. & Prorok, P. C. (1995). Non-parametric estimation of the post-lead-time survival distribution of screen-detected cancer cases, *Stat Med* 14: 2715–2725.
Zahl, P. H., Maehlen, J. & Welch, H. G. (2008). The natural history of invasive breast cancers detected by screening mammography, *Arch Intern Med* 168: 2311–6.
Zelen, M. & Feinleib, M. (1969). On the theory of screening for chronic diseases, *Biometrika* 56: 601–614.
Zelen, M. & Lee, S. J. (2002). Models and the early detection of disease: methodological considerations, *Cancer Treat Res* 113: 1–18.

4

Effects of Health Belief and Cancer Fatalism on the Practice of Breast Cancer Screening Among Nigerian Women

Adenike Akhigbe and Kingsley Akhigbe
University of Benin Medical School
Nigeria

1. Introduction

Breast cancer has been reported as the highest cause of cancer deaths amongst women worldwide. The incidence and prevalence of cancer is rapidly increasing in the developed and developing countries. More than 10 million people are diagnosed with cancer every year. It is estimated that there will be 15 million new cases every year by 2020 (Horton, 2006)

Rising incidence of breast cancer as well as earlier age of presentation has been reported in developing countries. Since no cure has been found for breast cancer, early diagnosis and early treatment have been found to yield a better survival rate.

There is now strong evidence that an individual's risk of developing cancer can be substantially reduced by healthy behavior such as participating in cancer screening according to recommended guidelines. The American Cancer Society posits that if we can effectively promote healthy behaviors, much of the suffering and death from cancer can be prevented or reduced (American Cancer Society, 2002).

However, poor practice of breast cancer screening methods has been reported in many studies in Nigeria (Akhigbe & Omuemu, 2009; Okobia *et al*, 2006). Beyond poor knowledge, or ignorance, several other factors have been found to influence the practice of breast cancer screening in different countries, including Nigeria.

In Nigeria, late presentation has been described as the hallmark of breast cancer and reasons given include poverty, under-education, lack of knowledge and poor access to care (Akhigbe & Omuemu, 2009; Okobia *et al*, 2006; Atoyebi *et al*, 1997). However, studies have shown that even when these factors are statistically controlled, African-Americans are still less likely to participate in cancer screening (Powe 1996). It was therefore concluded that other factors such as cultural values and beliefs may operate independent of variables such as poverty and education in affecting the decision to go for screening.

Health beliefs differ from culture to culture. In Nigeria, beliefs are usually influenced by cultural and religious values, which in turn influence health behavior such as response to screening awareness campaigns.

The Health Belief Model (HBM) has been used as a theoretical framework to study Breast Self-Examination and other breast cancer detection behaviors. The model stipulates that health-related behavior is influenced by a person's perception of the threat posed by a health problem and by the value associated with his or her action to reduce that threat (Champion *et al,* 1997).

Cancer fatalism, the belief that death is inevitable when cancer is present has also been identified as a barrier to participation in cancer screening, detection and treatment. Cancer fatalism is believed to be the result of cultural, historical and socioeconomic factors that have influenced the lived experience of African-Americans (Powe, 1996).

Nigeria is the most populous black African nation and breast cancer screening practice has been extremely poor. As has been found in other parts of the world, people of African origin are less likely to participate in cancer screening programs. (Powe, 1996) Breast cancer tends to be discovered in the later stages, when treatment options are limited and mortality rates increase, which is similar to reports in Nigeria.

If we are to develop materials for educational intervention, they have to be culturally sensitive as the goal of such a drive will be to increase breast cancer knowledge, decrease cancer fatalism and improve participation in breast cancer screening among Nigerian women.

Health beliefs and fatalism have been studied in various populations as means of identifying other strategies to help promote positive health behaviors, such as cancer screening. There is limited information concerning such a study in Nigeria.

1.1 Health belief model

The Health Belief Model (HBM) is by far the most commonly used theory in health education and health promotion (Glanz, Rimer, & Lewis, 2002).

The HBM is a method used to evaluate and explain individual differences in preventative health behavior (Janz *et al,* 2002). The HBM has had the greatest influence in research related to prediction associated with breast cancer screening behaviors; several studies have used the HBM to understand breast cancer screening behaviors. The HBM model subscales measure six concepts, including perceived susceptibility, perceived seriousness, barriers, benefits, health motivation, and confidence (Champion 1999).

1.1.1 Perceived susceptibility

As the first component of the HBM, perceived susceptibility is defined as a subjective perception of the risk of an illness. One's belief regarding the chances of being diagnosed with a medical condition can be applied by defining populations at risk and risk levels (Janz et al., 2002). Individual risk may be based on personal characteristics or behavior. Comparisons of perceived susceptibility with action risk can also be conducted (Janz et al., 2002). Related to breast cancer screening behaviors, perceived susceptibility may include the risk of a breast cancer diagnosis in the long term or immediate future.

1.1.2 Perceived severity

Perceived severity, formerly called perceived "seriousness" is the second construct of the HBM. Perceived severity speaks to an individual's belief about the severity or seriousness of a disease and the sequence of events after diagnosis and personal feelings related to the consequences of a specific medical condition (Janz,Champion, & Stretcher, 2002). Possible medical consequences may include death, disability, and pain; possible social consequences consist of effects on work, family life, and social relations (Janz et al., 2002).The combination of perceived susceptibility and perceived severity has been labeled perceived threat.

1.1.3 Perceived benefits

The construct of perceived benefits is a person's opinion of the value or usefulness of a new behavior in decreasing the risk of developing a disease. Also termed as perceived benefits of taking health action, the attitudes of health behavior changes are reliant on one's view of the health benefits for performing a health action (Janz et al.,2002). Perceived benefits play a significant role in the adoption of secondary preventive behaviours, such as screenings. It is widely known and accepted that the earlier breast cancer is found, the greater the chances of survival. It is also known that breast self-examination (BSE), when done regularly, can be an effective means of early detection. But not all women do BSE regularly. They have to believe there is a benefit in adopting this behavior, which is exactly what was found to be true among black women: those who believed breast self-examinations were beneficial did them more frequently (Graham, 2002).

1.1.4 Perceived barriers

Perceived barriers refer to the potential negative aspects of or obstructions to taking a recommended health action. This is the belief about physical and psychological costs of taking health action (Janz et al., 2002). An internal cost benefit analysis occurs, weighing the health action's expected effectiveness against perceptions that it may become an obstacle. Potential barriers may include financial expense, danger, pain, difficulty, upset, inconvenience, and time-consumption (Janz et al., 2002). Perceived barriers to performing breast cancer screening behaviors were emotional, social, and physical.

Even when women know that breast cancer is a serious disease, and one for which women are at risk and one for which the perception of threat is high, the barriers to performing BSE exert a greater influence over the behavior than does the threat of cancer itself (Champion, 1993; Champion & Menon, 1997; Umeh & Rogan-Gibson, 2001). Some of these barriers include difficulty with starting a new behavior or developing a new habit, fear of not being able to perform BSE correctly, having to give up things in order to do BSE, and embarrassment (Umeh & Rogan-Gibson, 2001).

1.1.5 Self-efficacy

Self-efficacy was added to the original four beliefs of the HBM in 1988 (Rosenstock, Strecher, & Becker, 1988). Self-efficacy is the belief in one's own ability to do something (Bandura, 1977). If a person believes a new behavior is useful (perceived benefit), but does not think he or she is capable of doing it (perceived barrier), chances are that it will not be tried. According to Umeh & Rogan-Gibson (2001), a significant factor in not performing BSE is fear of being unable to perform BSE correctly. In other words, unless a woman believes she is capable of performing BSE (that is, has BSE self-efficacy), this barrier will not be overcome and BSE will not be done.

1.1.6 Cues to action

Cues to action, formerly known as motivation, are events, people, or things that move people to change their behavior. Examples of cues include media reports about preventing breast cancer, illness of a family member, and perceived benefits (Graham, 2002).

1.2 Cancer fatalism

Studies have revealed that fatalism may be a deterrent to participation in health promoting behaviours. Fatalism is the belief that all things in the world are under the control of some invisible force, and we are powerless to do anything about it. Fatalism is in general the view which holds that all events in the history of the world, and, in particular, the actions and incidents which make up the story of each individual life are determined by fate (Knight, 2003). Fatalism is the belief that situations, such as illnesses or catastrophic events, happen because of a higher power (such as God), or they are just meant to happen, and cannot be avoided (Talbert PY, 2008). Indeed, fatalism has a strong tie with religion.

Religious beliefs are particularly dominant among Nigerians, and together with a passionate confidence in God are such beliefs in fatalism, magic, witchcraft, and demons. Although Christianity and Islam have replaced traditional religions, the thoughts of the people about life, and their attitude to it, are still shaped by the old worldview. They exhibit this in their day-to-day interpersonal interactions (Jegede, 2002). These beliefs therefore remain, even in educated people long after their possible conversion to Christianity or Islam. As a result, fatalism remains a part of the average Nigerian's worldview. Worldview may be defined as the mental grid through which one sees the world (Sarma, 2007).

Cancer fatalism is a situational manifestation of fatalism in which individuals may feel powerless in the face of cancer and may view a diagnosis of cancer as a struggle against insurmountable odds (Powe & Johnson, 1995).

This study therefore seeks to understand the perception of Nigerian women about breast cancer screening using the health beliefs model with the subscales of perceived susceptibility, perceived severity, perceived benefits and barriers as well as self-efficacy and cues to action, including cancer fatalism.

1.3 Hypotheses

1. There is no significant relationship between the practice of breast self-examination and perceived barriers.
2. There is no significant relationship between participants' use of mammography and perceived barriers.
3. There is no significant association between breast cancer fatalism and breast self-examination.

2. Methodology

This study employed a descriptive correlation design, with health beliefs and cancer fatalism operationalized by the participants' responses to Champion's Health Belief Model Scale and Powe's Cancer Fatalism Scale respectively.

The study evaluated the effects of health belief and cancer fatalism on the practice of breast cancer screening among educated Nigerian women. The dependent variables were breast self-examination and mammography. The independent variables were the components of the health belief model, and cancer fatalism.

2.1 Data collection

Purposive sampling was employed in recruiting two hundred and twenty five participants from among female health professionals (consisting of medical doctors, nurses, pharmacists and radiographers) in the Teaching Hospital and female teachers in secondary schools in the Benin City metropolis, aged between 30 and 60. The choice of purposive sampling technique "ensures that only elements relevant to the research are included and guarantees that extra care is taken to select those elements that satisfy the requirements of the research" (Nworgu, 1991). Informed consent was obtained and participants were assured confidentiality of responses. Participation meant responding to a questionnaire soliciting demographic information as well as the Champion's Health Belief Model Scale and the Powe Cancer Fatalism Scale.

2.2 Instruments

Champion's Health Belief Model Scale: HBM scales for measuring beliefs related to breast cancer were assessed for content validity by a panel of three health educators who are familiar with the HBM and breast cancer screenings. It was agreed that the first item in the subscale of perceived susceptibility (*It is extremely likely I will get breast cancer in the future*) might meet with a strong denial by the average Nigerian woman. A pilot testing of the instrument subsequently revealed two items in the Health Belief Model scale that considerably lowered the internal consistency of the subscales. Together with an item in the Cues to action subscale (*I have regular health check-ups even when I am not sick*), these two items were excluded. All HBM scales were measured on a five-point Likert type scale with the following coding: strongly disagree (1); disagree (2); neutral (3); agree (4); and strongly agree (5).

Powe Cancer Fatalism Scale: Participants' level of breast cancer fatalism was assessed with the Powe Cancer Fatalism Scale (Powe, 1995). The Inventory is a 15-item questionnaire based on the philosophic origins and attributes of cancer fatalism (fear, predetermination, pessimism, inevitable death), with a Yes or No response. Each "Yes" response was scored as one point and a "No" response as zero, giving the possible range of scores from 0 to 15.

Higher scores on the Powe Scale reflect higher degrees of fatalism. A score of zero to five indicates a low degree of fatalism, scores from six to ten indicate a moderate degree of fatalism, and scores from eleven to fifteen reflect a high degree of fatalism. In a study aimed at differentiating higher versus lower levels of cancer fatalism among a sample of African American women, Powe (2001) selected a mean score of 8 as a cut-off point, coding scores of 0 to 8 as low cancer fatalism and scores 9 to 15 as high cancer fatalism. In this study, a cut-off point determined by median split was used to classify participants as "High" and "Low" Breast Cancer Fatalism individuals. Participants with scores equal to or greater than 13 were categorized as "High Fatalism" individuals and those whose scores on this scale were below 13 were classified as "Low Fatalism" individuals.

The Statistical Package for the Social Science (SPSS) computer software programme (version 16 for Windows) was used to conduct frequency analyses and correlations.

3. Results

Cronbach's alpha tests of reliabilities, conducted to assess the internal consistency of the six HBM subscales (i.e., susceptibility, severity, benefits, barriers, self-efficacy, and cues to action) and the fatalism scale are presented in Table 1. All alpha coefficients were in the .82 to .97 which suggests the instrument had acceptable to excellent internal consistency (DeVillis, 2003).

Subscales/Scale	Alpha Coefficient, α	No. of Items
Susceptibility	.90	4
Severity	.82	5
Benefits BSE	.85	4
Benefits MAMMO	.82	5
Barriers BSE	.97	11
Barriers MAMMO	.93	11
Cues to action	.94	4
Self-Efficacy	.82	7
Powe Fatalism Scale	.94	15

Table 1. Cronbach's Alpha Reliabilities.

Demographic data

The survey population consisted of 225 women aged between 30 and 60 years who completed the survey instrument. Majority of the respondents (83.1%) were between 30 - 49 years of age. Most (95.1%) were married.

Educationally, 55.1% had completed University education while 44.9% had post-secondary but not university education. Post-secondary education includes training schools for nursing, medical laboratory science, radiography as well as colleges of education. Until recently, most of these schools offered certificate or diploma courses. Their products work as nurses, laboratory scientists, radiographers and teachers in primary and junior secondary schools. Health professionals, including doctors, pharmacists, nurses, medical laboratory scientists and radiographers accounted for 24.9% of the study population, while the remaining 75.1% were secondary school teachers. Nigeria is a multi-ethnic nation and Benin City is the capital of Edo State where the Binis and Ishans constitute a sizable proportion of the population. The Binis/Ishans constitute 56.4% with the Igbos and Yorubas together with a string of closely related ethnic groups contributing almost equally to the study population. The southern part of Nigeria is predominantly Christian, hence 88.4% professed Christianity as their religion.

None of the respondents has ever been diagnosed with breast cancer but 7.1% reported that a family member or friend has experienced breast cancer. 35.6% of the respondents regularly do breast self-examination while 64.4% do not. Only a minute proportion of the study population (6.7%) has ever had a mammogram done, an overwhelming percentage has never had a mammogram done.

Characteristics	Number N = 225	Percent
Age (Years)		
30-34	59	26.2
35-39	46	20.4
40-44	52	23.1
45-49	30	13.3
50-54	20	8.9
55-59	18	8.0
Marital Status		
Single	34	15.1
Married	180	80.0
Divorced	5	2.2
Separated	2	.9
Widowed	4	1.8
Ethnicity		
Bini/Ishan	127	56.4
Igbo	31	13.8
Yoruba	35	15.6
Urhobo/Itsekiri/Isoko	32	14.2
Education		
Secondary	101	44.9
Post-secondary/University	124	55.1
Occupation		
Health Professional	56	24.9
Teacher	169	75.1
Religion		
Christian	199	88.4
Muslim	26	11.6
Has a family member or friend experienced breast cancer?		
Yes	16	7.1
No	209	92.9
Do you regularly do breast self-examination?		
Yes	80	35.6
No	145	64.4
Have you ever had a mammogram done?		
Yes	15	6.7
No	210	93.3

Table 2. Demographic Characteristics of Study Respondents (n = 225).

3.1 Health belief model characteristics

Participants were asked to indicate the degree to which they agreed or disagreed with statements related to perceived susceptibility, perceived severity, perceived benefits, perceived barriers, cues to action and self-efficacy of breast cancer screening.

3.1.1 Perceived susceptibility

Majority of the respondents had high scores on the Perceived Susceptibility subscale. 79.5% either agreed or strongly agreed that their chances of getting breast cancer in the next few years are great. Similarly, majority either agreed or strongly agreed they feel they will get breast cancer sometime in their lifetime (77.3%), and concerned about the likelihood of developing breast cancer (53.3%). Table 3 shows a profile of perceived susceptibility.

3.1.2 Perceived severity

Although majority of participants agreed with the statements: *Breast cancer would threaten a relationship with my boyfriend, husband or partner* (39.6%); and *If I developed breast cancer, I would not live longer than 5 years* (69.3%), many neither agreed nor disagreed with most of the perceived severity subscale items.

3.1.3 Perceived benefits of breast self-examination

An overwhelming majority of the participants either disagreed or strongly disagreed with the statements: *When I do breast self-examination, I am doing something to take care of myself* (75.5%); *Completing breast self-examination each month may help me to find breast lumps early* (77.1%); *Completing breast self-examination each month may decrease my chances of dying from breast cancer* (68%); and *If I find a lump early through breast self-examination, my treatment for breast cancer may not be as bad* (69.3%). This reflects low perceived benefits to all the items in this subscale.

3.1.4 Perceived benefits of mammogram

Majority of the respondents do not agree that mammography has benefits as follows: *When I get a recommended mammogram or x-ray of the breast, I feel good about myself* (54.3%); *When I get a mammogram or x-ray of the breast, I don't worry as much about breast cancer* (52.9%); *Having a mammogram or x-ray of the breast will help me find lumps early* (60.9%); *Having a mammogram or x-ray of the breast will decrease my chance of dying from breast cancer* (51.5%); and *Having a mammogram will help me find a lump before it can be felt by me or a health professional* (58.2%). Very few participants agreed with the statements, while many others neither agreed nor disagreed, as seen in Table 4

3.1.5 Perceived barriers to BSE

Participants were asked to indicate to what degree they agreed or disagreed with statements related to perceived barriers of breast cancer screening. On all the items in this subscale, participants were more in agreement with each statement. However, five items received remarkably higher agreement: *I do not feel I can do breast self-examination correctly* (50.2%); *Doing breast self-examination will make me worry about what is wrong with my breast* (52.3%); *My breasts are too large for me to complete breast self-examination* (83.1%); *My breasts are too lumpy for me to complete breast examination* (81.8%); and *I have other problems more important than doing breast self-examination* (57.8%).

Questions (N = 225)	Strongly Disagree / Disagree		Neither Agree / nor Disagree		Strongly Agree / Agree	
	N	%	N	%	N	%
Susceptibility						
My chances of getting breast cancer in the next few years are great.	37	16.4	9	4.0	179	79.5
I feel I will get breast cancer sometime during my life.	49	21.8	2	0.9	174	77.3
Developing breast cancer is currently a possibility for me	38	16.9	33	14.7	154	68.4
I am concerned about the likelihood of developing breast cancer.	67	29.8	38	16.9	120	53.3
Severity						
I am afraid to think about breast cancer.	81	36.0	65	28.9	79	35.1
Problems I would experience with breast cancer would last a long time.	72	32.0	63	28.0	90	40.0
Breast cancer would threaten a relationship with my boyfriend, husband or partner.	57	25.3	79	35.1	89	39.6
If I had breast cancer my whole life would change.	86	38.2	63	28.0	76	33.8
If I developed breast cancer, I would not live longer than 5 years.	42	18.7	27	12.0	156	69.3

Table 3. Frequency and Percentages of Participants Susceptibility and Severity Responses.

3.1.6 Perceived barriers to mammogram

Majority of respondents agree or strongly agree with most of the statements in this subscale but those who neither agree nor disagree were in the majority on the following: *It is difficult to get transportation for a mammogram or X-ray of the breast* (50.2%); *Having a mammogram or X-ray of the breast costs too much money* (42.2%); *I cannot remember to schedule an appointment for a mammogram or X-ray of the breast* (57.3%).

3.1.7 Self-efficacy

Majority of the participants disagreed with the following statements: *I am sure of the steps to follow for doing breast self-examination* (44.9%); *I am able to tell something is wrong with my breasts when doing breast self-examination* (49.7%); and *I can use the correct part of my fingers when examining my breasts* (50.7%). Fifty-four percent neither agree nor disagree that they could find a breast lump by performing breast self-examination (54.2%).

Questions (N = 225)	Strongly Disagree/ Disagree		Neither Agree/nor Disagree		Strongly Agree/ Agree	
	N	%	N	%	N	%
Benefits of Breast Self-Examination						
When I do breast self-examination, I am doing something to take care of myself	170	75.6	36	16.0	19	8.4
Completing breast self-examination each month may help me to find breast lumps early.	196	87.1	8	3.6	21	9.3
Completing breast self-examination each month may decrease my chances of dying from breast cancer.	153	68.0	30	13.3	42	18.7
If I find a lump early through breast self-examination, my treatment for breast cancer may not be as bad.	156	69.3	43	19.1	26	11.6
Benefits of Mammography						
When I get a recommended mammogram or x-ray of the breast, I feel good about myself.	122	54.2	71	31.6	32	14.2
When I get a mammogram or x-ray of the breast, I don't worry as much about breast cancer.	119	52.9	79	35.1	27	12.0
Having a mammogram or x-ray of the breast will help me find lumps early.	137	60.9	66	29.3	22	9.8
Having a mammogram or x-ray of the breast will decrease my chance of dying from breast cancer.	116	51.6	77	34.2	32	14.2
Having a mammogram will help me find a lump before it can be felt by [me] or a health professional.	131	58.2	47	20.9	47	20.9

Table 4. Frequency and Percentages of Participants Perceived Benefits Responses.

3.1.8 Cues to action

An overwhelming majority of the participants disagreed or strongly disagreed with all the statements in Cues to action subscale: *I want to discover health problems early* (71.5%); *Maintaining good health is extremely important to me* (80.5%); *I search for new information to improve my health* (85%); and *I feel it is important to carry out activities which will improve my health* (75.1%).

Questions (N = 225)	Strongly Disagree/ Disagree		Neither Agree/nor Disagree		Strongly Agree/ Agree	
	N	%	N	%	N	%
Barriers of Breast Self-Examination						
I do not feel I can do breast self-examination correctly.	50	22.2	62	27.6	113	50.2
Doing breast self-examination will make me worry about what is wrong with my breast.	88	39.1	42	18.7	95	42.2
Breast self-examination is embarrassing to me.	88	39.1	42	18.7	95	42.2
Breast self-examination takes too much time.	91	40.4	56	24.9	78	34.7
It is hard to remember to do breast examination.	103	45.8	40	17.8	82	36.4
I don't have enough privacy to do breast examination.	64	28.4	61	27.1	100	44.4
Breast self-examination is not necessary if you have a breast exam by a health professional.	43	19.1	79	35.1	103	45.8
Breast self-examination is not necessary if you have a routine mammogram.	62	27.6	68	30.2	95	42.2
My breasts are too large for me to complete breast self-examination.	22	9.8	16	7.1	187	83.1
My breasts are too lumpy for me to complete breast examination.	12	5.3	29	12.9	184	81.8
I have other problems more important than doing breast self-examination.	86	38.2	9	4.0	130	57.8
Barriers of Mammography						
I am afraid to find out there is something wrong when I have a mammogram or X-ray of the breast.	68	30.2	47	20.9	110	48.9
I am afraid to have a mammogram or X-ray of the breast because I don't understand what will be done.	38	16.9	56	24.9	131	58.2
I don't know how to go about scheduling a mammogram or X-ray of the breast	20	8.9	81	36.0	124	55.1
Having a mammogram or X-ray of the breast would be embarrassing.	25	11.1	67	29.8	133	59.1
Having a mammogram or X-ray of the breast would take too much time.	27	12.0	78	34.7	120	53.3
Having a mammogram or X-ray of the breast would be painful.	39	17.3	86	38.2	100	44.4
Having a mammogram or X-ray of the breast would expose me to unnecessary radiation.	58	25.8	82	36.4	85	37.8
It is difficult to get transportation for a mammogram or X-ray of the breast.	21	9.3	113	50.2	91	40.4
I have other problems more important than getting a mammogram or X-ray of the breast.	44	19.6	72	32.0	109	48.4

Questions (N = 225)	**Strongly Disagree/ Disagree**		**Neither Agree/nor Disagree**		**Strongly Agree/ Agree**	
	N	%	N	%	N	%
Having a mammogram or X-ray of the breast costs too much money.	67	29.8	95	42.2	63	28.0
I cannot remember to schedule an appointment for a mammogram or X-ray of the breast	26	11.6	129	57.3	70	31.1

Table 5. Frequency and Percentages of Participants Perceived Barriers Responses.

Questions (N = 225)	**Strongly Disagree/ Disagree**		**Neither Agree/nor Disagree**		**Strongly Agree/ Agree**	
	N	%	N	%	N	%
Self-Efficacy						
I know how to perform breast self-examination	94	41.8	66	29.3	65	28.9
I can perform breast self-examination correctly.	65	28.9	76	33.8	84	37.3
I could find a breast lump by performing breast self-examination	63	28.0	122	54.2	40	17.8
I am sure of the steps to follow for doing breast self-examination.	101	44.9	51	22.7	73	32.4
I am able to tell something is wrong with my breasts when doing breast self-examination.	112	49.8	31	13.8	82	36.4
I am able to tell something is wrong with my breasts when I look in the mirror.	92	40.9	56	24.9	77	34.2
I can use the correct part of my fingers when examining my breasts.	114	50.7	60	26.7	51	22.7
Cues to Action						
I want to discover health problems early.	161	71.6	53	23.6	11	4.9
Maintaining good health is extremely important to me.	181	80.4	41	18.2	3	1.3
I search for new information to improve my health.	193	85.8	32	14.2	0	0
I feel it is important to carry out activities which will improve my health.	169	75.1	36	16.0	20	8.9

Table 6. Frequency and Percentages of Participants Self efficacy and Cues to action Responses.

3.2 Fatalism scores

Majority of the participants were in agreement with all the items of the fatalism scale, with the following items having seventy-five percentile "Yes" scores: *I believe if someone is meant to have cancer, it doesn't matter what they eat, they will get cancer anyway* (69.3%); *I believe cancer will kill most people who get it* (76.4%); *I believe someone can smoke all their life, and if they are not meant to get cancer, they won't get it* (77.8%);and *I believe some people don't want to know if they have cancer because they don't want to know they may be dying from it* (82.2%). Total scores on the Fatalism Scale ranged from 0 -15, with means of 10.82 (SD = 4.35). Table 7 shows a profile of Fatalism scores.

	ITEM (N = 225)	**YES**		**NO**	
		N	%	N	%
1	I believe if someone is meant to have cancer, it doesn't matter what they eat, they will get cancer anyway.	156	69.3	69	30.7
2	I believe if someone has cancer, it is already too late to do anything about it.	135	60.0	90	40.0
3	I believe someone can smoke all their life, and if they are not meant to get cancer, they won't get it.	175	77.8	50	22.2
4	I believe if someone is meant to get cancer, they will get it no matter what they do.	146	64.9	79	35.1
5	I believe if someone gets cancer, it was meant to be.	138	61.3	87	38.7
6	I believe if someone gets cancer, their time to die is near.	115	51.1	110	48.9
7	I believe if someone gets cancer, that's the way they were meant to die.	105	46.7	120	53.3
8	I believe getting checked for cancer makes people think about dying.	136	60.4	89	39.6
9	I believe if someone is meant to have cancer, they will have cancer.	146	64.9	79	35.1
10	I believe some people don't want to know if they have cancer because they don't want to know they may be dying from it.	185	82.2	40	17.8
11	I believe if someone gets cancer, it doesn't matter when they find out about it, they will still die from it.	155	68.9	70	31.1
12	I believe if someone gets cancer a lot of different treatments won't make any difference.	144	64.0	81	36.0
13	I believe if someone was meant to have cancer, it doesn't matter what the doctor tells them to do, they will get cancer anyway.	143	63.6	82	36.4
14	I believe if someone is meant to have cancer, it doesn't matter if they eat healthy foods, they will still get cancer.	153	68.0	72	32.0
15	I believe cancer will kill most people who get it.	172	76.4	53	23.6

Table 7. Scores on the Fatalism Scale.

Hypotheses

Model	R	R Square	Adjusted R Square	Std. Error of the Estimate	Change Statistics				
					R Square Change	F Change	df1	df2	Sig. F Change
1	.478[a]	.229	.189	.43206	.229	5.744	11	213	.000

Table 8. Summary of regression analysis on breast self-examination and perceived barriers.

From Table 8 r = .478, f = 5.744, p > .001. This indicates a significant correlation. Therefore the hypothesis which stated that perceived barriers will have no effect on breast self-examination practice is rejected.

Mode 1	R	R Square	Adjusted R Square	Std. Error of the Estimate	Change Statistics				
					R Square Change	F Change	df1	df2	Sig. F Change
1	.415[a]	.172	.129	.23330	.172	4.020	11	213	.000

Table 9. Summary of regression analysis on mammography practice and perceived barriers.

From Table 9 r = .415, f = 4.020, p > .001. This indicates a significant correlation. Therefore the hypothesis which stated that perceived barriers will have no effect on mammography practice is rejected.

Lastly, there is no significant association between breast cancer fatalism and the practice of breast self-examination. These results indicate that there is no statistically significant relationship between breast cancer fatalism and breast self-examination practice X^2 (1, n = 225) = 2.39, p = .122, phi = .113 There is no association between breast cancer fatalism and breast self-examination.

4. Discussion

Majority of women see themselves as susceptible to having breast cancer and yet an abysmally low proportion does nothing to prevent breast cancer by adopting the standard screening practices. Lack of knowledge about preventative measures has been a frequent finding from studies in this environment (Akhigbe & Omuemu, 2009).

The scores on the perceived benefits of breast self-examination subscale reflect low perceived benefits. A low knowledge of screening methods for breast cancer, even among final year medical students had been reported in this environment (Akhigbe *et al*, 2009). The finding of low perceived benefits in the present study is therefore not surprising.

Participants generally do not recognise the perceived benefits of screening mammography. This may explain why mammography use is very low in the study population (6.7%). Previous studies (Odusanya & Tayo, 2001; Akhigbe & Omuemu, 2009; Akhigbe & Igbinedion 2010) have confirmed this low mammography usage in other populations in

Nigeria. There is as yet no national health policy concerning breast cancer screening but several health and advocacy groups have been calling on the relevant health authorities to formulate and implement such a policy. However, appropriate health policy even with government funding will not necessarily increase mammography usage; awareness has to be created and populaton at risk have to know what benefits they stand to gain from having screening mammography done.

The present study has revealed a high level of breast cancer fatalism among Nigerian women. It is therefore not surprising that the respondents who have shown high levels of perceived susceptibility still do not take preventative measures. It is like 'If it will happen, nothing can stop it from happening'. Powe (1996) observed that many factors affect a person's decision to participate in cancer screening; poor access to care, poverty, under-education, and lack of knowledge regarding cancer have a negative relationship to participation in cancer screening. Studies have shown that being African American is positively correlated with these factors, and that even when these factors are statistically controlled, African Americans are still less likely to participate in cancer screening. Could the findings among African Americans be a 'cultural carry-over' from their roots?

The present study appears to be highly supportive of the preceding conclusion. The academic and professional background of the study participants is clearly remarkable and above average, all of them working as either health professionals or secondary school teachers. They however have high scores in perceived susceptibility subscale of the HBM and very low score in the perceived benefits subscale; besides the practice of BSE and mammography is pitiably low. This poses a problem for working out appropriate, culturally relevant educational protocol for increasing breast cancer screening practices among Nigerian women. Having adequate knowledge of breast cancer and breast cancer screening methods is clearly not enough. Cultural barriers such as breast cancer fatalism will need to be overcome using appropriate educational intervention.

Three hypotheses were tested. The rejection of the first hypothesis shows that perceived barriers have a direct negative effect on the practice of breast self-examination among the study population. Previous studies have noted poor knowledge of breast self-examination practice as a screening method among Nigerian women irrespective of their level of education or professional status (Odusanya & Tayo 2001; Akhigbe & Omuemu 2009). From the item responses on the perceived barrier subscale, such factors as large breast size and inadequate self-efficacy in performing a breast self-examination constitute major barriers. Focused educational intervention remains the obvious solution.

The rejection of the second hypothesis shows that perceived barriers have a direct negative effect on mammography practice among the study population. There is a technology requirement for mammography practice. This makes economic consideration a veritable factor to overcoming this barrier. Unfortunately, health professional do not seem to fare better in their knowledge and practice of mammography, as this study and previous studies have consistently shown. There is therefore an urgent need for a review of training curricula by health institutions to include cancer awareness and screening methods. This may positively impact on the health behavior of those who are expected to teach others.

The third hypothesis was accepted, that is, there is no significant relationship between cancer fatalism and the practice of breast self-examination. Cancer fatalism is deeply rooted in ethno religious beliefs of the people. The individual, having resigned herself to fate or luck does nothing as prevention. Cancer fatalism, however, is a complex phenomenon with far-reaching implications (Powe & Finnie, 2003).

5. Conclusion

There is paucity of research publications on the effects of health belief model and cancer fatalism with regards to breast cancer among Nigerian women.

There is need to for us to understand the psychological and psychosocial barriers that deter Nigerian women from having adequate breast cancer awareness as well as routine screening. Such information will be useful in putting together culturally relevant awareness literature and media content that address these barriers.

From the health belief model, there are significant barriers that impact negatively on the practice of the two main screening methods, breast self-examination for which no tools or economic input is required, and screening mammography with the obvious advantages. Another significant finding is the high level of breast cancer fatalism among the study population. This represents a helpless resignation to accepting whatever the "death sentence" of breast cancer brings to the afflicted. Fatalism has remained a major cultural setback in this setting.

This study therefore represents preliminary findings that should form the basis for further research.

6. Acknowledgement

This research received no specific grant from any funding agency in the public, commercial, or non-profit sectors. Both authors declare that they do not have conflict of interests with this manuscript publication and gratefully acknowledges the women who participated in the study.

7. References

Akhigbe AO, Omuemu VO.(2009) Knowledge, attitudes and practice of breast cancer screening among female health workers in a Nigerian urban city. *BMC Cancer.* 2009 Jun 25;9:203

Akhigbe AO, Igbinedion BO, Ogbeide UO & Ikubor JE (2009) Final year medical students' knowledge about breast cancer risk factors and screening methods. *Journal of Medicine & Biomedical Research* 2009; 8(1): 49-57

Akhigbe AO & Igbinedion BO (2010) Pattern of utilization of mammography: experience from Benin City, Nigeria. *Nigerian Journal of Surgical Sciences.* 2010; 20(2):61-68

American Cancer Society. Cancer Statistics. CA: *Am Cancer J Clin* 2002; 52: 10-11

Atoyebi OA, Atimomo CE, Adesanya AA, Beredugo BK, da Rocha-Afodu JT: An appraisal of 100 patients with breast cancer seen at the Lagos University Teaching Hospital. *Nig. Qt J. Hosp. Med.* 1997: 7: 104-8.

Champion, V. (1993). Instrument for breast cancer screening behaviors. *Nursing Research*, 42, 139–143.

Champion, V., & Menon, U. (1997). Predicting mammography and breast self-examination in African-American women. *Cancer Nursing*, 20 , 315–322.

Champion VL (1999). Revised susceptibility, benefits, barrier scale for mammography screening. *Research in Nursing & Health*, 1999, 22, 341-348

Corsini, R. J. (1999). The dictionary of psychology. Philadelphia: Taylor & Francis Group.

DeVellis, RF (2003). Scale development: Theory and applications (2nd ed.) Thousand Oaks, California:Sage.

Glanz, K, Rimer, BK, Lewis, FM.. Eds. *Health behavior and health education: theory, research, and practice.* 3rd Edition. Jossey-Bass publishing, San Francisco, CA. 2002.

Graham, ME (2002) Health beliefs and self breast examination in black women. *J Cult Divers.*; 9(2):49-54

Horton J (2006). Breast cancer in 2020: What can we expect? *Cancer Detect Prev*, 30, 109-10

Janz, N. K., Champion, V. L., & Strecher, V. J. (2002). The Health Belief Model. In K.Glanz, B.K. Rimer, & F.M. Lewis (Eds.), *Health Behavior and Health Education:Theory, Research, and Practice 3rd Edition* (pp.45-66). Jossey-Bass. San Francisco,CA 2002.

Jegede, AS (2002) The Yoruba Cultural Construction of Health and Illness *Nordic Journal of African Studies* 11(3): 322-335

Knight, K. (2003). *The Catholic Encyclopaedia* (Vol.5), New York: Robert Appleton.

Nworgu BG (1991). *Educational Research: Basic Issues and methodology.* Wisdom Publishers Ltd. Ibadan

Odusanya OO, Tayo OO (2001) Breast cancer knowledge, attitude and practice among nurses in Lagos, Nigeria. *Acta Oncol.* 2001; 40(7):844-848

Okobia MN. Bunker CH, Okonofua FE, Osime U. Knowledge attitude and practice of Nigerian women towards breast cancer; a cross sectional study. *World journal of surgical oncology*, 2006: 4:11.

Powe BD (1995) Fatalism among elderly African Americans: Effects on colorectal screening. *Cancer Nursing*, 18(5), 385-392.

Powe BD & Johnson A (1995) fatalism among African Americans: philosophical perspectives. *J. Religion Health.* 1995;34(2):18-21

Powe BD (1996) Fatalism among African Americans: A review of the literature. *Nursing Outlook*, 44(1), 18-21.

Powe BD (1997) Cancer Fatalism – Spiritual Perspectives *Journal of Religion and Health*, 36 (2), 135-144

Powe BD (2001) Cancer fatalism among African American women: predictors of the intensity of the perceptions. *J Psychosoc Oncol.* 2001; 19(3/4):85-96

Powe BD & Finnie R (2003) Cancer fatalism -the state of the science. Cancer Nursing, 2003; 26(6):454-465

Rosenstock, I.M, Strecher, V.J., & Becker, M.H. (1988). Social learning theory and the Health Belief Model. *Health Education Quarterly*, 15 (2), 175–183.

Sarma BA (2007) Belief and Character: Theology and Ethics of Road Safety in Nigeria , *TCNN Research Bulletin* 48,13-27

Talbert PY (2008) The Relationship of Fear and Fatalism with Breast Cancer Screening Among a Selected Target Population of African American Middle Class Women *Journal of Social, Behavioral, and Health Sciences*,2008,2,96-110

Umeh K, Rogan-Gibson(2001) J Perceptions of threat, benefits, and barriers in breast self-examination amongst young asymptomatic women *British Journal of Health Psychology* (2001), 6, 361-372

5

Screening Mammography Need, Utilization and Capacity in Chicago: Can We Fulfill Our Mission and Our Promises?

Kristi L. Allgood[1], Garth H. Rauscher[2] and Steve Whitman[1]
[1]*Sinai Urban Health Institute, Sinai Health System, Chicago, Illinois,*
[2]*Division of Epidemiology and Biostatistics, University of Illinois at Chicago Chicago, Illinois,*
United States of America

1. Introduction

There is a widening Black:White breast cancer mortality disparity in Chicago (Figure 1). In 1980 the mortality rates were equal; by 2005 Black women were nearly twice as likely to die from breast cancer (Ansell et al, 2009; Whitman et al, 2011). This disparity has been increasing since the early 1990's because the breast cancer mortality rates for Black women in Chicago have remained constant while the rates for White women have decreased substantially (Whitman et al, 2011). Additionally, this disparity in Chicago is unusually high. For example, in 2005 the breast cancer mortality rate for Black women in Chicago was 43.2 per 100,000 population and the rate for White women was 21.8 per 100,000 population (Whitman et al, 2011). This equates to a rate ratio of 1.98 (43.2/21.8) which is interpreted by stating that in 2005 Black women were 98% more likely to die from breast cancer than White women in Chicago. More recent data suggests that Black women in Chicago are 62% more likely to die from breast cancer using the 2005-2007 three-year average (38.3/23.6=1.62) (Figure 1). Disparities are seen in other cities as well. For example, in New York City the Black:White breast cancer disparity in 2005 was 37% (Whitman et al, 2011). These data suggest that Black women in Chicago are not benefiting from the technological advancements that have been made in early detection and treatment over the last two decades (Berry et al, 2005; Smith-Bindman et al, 2006; Tehranifar et al, 2009).

In response to such data, health care providers, researchers, community leaders, educators, administrators and breast cancer survivors joined efforts to devise a strategy to eliminate the breast cancer mortality disparity in the Chicago area. As a result of a call to action, 111 individuals from 74 local institutions formed three working groups focusing on access to mammography, quality of the diagnostic process, and access and quality of breast cancer treatment. These three groups formed the Metropolitan Chicago Breast Cancer Task Force and outlined a plan consisting of 37 actionable recommendations to decrease breast cancer mortality for the metropolitan area of Chicago (Ansell et al, 2009; Metropolitan Chicago Breast Cancer Task Force [Task Force], 2007).

One of the three main goals of the Task Force was to implement interventions to increase the number of age-eligible women in Chicago who obtain regular screening mammograms. At

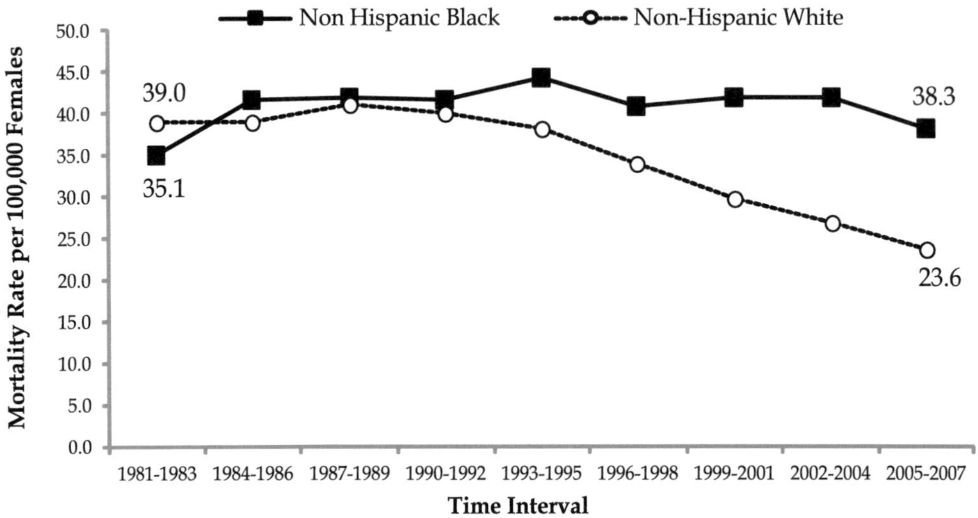

Fig. 1. Age Adjusted Female Breast Cancer Mortality Rates, Chicago, By Race, 1981-2007.

an early point we asked ourselves: If our efforts were successful in increasing the number of women who wanted to obtain mammograms, would there be adequate capacity? We thus began an inquiry to determine what this capacity was in Chicago. Researchers in the city did not know the answer to this question. Neither did advocacy groups. We were surprised that such a number was not even partially established for Chicago so we turned to other large cities. We were then more surprised that we were not able to find even one city that had an estimate of mammography capacity that might be useful in understanding the situation in Chicago.

Given this general lack of information the Task Force thus decided to undertake a study of mammography screening capacity in Chicago. The purpose of this chapter is to report the results from a survey of such mammography facilities in order to estimate and compare potential need for screening mammography, utilization, and current capacity for screening mammography in the third largest city in the United States. To our knowledge this is the first such analysis of capacity for a major urban area in the United States.

2. Methods

2.1 The survey instrument

The mammography capacity survey, which was conducted July - September 2007, contained 31 questions (Figure 2.), and was designed to take about 10 minutes to complete for someone familiar with the information. We asked facilities to provide information related to 2007 capacity, including the number of screening and diagnostic mammograms performed per month, hours of operation, number of machines, number of imaging technologists and radiologists interpreting mammograms, and the level of difficulty maintaining staffing.

2.2 Recruitment of mammography centers

In order to determine what mammography facilities existed in Chicago, we compiled a list of certified mammography facilities (U.S. Food and Drug Administration [FDA], 2007). We searched the FDA website by zip codes beginning with "606" which designates the city of Chicago. At the time of the survey there were no operating mobile mammography units, thus none were surveyed.

Each facility received a cover letter stating the purpose of the Task Force, the purpose of the survey and the expectation of confidentiality. We mailed the letter along with a copy of the survey and waited two weeks. As expected few centers responded to an unsolicited letter requesting information about their mammography facility. For facilities that did not respond within the 2 weeks, we recruited partners in the Task Force to distribute the survey to their contacts or colleagues in the radiology departments on the list. This round of efforts improved the response rate substantially but still not enough. We next solicited the help of three prominent health care leaders in the city who also serve as the co-chairs of the Task Force. They were able to stimulate several more institutions to complete the surveys.

In the end we identified and attempted to survey all 49 FDA certified mammography centers located in Chicago. The overall response rate was 88% (43 out of 49). Every major institution responded. There were 6 non-responding sites according to state inspection records obtained by the authors each of which operated a single licensed mammography machine.

2.3 Estimating potential need for screening mammography

We estimated potential need for screening mammography as a function of the estimated number of female residents of Chicago aged 40 or older according to the 2000 United States Census (http://factfinder.census.gov) (577,609) (Unites States Census Bureau, n.d.), and current guidelines which typically recommend a screening mammogram every year or every other year for women aged 40 and above (American Cancer Society, 2009; Lee et al, 2010; Humphrey et al, 2002; U.S. Preventive Services Task Force, 2009). Need according to the recommendation for annual mammography was simply the number of age-eligible women residing in Chicago, and need according to biennial recommendation was equal to the number of age-eligible women divided by two.

2.4 Estimating mammography utilization (volume)

Facilities were asked to report separately on the number of screening and diagnostic mammograms performed in an average month. For the six non-responding Chicago sites, we estimated the numbers of screening and diagnostic mammograms based on the mean values for participating facilities obtained after excluding the larger academic centers.

Mammography volume was calculated based on the responses to the question: "How many screening mammograms does this facility perform approximately per month?" This number was then divided by the site specific number of days open for mammograms. Consistent with previous reports, volume was then sub-divided into 3 categories: High, Medium and Low. High Volume was defined as 15 or more mammograms performed each day, Medium Volume was 5-14 mammograms per day and Low Volume included centers that performed 4 or fewer mammograms per day (Houn & Brown, 1994; Hendrick et al, 2005).

2.5 Estimating mammography maximum capacity

We estimated each facility's maximum capacity by using the 2006 Government Accountability Office (GAO) definition of maximum capacity that assumes that three mammograms can be performed per machine per operating hour (U.S. Government Accountability Office [GAO], 2006). We defined "maximum GAO screening capacity" as three times the number of mammography machines, times the number of hours open, multiplied by the proportion of all mammograms that were for screening. For non-responding facilities, we estimated the number of machines, number of hours open, and maximum capacity based on information available on participating non-academic facilities.

2.6 Staffing difficulties

Our survey also asked questions about difficulties in staffing open positions in imaging. Difficulty was categorized as such: much, moderate, none, and did not have to recruit new staff).

2.7 Classifying mammography centers

We asked the affiliation of every site filling out the survey. Sites were classified as academic if they reported a university affiliation with a medical school. Academic institutions in Chicago are larger and may have more resources than non-academic institutions due to grant opportunities, endowments, payer mix, etc. The survey also requested information on whether each facility made available a variety of breast screening and diagnostic procedures, imaging staff, the ability to interpret mammograms on site, the ability to offer same day results or procedures and general demographics of patients such as insurance status and race/ethnicity.

2.8 Statistical analysis

Data were entered into a Microsoft Access database and then analyzed in SAS (v. 9.0).

3. Results

In most cases (77%) the surveys were completed by staff members who were directly involved with the day to day workings of the imaging departments. Of the n=43 completed surveys, 12% of the sites (n=5) had senior management, consisting of executive directors and department heads, complete the survey. Forty-seven percent were directors or managers of breast imaging or general imaging (n=20), 14% were either radiologists or nurse practitioners (n=6), 9% were lead technologists (n=4), 7% were non-lead technologists (n=3), and 12% were data analysts or clerks (n=5). (Data not Shown).

3.1 Potential need for screening mammography

According to the 2000 U.S. Census, there were approximately 578,000 female residents of Chicago aged 40 or older. In order for every age-eligible woman in Chicago to obtain annual screening mammography there would need to be 578,000 screening mammography slots or appointments available, and one half of that or 289,000 slots or appointments in order for every age-eligible woman in Chicago to obtain a mammogram every two years.

	Total For Chicago
Number of Centers	49 [a]
Annual Screening Mammographic Need [b]	577,609
Biennial Screening Mammographic Need [c]	288,805
Number of Screening Mammograms (Utilization/Volume)	176,214
Number of Total Mammograms (Utilization/Volume)	254,850
Maximum Capacity for Screening using GAO (2006) Estimation [d]	492,879

[a] 43 facilities responded to the survey; totals for the remaining 6 were estimated
[b] defined as female residents of Chicago aged 40 and over
[c] defined as female residents of Chicago aged 40 and over divided by 2
[d] Government Accountability Office

Table 1. Estimated Mammography Utilization, Capacity, and Need for Chicago, 2007.

3.2 Mammography utilization (volume) compared with potential need

Table 1 presents the screening mammography need, utilization, and capacity. In 2007, an estimated 176,214 screening mammograms were provided by Chicago facilities. If one assumes, consistent with several recommendations (American Cancer Society, 2009; Lee et al, 2010), that all women 40 years of age and older should have an annual mammogram then the estimated screening mammography volume (176,214) represents 31% of eligible women or "need" (577,609). If one instead assumes, consistent with other recommendations (Humphrey et al, 2002), that all women age 40 and over should have a mammogram every two years then the "need" is halved (288,805) and the estimated screening mammography volume represents 71% of eligible women or "need".

3.3 Mammography capacity compared with potential need

According to the GAO-defined maximum capacity based on their 2006 revised definition that assumes 3 mammograms can be performed on one machine in an hour (GAO, 2006), there are 492,879 available screening mammography slots or appointments in the City of Chicago. This represents roughly 85% the "need" or number of age-eligible for annual screening (women 40 and over) women in Chicago (approximately 578,000) and 170% of the "need" or age eligible women for biennial screening (all women 40 and over divided by 2).

3.4 Difficulty recruiting mammography staff

More than one third (37%) of all facilities reported some difficulty in recruiting mammography technologists or radiologists, corresponding to one third (32%) of screening mammograms performed across these facilities (Table 2). One quarter of facilities representing one of every five screening mammograms reported difficulty hiring technologists, while a fifth of all facilities representing one quarter of screening mammograms reported difficulty hiring radiologists. Most notably, while only 1 in 10 facilities reported difficulties recruiting breast imaging specialists, they accounted for nearly one of every 5 mammograms performed (Table 2).

A city wide task force was assembled in March of this year to address the unacceptable disparity in breast cancer mortality by race in Chicago. This task force is compiling a list of recommendations to be released on October 17, 2007 to address the issues related to Access to and Quality of Mammography as well as Access and Quality of Treatment for breast cancer. In order to ensure that our recommendations are in line with mammography capacity in Chicago we need your help. We are asking you or someone knowledgeable within your institution to complete this brief survey and return this form as soon as possible.

These data will be used to further guide our recommendations to improve breast health for all women in Chicago. We will not present or publish information from individual facilities or institutions either as part of the task force or elsewhere. Your name and the names of any colleagues will not be published in this report and will remain confidential. We will only use your name and contact information if we have further follow-up questions.

Thank you in advance for helping to fill in this important picture of access to mammography in Chicago.

Instructions: Please fill out ONE form for EACH mammography facility at your institution, for your convenience we have typed in the names of the facilities which we are interested in learning more about.

Facility name: ____
Address: ____
City: _______________________________ ZIP: ________________
Institution affiliation (if any): ______________________________
Name of person(s) completing this questionnaire: ____________________
Position or title(s): _______________________________________

Capacity:

1. How many hours is this facility open Monday-Friday? ________
2. How many hours is this facility open on the weekend? ________
3. How many mammography machines do you have at this facility? ________
4. How many imaging techs do you have who are dedicated to mammography (>75% of time spent on mammograms)? ________
5. How many imaging techs does this facility have who spend <75% of their time on mammography? ________
6. How many radiologists who specialize in mammography (e.g. dedicated to mammography) does this facility have? ________
7. How many general radiologists who read mammograms does this facility have? ________
8. How many screening mammograms does this facility perform:
9. approximately ______ per month?
10. How many diagnostic mammograms does this facility perform: approximately ______ per month?

Fig. 2. Mammography Facility Survey.

11. Roughly what percentage of your patients have private insurance?
☐ <25% ☐ 25-49% ☐ 50-75% ☐ >75%
12. Roughly what percentage of your patients are African American?
☐ <25% ☐ 25-49% ☐ 50-75% ☐ >75%
13. Roughly what percentage of your patients are Latina/Hispanic?
☐ <25% ☐ 25-49% ☐ 50-75% ☐ >75%
14. Roughly what percentage capacity is your facility at now?
☐ <25% ☐ 25-49% ☐ 50-74% ☐ 75-89% ☐ 90-99% ☐ 100%

Does your facility routinely	Never	Rarely	Sometimes	Often	Always
15. Read mammograms on site at your facility?	☐	☐	☐	☐	☐
16. Read films on the same day so that the patient can leave with the results?	☐	☐	☐	☐	☐
17. Routinely double-read mammograms with suspicious findings?	☐	☐	☐	☐	☐
18. Routinely double-read all mammograms?	☐	☐	☐	☐	☐
19. Provide computer-aided detection (CAD) for suspicious mammograms findings?	☐	☐	☐	☐	☐
20. Provide computer-aided detection (CAD) for all screening mammograms?	☐	☐	☐	☐	☐

Does your facility offer:

21. Diagnostic mammography?	☐ Yes	☐ No
22. Breast ultrasound?	☐ Yes	☐ No
23. Digital mammography?	☐ Yes	☐ No
24. Breast magnetic resonance imaging?	☐ Yes	☐ No
25. Breast nuclear medicine scanning?	☐ Yes	☐ No
26. Biopsies after a diagnostic mammogram?	☐ Yes	☐ No
27. Biopsies carried out during the same visit?	☐ Yes	☐ No

Over the last year how much difficulty have you had staffing...	Much difficulty	Moderate Difficulty	No difficulty	Did not have to recruit new staff
28. Dedicated mammography technicians	☐	☐	☐	☐
29. X-ray technicians who perform some mammograms	☐	☐	☐	☐
30. Dedicated mammography radiologists	☐	☐	☐	☐
31. General Radiologists who read mammograms	☐	☐	☐	☐

If we need to ask follow-up questions, please provide the name and phone number of the person we should contact:

Name:____________________________Phone number:______________________

Fig. 2. Mammography Facility Survey (continued).

Difficulty Hiring	% Facilities (N=43)	% Screening Mammograms (N=159,612)[b]
Mammography Technicians or Radiologists	37	32
Mammography Technicians	26	19
Dedicated Mammography Technicians	12	10
General Mammography Technicians	23	12
Breast Radiologists	19	26
Dedicated Breast Radiologists	10	19
General Breast Radiologists	14	13

[a] Difficulty defined as much/moderate difficulty vs. no difficulty/did not need to recruit staff.
[b] Does not include non-responding sites (n=6)

Table 2. Difficulty[a] Recruiting Mammography Staff for Chicago, 2007.

3.5 Characteristics of mammography centers

Table 3 presents the characteristics of the Chicago facilities with completed surveys and also demonstrates how these characteristics are distributed according to facility volume (Low, Medium, High; see Methods). Because the number of facilities in each category is small we omit tests of significance. However, several of the trends suggest strong relationships.

As Table 3 indicates, in 2007 the 43 responding Chicago facilities (out of a total of 49) performed about 160,000 screening mammograms. Sixty-eight percent of the mammograms performed by the 43 responding Chicago facilities were performed at High Volume facilities. On average the High Volume centers performed 8,400 screening mammograms per site, whereas the Medium Volume centers performed 2,704 and the Low Volume centers performed 785.

The facilities are open for an average of 45 hours per week (range = 4 hrs - 90 hrs) and more than half offer weekend hours. They reported employing a total of 160 radiologists who read screening mammograms, of whom 36% are dedicated mammography radiologists (interpreting mammograms or conducting breast procedures for >75% of working hours). The mean number of dedicated radiologists per institution (1.3 overall) was highest for High Volume facilities (2.6). These institutions reported the use of 84 mammography machines with the highest average per institution again being for High Volume facilities.

About 16% of these facilities reported an academic affiliation, more than half of them occurring at High Volume facilities. A majority of facilities offer diagnostic services (67%) and interpret mammograms on site (79%) while smaller proportions offer same day results (23%) or same day biopsies (30%).

About a quarter of these facilities serve a high proportion (>75%) of patients with private insurance, including almost half of the High Volume facilities. Forty-two percent of the facilities serve a majority Black population and this proportion is highest at Low Volume facilities. Nineteen percent of the facilities serve a majority Hispanic population and this proportion is highest at Medium Volume facilities.

4. Discussion

The results of this unique survey show that the current available capacity for screening mammography in Chicago, as measured in terms of available mammography machines, is not adequate to meet the need of screening all Chicago residents (Table 1). In addition, there appear to be substantial issues pertaining to recruitment of staff needed to perform activities necessary to achieve this capacity (Table 2).

The other important set of observations (Table 3) revolves around the many differences in the characteristics of Low, Medium and High Volume facilities. High Volume facilities (those doing ≥ 15 screening mammograms/day) were different in many ways from Low (≤4/day) and Medium (5-14/day) Volume facilities (Table 2). High Volume facilities are open more hours, have a greater proportion of radiologists who are dedicated to mammography, more often have academic affiliations and serve a greater proportion of patients with private insurance. They are also less likely to serve patient populations who are majority Black or Hispanic. These differences are most stark when comparing High Volume facilities with Low Volume (≤ 4/day) facilities. Literature suggests that both volume and academic affiliation may be associated with higher quality (Esserman et al, 2002; Barlow et al, 2004; Woodward et al, 2002; Sickels et al, 2002; Miglioretti et al, 2007).

There is some confusion in vocabulary in the few existing capacity studies and we would thus like to spell out some concepts and terminology before proceeding with a contextualization of our findings. *Need* for screening mammography is both a function of the number of women aged 40 or over (which is a function of the size of the population and its age structure), the screening rate and the accepted recommendation for the frequency of screening mammography (e.g., every year or every two years). *Utilization (Volume)* is in turn a function of capacity, education and outreach, geographic distribution of machines, financial barriers and opportunities, etc. (Etling et al, 2009; Elkin et al, 2010; Schueler et al, 2008; Masi et al, 2008). Finally, *Capacity* refers to the potential supply of screening mammography and is a function of the number of available machines, the technology of the machines (e.g., analog or digital), and the numbers of available technologists and interpreters. Curiously, the number of mammography facilities is a frequently studied topic (Etling et al, 2009) but this is irrelevant to capacity and would be subsumed by consideration of the available number of machines.

Given this terminology let us examine in greater detail the screening mammography situation in Chicago. In 2007, 206,000 women received (utilized) screening mammograms. Depending upon which screening frequency recommendation one employs, this number may be compared with a potential annual need of 578,000 mammograms or 289,000 mammograms (Table 1). We see that the utilization of screening mammography in Chicago is far less than what is theoretically possible given that Chicago facilities can perform approximately 493,000 mammograms at full capacity.

We have been able to locate only a few peer-reviewed journal articles on the topic of capacity and utilization of screening mammography. Brown and colleagues published an economic analysis which was conducted in 1990 (Brown et al, 1990). This study concluded that there was an excess supply of mammograms for the utilization at that time. However, two major events occurred since this publication that affect capacity. First, the Mammography Quality Standards Act (MQSA) was enacted in 1993 creating an infrastructure for quality (FDA, 2002). After the enactment of MQSA several facilities closed due to not being able to keep up with the standards (Eastern Research Group, 2001). Second, insurance companies began covering screening mammograms as part of routine care. Thus, mammography became available to more women (Institute of Medicine, 2005). The conclusion of this study is now 20 years old and has only decreasing relevance to the field.

The most prominent studies of capacity data revolve around the two main reports on this topic which are authored by the Government Accountability Office (GAO) in formats prepared for Congress. In 2002 the GAO (GAO-2002) prepared a report that evaluated capacity for the U.S. as a whole between 1998 and 2001 following the enactment of the Mammography Quality Standards Act (MQSA) (FDA, 2002).

The GAO-2002 report noted that even while the number of mammography facilities had decreased during this interval the number of technologists and machines had increased (GAO, 2002). At the same time the GAO cited signs that these increases were coming to a halt. The GAO also noted, "Although mammography services are generally available, women have problems obtaining timely mammography services in some locations. Most of the availability problems are in certain metropolitan areas . . ." (GAO, 2002, pp. 3). Chicago may be one of these areas but that remains unknown since the GAO did not present any estimates for cities.

The GAO issued the second report in 2006 (GAO-2006) to evaluate the potential capacity issues with possible facility closures related to MQSA that may have occurred between 2001 and 2004 and found that capacity was adequate in most places (GAO, 2006). In the GAO-2006 report facilities performing mammography, machines, and staff had all decreased since 2001 yet capacity remained sufficient (GAO, 2006). In addition, the GAO-2006 report noted that Illinois, and Cook County (which contains Chicago) in particular, was one of the areas which had significant facility closures. The reports conclude that low-income women may be most affected by these closures.

The picture painted in this report was more pessimistic than its predecessor. It noted that, "The numbers of mammography facilities, machines, radiologic technologists, and interpreting physicians decreased from 2001 to 2004" (GAO, 2006, pp. 4) even as the number of women seeking and receiving mammograms increased. The declines were 4% for machines, 3% for technologists, and 5% for physician mammogram interpreters, "usually radiologists." The report thus notes: "Although experts believe the nation's current overall capacity to provide mammography services is adequate, they are concerned that the numbers of radiologic technologists and radiologists entering the field might not be sufficient to serve the increasing population that will need mammography services" (GAO, 2006, pp. 21).

Indeed, other research has shown evidence of a shortage of radiologists who interpret mammograms and mammography technicians (D'Orsi et al, 2005; Lewis et al, 2006; D'Orsi, 2004). Our survey indicates that there was substantial difficulty filling open positions in breast imaging. For instance, nearly 20% of the responding facilities had difficulty filling open positions for any type of radiologist, 10% had some difficulty hiring dedicated radiologists and 14% had difficulty hiring general radiologists. In addition, nearly 30% of the sites had difficulty filling open positions for dedicated mammography technicians or x-ray technicians (Table 2).

Although there are few studies in this field some have recently emerged in the literature indicating a potential growing interest in the topic. For instance Etling and colleagues conducted a study in Texas. This group researched mammography facility proximity by county and the correlates of self-reported mammography utilization and reported that there was unequal distribution of mammography facilities in Texas counties which impacted utilization of screening mammography in some areas (Etling et al, 2009). In Texas, the rural counties had fewer facilities within them and this in turn was correlated with higher late-stage breast cancers (Etling et al, 2009). The main limitations to this study are that the researchers did not analyze machine availability, just facilities, and the results are mainly applicable to a more rural population. Although the methods are different this study does illuminate a potential capacity issue locally.

Another way to examine Chicago's capacity for screening mammograms comes from a study by Elkin and colleagues. This study concludes that in order to have adequate capacity to meet the recommendation of annual screenings there needs to be more than 1.7 mammography machines for every 10,000 age-eligible women. The study further estimated that if the screening rate of 70% of the target population is the goal (per Healthy People 2010) then 1.2 machines per 10,000 age eligible women would be needed (Elkin et al, 2010; U.S. Department of Health and Human Services, 2001). As Table 3 indicates, there are 84 mammography machines serving Chicago. In addition, there are approximately 578,000 age eligible women in Chicago equating to 58 groups of 10,000 women (578,000/10,000=57.8). In order to provide mammograms to 100% of the age eligible women Chicago would need 99 machines (58*1.7 machines). If Chicago were to accomplish screening 70% of age eligible women (which is recommended by the U.S. Healthy People 2010) then 70 machines (58*1.2) would be needed according to Elkin and colleagues' calculations (U.S. Department of Health and Human Services, 2001; Elkin et al, 2010). If one assumes that all age eligible women should receive mammograms annually, then it seems clear that the current capacity in Chicago is not adequate. If however, one assumes biennial mammography for age eligible women, then capacity in Chicago is adequate.

Of course in this chapter we have only been analyzing the issue of capacity. Even if there were adequate capacity to screen all women in Chicago, and our findings suggest that there is not, many other questions arise with respect to utilization. These include issues of health insurance, outreach, education, etc. All in all the breast cancer screening capabilities seem hardly up to the task of accommodating all women for screening, which is the goal of many advocates and physicians in the city.

The question must then be posed whether we will soon be doing a disservice to women by urging them to obtain a mammogram only to be turned away because there are no appointments available for several months. The problem is already at hand in some cases in Chicago. For example, the waiting time for a screening mammogram appointment at one of the most prominent academic medical centers in the city is between 7-10 months (Deardorff, 2008a, 2008b). At the same time the city's only public hospital has stopped doing screening mammograms altogether, a loss of about 10,000 mammograms per year which were obtained by the most vulnerable women in the city. Access is thus being challenged at both ends of the socioeconomic spectrum.

	Low ≤4/day	Medium 5-14/day	High ≥15/day	Total
Facilities, n	16	14	13	43
Screening mammograms provided*, n (mean)	12,552 (785)	37,860 (2,704)	109,200 (8,400)	159,612 (3,712)
Screening mammograms provided to Chicago residents, %	7.9%	23.7%	68.4%	100.0%
Maximum capacity for screening using GAO (2006), sum (mean)	5,379 (5,355)	113,573 (8,112)	231,684 (17,822)	431,319 (10,031)
Screenings per machine, mean (median)	761 (720)	1,992 (1,800)	2,980 (2,400)	1,833 (1,578)
Hours open per week, mean	36.8 hrs	44.4 hrs	56.5 hrs	45.4 hrs
Sites with weekend hours, n	4 (25.0%)	9 (64.3%)	10 (77.0%)	23 (53.5%)
Dedicated radiologists, n (mean)	9.0 (0.6)	15.0 (1.1)	33.5 (2.6)	57.5 (1.3)
General radiologists who read mammograms, n (mean)	27.0 (1.7)	47.5 (3.4)	28.0 (2.2)	102.5 (2.4)
Dedicated mammography technologists, n (mean)	17.0 (1.1)	26.0 (1.9)	101.5 (7.8)	144.5 (3.4)
X-Ray technologists who perform mammograms, n (mean)	18.0 (1.3)	19.5 (1.4)	62.0 (4.8)	99.5 (2.3)
Machines, n (mean)	17.0 (1.1)	20.0 (1.4)	47.0 (3.6)	84 (2.0)
Academic affiliation, n (%)	0 (0%)	3 (21.4%)	4 (30.8%)	7 (16.3%)
Offers diagnostic breast services (e.g.) diagnostic mammograms, Ultrasounds, MRI or Image Guided biopsy	7 (43.8%)	11 (78.6%)	11 (84.6%)	29 (67.4%)
Reads/interprets mammograms on site	8 (50%)	13 (92.9%)	13 (100%)	34 (79.1%)
Offers same day results (often or always)	2 (12.5%)	2 (14.3%)	6 (46.2%)	10 (23.3%)
Offers same day biopsy, n (%)	2 (12.5%)	0 (0%)	6 (46.2%)	8 (18.6%)
Patients with >75% with private insurance [a]	1 (6.7%)	3 (21.4%)	6 (46.2%)	10 (23.3%)
50% or more African American/Black patients [a]	9 (56.3%)	4 (28.6%)	5 (38.5%)	18 (41.9%)
50% or more Hispanic/Latino patients [a]	3 (18.8%)	4 (28.6%)	1 (7.7%)	8 (18.6%)

[a] Some responses were missing, thus not included in the denominator

Table 3. Distribution of Indicators by Capacity Category, n=43.

4.1 Limitations

There are some methodological limitations to consider. First, we had to estimate important measures for non-responders such as mammography volume and capacity indicators (e.g., machines and hours of operation). However, the non-response accounted for only 9% of the Chicago screening volume. In addition, all non-responding sites were smaller community based hospitals (e.g., none were larger academic institutions). Thus, our estimation techniques could not have affected the contours of our analysis.

Second, all surveys were self-reported by facility representatives. There was thus a chance that some of the questions may have been interpreted in an idiosyncratic manner but it is not obvious how the summation of these interpretations would have influenced our results.

4.2 Recommendations for further consideration

It has been suggested that with looming staff shortages in the field of mammography, one may need to begin looking for ways to improve quality or efficiency. Some possible areas to explore are as follows:

- The Metropolitan Chicago Breast Cancer Task Force recommends that the state of Illinois offer some tuition reimbursement for the medical training of physicians willing to practice radiology, and specifically mammography, in underserved communities, where fellowship trained radiologists are lacking. Perhaps an incentive for repaying medical school loans for physicians choosing to practice in underserved areas in mammography may increase the dwindling mammography workforce (Bärnighausen & Bloom, 2009).
- Literature notes that independent double reading of mammograms improves the performance of a screening mammography program (Harvey et al, 2001). However, in the United States, it has been suggested that there is a radiologist shortage willing to interpret screening mammograms (D'Orsi et al, 2005; D'Orsi, 2004). One way to increase the workforce in mammography and improve quality is to increase the use of physician assistants, trained breast cancer nurses or highly skilled mammography technologists into a mammography practice. The literature suggests that these staff could be used as second readers or to complete administrative work such as communicating results with primary care clinics or following up with patients who have abnormal findings under the supervision of a radiologist (IOM, 2005; Duijum, 2007; Tonita, 1999). These staff may be able to increase the time a radiologist has to interpret mammograms and perform breast procedures, thus allowing each site to provide more mammograms.
- Centralizing or regionalizing either interpreting radiologists and/or a film library may begin to solve some of the bottlenecks in Chicago, thus freeing up machine space for more mammograms. Having radiologists interpreting mammograms in a centralized location allows sites that do not have access to a fellowship trained radiologist to have their mammograms interpreted by the best possible radiologist. In addition, having a universal film library will allow sites to gain access to their patients' prior films. Having prior films available for comparison to current films could prevent unneeded additional imaging (Burnside et al, 2002).
- Some facilities have reputations for high quality care and thus have high demand for all services they provide, including mammograms. This can lead to long wait times at

facilities to obtain a simple screening mammogram. In Chicago those wait times have been as high as 10 months for a screening mammogram appointment. A way to combat this problem is to have a centralized scheduling database that allows referring physicians to find open appointments for mammograms across the city. Although it is not ideal to have women obtain mammograms at multiple sites, coupled with centralized interpretations and storage this should make it easier on both physicians and patients. In addition, mammograms can be distributed throughout the city rather than clustered at a few facilities, thus utilizing all available capacity throughout Chicago.

- The only public hospital system in the Cook County area no longer provides screening mammograms due to budget cuts. This leaves about 10,000 uninsured and underinsured women without a mammogram. In addition, public clinics operated by the city of Chicago are not nearing capacity. If they do operate at capacity an additional 25,000 mammograms could become available to the most underserved women in Chicago and Cook County. Safety-net providers have stepped up to absorb the uninsured women into their routine screening population. However this places a large financial burden on these facilities, rather than spreading the burden to other area facilities. We propose that the Cook County public hospital system reopen screening mammograms for its patients and that other public facilities begin to operate at capacity. In addition, other area facilities must also begin managing these patients for breast and other services.
- Finally, insurance carriers reimburse at various rates, and most hover around the cost of the image. Public insurances also differ in how they reimburse for mammograms. Medicare, the insurance plan that older Americans use, reimburses slightly below the cost of a mammogram, whereas Medicaid, the insurance provided to the poorest Americans, reimburses at about half to three-quarters of the cost. For those who have no insurance, either the facility must enroll them in a state program which reimburses at the Medicaid rate or the facility must absorb the total cost. Most mammography facilities operate in a deficit or break even, thus leaving little room for upgrades or departmental improvements including upgrading equipment, elective training for staff or hiring assistants (Chen et al, 2004). All insurance carriers (including government insurance plans) must reimburse for the costs of these services so that these departments can be profitable enough to improve care and efficiency. Once mammography facilities become more fiscally sustainable, they may be able to absorb more patients without health insurance and thus provide more mammograms.

Without testing or implementing some of these strategies, we will constantly run up against limited capacity as a barrier to receiving mammograms.

5. Conclusions

The findings in this chapter suggest that there is currently inadequate screening mammography capacity in Chicago to screen all age eligible women annually. However there is adequate capacity to screen all age eligible women biennially. Given the existence of programs to increase access and the work of the Metropolitan Chicago Breast Cancer Task Force and other advocacy organizations seeking to increase education and outreach, women may continue to confront barriers when scheduling their annual mammograms.

This brings us back to the motivation for this survey - the large and growing racial disparity in breast cancer mortality in the city. There may be two driving forces with respect to screening mammography that are perpetuating this disparity. First, women may be delaying care for various reasons (usually financial or lack of insurance) leading to larger tumors being discovered at screening mammography (Rauscher et al, 2010). Not having insurance may also lead to women waiting for diagnostic services because they have no other choice. The second is that facilities may not have enough appointments available for the demand. As noted above, we know that two major institutions are already experiencing such problems. Community-based organizations and other agencies spend a lot of time and money navigating women to screening and working towards women receiving routine breast services. There are things facilities can do to promote regular screening and some facilities employ these tactics. However, these efforts will fail unless there are enough appointments available for women to get timely mammography services.

The chicken and egg relationship between supply and demand must be understood in this context. Is utilization as low as it is because women do not yet desire screening mammograms or is it because they have pursued them and been turned away because of insurance difficulties? Or is it because of very long waits? Are we indeed inadvertently limiting utilization by limiting capacity? These are questions that require answers. More generally, this is a problem that demands a solution.

6. Acknowledgements

We would like to acknowledge the Metropolitan Chicago Breast Cancer Task Force and its affiliated members who took the time to distribute and complete the facility survey. This work was funded in part by the Avon Foundation (Grant ID# 05-2007-004 and The Avon Supporting the Safety-Net grant), the Sinai Urban Health Institute and Sinai Health System and by the National Cancer Institute, Grant # 5 P50 CA 106743 to the University of Illinois at Chicago Center for Population Health and Health Disparities. Finally we would like to acknowledge Teena Francois, MPH for her assistance in identifying the mammography facilities to survey.

7. References

American Cancer Society. (June 23,2011). Breast Cancer, In: *American Cancer Society guidelines for the early detection of cancer,* August 8, 2011, Available from: http://www.cancer.org/docroot/PED/content/PED_2_3X_ACS_Cancer_Detection_Guidelines_36.asp?sitearea=PED.

Ansell, D., Grabler, P., Whitman, S., Ferrans, C., Burgess-Bishop, J., Murray, L.R., Rao, R., & Marcus, E. A community effort to reduce the black/white breast cancer mortality disparity in Chicago. *Cancer Causes and Control,* Vol. 20, No. 9, (November 2009), pp.1681-1688.

Barlow, W.E., Chi, C., Carney, P.A., Taplin, S.H., D'Orsi, C., Cutter, G., Hendrick, R.E., & Elmore, J.G. Accuracy of screening mammography interpretation by characteristics of radiologists. *Journal of the National Cancer Cancer Institute, Vol.* 96, No. 24, (December 2004), pp.1840-1850.

Bärnighausen, T., & Bloom, D.E. Financial incentives for return of service in underserved areas: a systematic review. *BMC Health Services Research,* Vol. 9, No. 86, doi:10.1186/1472-6963-9-86.

Bassett, L.W., Monsees, B.S., Smith, R.A., Wang, L., Hooshi, P., Farria, D.M., Sayre, J.W., Feig, S.A., & Jackson, V.P. Survey of radiology residents: breast imaging training and attitudes. *Radiology,* Vol. 227, No. 3, (June 2003), pp. 862-869.

Berry, D.A., Cronin, K.A., Plevritis, S.K., Fryback, D.G., Clarke,L., Zelen, M., Mandelblatt, J.S., Yakovlev, A.Y., Habbema, J.D., Feuer, E.J., & Cancer Intervention and Surveillance Modeling Network Collaborators. Effect of screening and adjuvant therapy on mortality from breast cancer. *New England Journal of Medicine,* Vol. 353, No. (October 2005), pp. 1784-1792.

Brown, M.L., Kessler, L.G., & Rueter, F.G. Is the supply of mammography machines outstripping need and demand? *Annals of Internal Medicine,* Vol. 113, No. 7, (October 1990), pp. 547-552.

Burnside, E.S., Sickles, E.A., Sohlich, R.E., & Dee, K.E. Differential Value of Comparison with previous examinations in diagnostic versus screening mammography. *American Journal of Roentgenology,* Vol. 179, No. 5, (November 2002), pp. 1173-1177.

Chen, S.L., Clark, S., Pierce, L.J., Hayes, D.F., Helvie, M.A., Greeno, P.L., Newman, L.A., & Chang, A.E. An academic health center cost analysis of screening mammography: creating a financially viable service. *Cancer,* Vol. 101, No. 5, (September 2004), pp.1043-1050.

Deardorff J. (October 5, 2008). Want a mammogram? Get in line, In: *Chicago Tribune,* August 8, 2011, Available from: http://articles.chicagotribune.com/2008-10-05/features/0810010630_1_breast-imaging-radiologists-yearly-mammograms.

Deardorf J. (November 25, 2008). Northwestern apologizes for mammogram wait, In: *Julie's Health Club Blog,* August 8, 2011, Available from: http://featuresblogs.chicagotribune.com/features_julieshealthclub/2008/11/northwestern-ap.html.

Duijm, L.E., Groenewoud, J. H., Fracheboud, J., de Koning, H.J. Additional double reading of screening mammograms by radiologic technologists: impact on screening performance parameters. *Journal of the National Cancer Institute,* Vol. 99, No. 15, (August 2007), pp. 1162-1170.

D'Orsi, C.J. Mammography: will adequate manpower exist? *Radiologic Clinics of North America,* Vol. 42, No. 5, (September 2004), pp. 975-978.

D'Orsi C., Tu, S., Nakano, C., Carney, P.A., Abraham, L.A, Taplin, S. H., Hendrick, R.E., Cutter, G.R., Berns, E., Barlow,W., & Elmore J.G. Current realities of delivering mammography services in the community: do challenges with staffing and scheduling exist? *Radiology,* Vol. 235, No. 2, (May 2005), pp. 391-395.

Eastern Research Group, Inc. (December 18, 2001). Assessment of the availability of mammography services: final report, In: U.S. Food and Drug Administration-Radiation Emitting Products, Mammography Quality Standards Act and Program, Reports (MQSA), August 10, 2011, Available from: http://www.fda.gov/Radiation-EmittingProducts/MammographyQualityStandardsActandProgram/Reports/ucm124361.htm.

Elkin, E.B., Ishill, N.M., Snow, J.G., Panageas, K.S., Bach, P.B., liberman, L., Wang, F., & Schrag, D. Geographic Access and use of screening mammography. *Medical Care,* Vol. 48, No. 4, (April 2010), pp. 349-356.

Elmore, J.G., Jackson, S.L., Abraham, L., Miglioretti, D.L., Carney, P.A., Geller, B.M., Yankaskas, B.C., Kerlikowske, K., Onega, T., Rosenberg, R.D., Sickles, E. A., & Buist D.S.M. Variability in interpretive performance at screening mammography and radiologist's characteristics associated with accuracy. *Radiology,* Vol. 253, No. 3, (December 2009), pp. 641-651.

Elting, L.S., Cooksley, C.D., Bekele, B.N., Giordano, S.H., Shih, Y.C., Lovell, K.K., Avritscher, E.B., & Theriault, R. Mammography capacity-impact on screening rates and breast cancer stage at diagnosis. *American Journal Preventive Medicine,* Vol. 37, No. 2, (August 2009), pp. 102-108.

Essernan, L., Cowley, H., Eberle, C., Kirkpatrick, A., Chang, S., Berbaum, K., & Gale, A. Improving accuracy of mammography: volume and outcome relationships. *Journal of the National Cancer Institute,* Vol. 94, No. 5, (March 2002), pp. 369-375

FDA (U.S. Food and Drug Administration). (March 4, 2009). In: *Mammography Quality Standards Act Regulations,* August 8, 2011. Available from: http://www.fda.gov/Radiation-EmittingProducts/MammographyQualityStandardsActandProgram/Regulations/ucm110906.htm.

Government Accountability Office (GAO). (April 19, 2002). *Capacity generally exists to deliver services,* Government Accountability Office (US), Report no: GAO-02-532, Washington, D.C.

Government Accountability Office (GAO). (July 25, 2006). *Current nationwide capacity is adequate, but access problems may exist in certain locations.* Government Accountability Office (US), Report no: GAO-06-724, Washington, D.C.

Harvey, S.C., Geller, B., Oppenheimer, R.G., Pinet, M., Riddell, L., & Garra, B. Increase in cancer detection and recall rates with independent double interpretation of screening mammography. *American Journal of Roentgenology,* Vol. 180, No. 5, (May 2003), pp. 1461-1467.

Hendrick, R.E., Cutter, G.R., Berns, E.A., Nakano, C., Egger, J., Carney, P.A., Abraham, L., Taplin, S.H., D'Orsi C.J., Barlow, W., & Elmore, J.G.. Community based mammography practice: services, charges and interpretation methods. *American Journal of Roentgenology,* Vol. 184, No. 2, (February 2005), pp. 433-438.

Houn, F., & Brown, M.L. Current practice of screening mammography in the United States: data from the National Survey of Mammography Facilities. *Radiology,* Vol. 190, No. 1, (January 1994), pp. 209-215.

Humphrey, L.L., Helford, M., Chan, B.K.S., & Woolfe, S.H. Breast cancer screening: a summary of the evidence for the US Preventative Services Task Force. *Annals of Internal Medicine,* Vol. 137, No. 5 part 1, (September 2002), pp. 347-360.

Institute of Medicine. (2005). Chapter 4. Ensuring an adequate workforce for breast cancer screening and diagnosis, In: *Improving Breast Imaging Quality Standards.* Nass, S., & Ball, J., pp. 117-163, National Academies Press, 0-309-09648-0, Washington, D.C.

Lee, C.H., Dershaw, D.D., Kopans, D., Evans, P., Monsees, B., Monticciolo D., Brenner, R.J., Bassett, L, Berg, W., Feig, S., Hendrick, E., Mendelson, E., D'Orsi, C., Sickles, E., & Burhenne, L.W. Breast cancer screening with imaging: recommendation from the Society of Breast Imaging and the ACR on the use of mammography, breast MRI, breast ultrasound, and other technologies for the detection of clinically occult breast cancer. *Journal of the American College of Radiology,* Vol. 7, No. 1, (January 2010), pp. 18-27.

Lewis, R.S., Sunshine, J.H., & Bhargavan, M. A portrait of breast imaging specialists and the interpretation of mammography in the United States. *American Journal Roentgenology,* Vol. 187, No. 5, (November 2006), pp. W456-W468.

Masi, C.M., Blackman, D.J., & Peek, M.E. Interventions to enhance breast cancer screening among racial and ethnic minority women. *Medical Care Research & Review,* Vol. 64, No. (5 suppl.), (October 2007), pp. 195S-242S.

Metropolitan Chicago Breast Cancer Task Force. (October 2007). *Improving quality and reducing disparities in breast cancer mortality in metropolitan Chicago.* Chicago, IL. Retrieved from:

http://www.sinai.org/urban/summit/docs/Task%20Force%20Rpt_Oct%202007_FINAL.pdf.
Miglioretti, D.L., Smith-Bindman, R., Abraham L., Brenner, R.J., Carney, P.A., Boweles, E.J., Buist, D.S., & Elmore, J. Radiologist characteristics associated with interpretive performance of diagnostic mammography. *Journal of the National Cancer Institute,* Vol., 99, No. 24, (December 2007), pp. 1854-1863.
Rauscher, G.H., Ferrans, C.E., Kaiser, K., Campbell, R.T., Calhoun, E.E., & Warnecke, R.B. Misconceptions about breast lumps and delayed medical presentation in urban breast cancer patients. *Cancer Epidemiology, Biomarkers & Prevention,* Vol. 19, No. 3, (March 2010), pp. 640-647.
Schueler, K.M., Chu, P.W., & Smith-Bindman, R. Factors Associated with Mammography Utilization: A Systematic Quantitative Review of the Literature. *Journal of Women's Health,* Vol. 17, No. 9, (November 2008), pp. 1477-1498.
Sickles, E.A., Wolverton, D.E., & Dee, K.E. Performance parameters for screening and diagnostic mammography: specialist and general radiologists. *Radiology,* Vol. 224, No. 3, (September 2002), pp. 861-869.
Smith-Bindman, R., Miglioretti, D.L., Lurie, N., Abraham, L., Barbash, R.B., Strzelczyk, J., Dingan, M., barlow, W.E., Beasley, C.M., & Kerlikowske, K. Does utilization of screening mammography explain racial and ethnic differences in breast cancer? *Annals of Internal Medicine,* Vol. 144, No. 8, (April 2006), pp. 541-553.
Tehranifar, P., Neugut, A.I., Phelan, J.C., Link, B.G., Liao, Y., Desai, M., & Terry, M.B. Medical advances and racial/ethnic disparities in cancer survival. *Cancer Epidemiology, Biomarkers & Prevention,* Vol. 18, No. 1, (October 2009), pp. 2701-2708.
Tonita, J.M., Hillis, J.P., Lim, C-H. Medical radiologic technologist review: effects on a population-based breast cancer screening program. *Radiology,* Vol. 211, No. 2, (May 1999), pp. 529-533.
Unites States Census Bureau. (n.d.). In: *American Factfinder, decennial census,* August 8, 2011. Available from: http://factfinder.census.gov/servlet/DTTable?_bm=y&-context=dt&-ds_name=DEC_2000_SF1_U&-mt_name=DEC_2000_SF1_U_P012&-CONTEXT=dt&-tree_id=4001&-all_geo_types=N&-geo_id=16000US1714000&-search_results=16000US1714000&-format=&-_lang=en.
United States Department of Health and Human Services [HHS]. (January 30, 2001). In: *Healthy People 2010, Volume I (second edition), Objectives for Improving Health (Part A, Focus area 1-14), 3. Cancer,* August 8, 2011, Available from: http://www.healthypeople.gov/2010/Document/HTML/Volume1/03Cancer.htm.
United States Food and Drug Administration [FDA]. (July 29, 2011). Mammography Facilities Database, In: *Medical Devices,* August 8, 2011, Available from: http://www.accessdata.fda.gov/scripts/cdrh/cfdocs/cfMQSA/mqsa.cfm.
United States Preventive Services Task Force. Screening for breast cancer: U.S. Preventive Services Task Force recommendation statement. *Annals of Internal Medicine,* Vol. 151, No. 10, (November 2009), pp. 716-726.
Whitman, S., Ansell, D., Orsi, J., & Francois, T. The racial disparity in breast cancer mortality. *Journal of Community Health,* Vol. 36, No. 4, (August 2011), pp. 588-596.
Woodard, D.B., Gelfand, A.E., Barlow, W.E., & Elmore, J.G. Performance assessments for radiologists interpreting screening mammography. *Statistics in Medicine,* Vol. 26, No. 7, (March 2007), pp. 1532-1551.

Part 2

Quality Control

6

Comparison of Individual Doses During Mammography Screening Examinations with Screen – Film and DR Systems and Optimization Attempts of Exposure Parameters

E. Fabiszewska, K. Pasicz, I. Grabska, W. Bulski and W. Skrzyński
Maria Skłodowska - Curie Memorial Cancer Center and Institute of Oncology
Medical Physics Department
Warsaw,
Poland

1. Introduction

In Poland, the number of new installations of FFDM (Full - Field Digital Mammography) units is increasing every year. These increasing numbers of digital mammography systems (DR systems) were possible to be evaluated on the basis of the data provided by the facilities taking part in the mammography screening program organized by the Polish Ministry of Health.

In 2006, in the framework of the "Polish National Breast Cancer Early Detection Program for Women aged from 50 to 69" was initiated. In order to create a structure for administration of the screening program of the Ministry of Health, 16 regional Coordination Centres, covering the administrative regions of the country, were created. Also, a Central Coordination Centre, located at the Centre of Oncology in Warsaw was set up. Thanks to such organization it was possible to contact all mammography facilities involved in the screening program, to receive the necessary data from them and to evaluate their equipment. Furthermore, it was possible to curry out control of physical and technical parameters of the mammography equipment and to collect data concerning the individual woman exposures. The data, in the range necessary to calculate the doses received by the women during the examinations were collected. On this basis it was possible to evaluate that in 2007 in the whole country there were 320 mammography units used in the mammography screening program, and among them there were only 5 DR systems. On the other hand in 2010 and in 2011 only in the Mazovia region the screening was carried out with 7 (out of 48) and 9 (out of 51) DR mammography systems respectively. Two of them were installed at the Centre of Oncology in Warsaw. However, the increase of the DR systems in Poland is limited by the relatively high costs of such installations as compared with the screen - film mammography systems (SFM systems). Moreover, the facilities equipped with mammography systems complying with the quality control requirements, are replacing SFM systems with computed radiography systems (CR systems).

The literature data indicate the evident advantages of the application of digital detectors in mammography. Apart from advantages linked with much simpler procedures of computer systems as far as processing, presentation, archiving and transmission of digital images are concerned there are more important advantages of DR systems over SMF systems namely: better image quality and lower doses of radiation received by the examined women. According to the published data (Gennaro, 2004, 2006; Gosch, 2006; Hermann, 2002; Lawinski, 2008) the average glandular doses are within 2.0 mGy per exposure allowing for detection of the objects of 0.1 mm diameter which is very satisfying. However, the results of some authors (Fischmann et al., 2005) indicate that the doses received by women examined with the systems equipped with digital detector are higher than those when the screen - film detector is used. These discrepancies in the results called for further analysis of absorbed doses and image quality in mammography with DR systems. The authors of this chapter analysed and evaluated the values of absorbed doses received by women undergoing screening mammography examinations at 8 facilities in Poland equipped with DR systems from 4 different manufacturers. This made possible a comparison of the performance of different DR systems as far as image quality is concerned.

2. Doses in mammography

2.1 Average glandular dose

According to "Dosimetry in Diagnostic Radiology: An International Code of Practice" by International Atomic Energy Agency the average glandular dose (later called AGD) is the mean absorbed dose in the glandular tissue (excluding skin) in a uniformly compressed breast. The absorbed dose is the mean energy imparted to matter of mass. The unit of absorbed dose is gray (Gy).

The higher the AGD value the higher the probability of inducing a cancer in examined women. It is especially important in case of mammography screening when probably healthy women are examined. For this reason the determination of this dose is one of the elements of quality control of the mammography equipment. The direct determination of the AGD is rather impossible, therefore it is determined in practice by the multiplication of the air kerma at the upper surface of the breast (without taking into account the scattered radiation) by the appropriate conversion factors according to the following formula:

$$AGD = Kgcs \quad (1)$$

where:

AGD – average glandular dose, in mGy;
K - entrance surface air kerma (ESAK), in mGy;
g – factor taking into account breast thickness after compression, dependent on the half value layer of the X-ray beam;
c – factor taking into account the breast tissue composition, dependent on the half value layer of the X-ray beam and on the breast thickness after compression;
s – factor taking into account the X-ray spectrum, dependent on the anode material and on the additional filter.

The values of the above mentioned factors have been calculated by Dance using Monte Carlo methods for simple breast model and various X-ray spectra in mammography. They were presented, in the form of tables, in "Additional factors for the estimation of mean glandular breast dose using the UK mammography dosimetry protocol" by Dance et al. In this paper it was assumed that the breast tissue composition is dependent on the breast thickness after compression according to the following formula:

$$y = \alpha t^3 + \beta t^2 + \gamma t + \delta \quad (2)$$

where:

y – glandular tissue content of the breast, in %;
t - breast thickness after compression, in mm;
α, β, γ, δ – coefficients dependent on the age of women in two age groups: 40 - 49 years and 50 - 64 years, given in Table 1.

Coefficient	Age 40 to 49	Age 50 to 64
α	0,00005209	-0,0001118
β	0,00125494	0,03932
γ	-1,988	-4,544
δ	138,8	176,0

Table 1. Coefficients for polynomial fit of glandularity of breast, dependent on the age of women in two age groups: 40 - 49 years and 50 - 64 years (according to "Additional factors for the estimation of mean glandular breast dose using the UK mammography dosimetry protocol").

The above mentioned method of AGD determination is limited to the central part of the breast above the ionization chamber of the Automatic Exposure Control (AEC) system (in the SFM systems) and above the main region of detector of the AEC system (in DR systems).

The measurement of ESAK during the exposure requires the use of very small detectors such as thermoluminescence dosimeters which would be visible on mammography images. However, the thermoluminescence dosimeters require complicated and well calibrated read-out systems. Simpler method of determining of the ESAK, not influencing the mammography image, is the measurement of the dose with a dosimeter of larger dimensions than the TLDs at the tube voltage (in kV) and a combination of anode/filter (such as for the breast exposure during examination) with arbitrary tube load (in mAs) and focus-dosimeter distance. Subsequently, assuming the linear dependence of dose in air on tube load and inverse dependence on focus-detector distance squared, it is possible to calculate the ESAK on the basis of the measured dose for an exposure of the breast of determined thickness after compression and taking into account the parameters of the exposure. Therefore, in order to calculate the doses received by women during mammography examinations the following parameters have to be known: anode/filter combination, tube voltage, tube load, breast thickness after compression, and also the woman age. Subsequently, the measurements of the half-value layer and the air kerma for every tube voltage value and anode/filter combination used during examinations should be performed. On the basis of gathered data and performed measurements the values of AGD for single exposure for individual woman may be determined, later called the clinical breast dose.

For the maximal uncertainty of the AGD determination a value of 14% suggested in the „Patient dose in digital mammography" by Chevalier et al. may be adopted.

2.2 Doses for typical breast

According to „European guidelines for quality assurance in breast cancer screening and diagnosis Fourth edition" by European Commission, in the frame of quality control tests the AGD values for typical breast, simulated by the homogenous PMMA plates should be determined. The PMMA plates from 2.0 cm to 7.0 cm thick are equivalent to typical breast from 2.1 cm to 9.0 cm thick, as it is shown in Table 2. During the quality control tests the exposures of PMMA plates should be performed with the same settings as during the clinical exposures (the same choice of the AEC mode, the same choice of the anode and additional filters, the same exposure control step). Subsequently, the AGD values for the different PMMA thicknesses exposures should be determined as for the exposure of equivalent breast (as described in 2.1 above). The AGD values obtained in such way may be compared to the limiting values. In Table 2, two types of such limiting values are listed for various PMMA thicknesses and equivalent breast thicknesses after compression. The first one, acceptable level, is a minimum requirement which has to be fulfilled by every mammography system. The second one, achievable level, more restrictive, should be the aim to attain by every mammography facility.

PMMA thickness [cm]	Equivalent breast thickness [cm]	Maximum AGD for equivalent breast [mGy]	
		Acceptable level	Achievable level
2.0	2.1	< 1.0	< 0.6
3.0	3.2	< 1.5	< 1.0
4.0	4.5	< 2.0	< 1.6
4.5	5.3	< 2.5	< 2.0
5.0	6.0	< 3.0	< 2.4
6.0	7.5	< 4.5	< 3.6
7.0	9.0	< 6.5	< 5.1

Table 2. AGD limiting values for equivalent breast thicknesses according to "European guidelines for quality assurance in breast cancer screening and diagnosis Fourth edition".

2.3 Clinical breast doses

The authors of this chapter had an opportunity to determine the AGD values for exposures of individual women (clinical breast doses). These doses were determined for women examined with 10 mammography units equipped with full-field digital detectors (DR systems), installed at facilities taking part in the screening program in Poland.

Determination of the clinical breast doses required the collection of all exposure parameters for examined women. The collected data included the following parameters: anode material, additional filter type, tube potential value, tube load value, birth year of a woman and breast thickness after compression. For every mammography unit the data for 200 exposures (examination of 50 women) were collected. Subsequently, for every mammography unit the measurements of air kerma were performed (taking into account the linear dependence of air kerma on tube load) and also the measurement necessary for determination of half value layer for all tube potential values used during the exposures. The measurement were performed with a multimeter Piranha from RTI Electronics AB (type: 305; uncertainty: ± 5%) and with aluminium filters from Gammex (6x: 0.10 mm thickness and Al purity ≥ 99.9%). According to the methodology described in 2.1 above, the AGD values were calculated for every exposure. In this way the values of clinical breast doses were determined for 500 women (2000 exposures).

Subsequently, the estimated values of clinical breast doses for each exposure were compared to the levels listed in Table 2. To determine the clinical breast dose limit for each breast thickness after compression the second-degree polynomial, based on data contained in Table 2, was fitted. The polynomial for acceptable level is given by the formula (3), and for the achievable level by the formula (4):

$$y = 0.091x^2 - 0.2326x + 1.1786 \tag{3}$$

$$y = 0.059x^2 - 0.012x + 0.402 \tag{4}$$

where:

y - the clinical breast dose limit for each breast thickness, in mGy;
x - breast thickness after compression, in cm.

The correlation coefficient R^2 between the values given by the above formulas and the values listed in Table 2 was higher than 0.99 in every case.

In Table 3, for each of 10 DR systems (from 4 manufacturers indicated by consecutive numbers) the following parameters are given: material of image detector, the percentage of exposures performed with given anode/filter combination, the percentage of exposures for which the clinical breast doses did not exceed the acceptable an achievable limits. The presented results indicate that the maximal percentage of exposures for which clinical breast doses met the acceptable and achievable limits for DR systems for which all exposures were performed with the W/Rh combination. However, the case of the mammography unit 8 does not confirm it. Furthermore, the analysis of the results of mammography units 2, 3, 6, 8 (from the same manufacturer) indicate that the doses received by the women depend not only on the type of the unit and the manufacturer of the unit but first of all on that how the particular mammography system was calibrated by manufacturer service.

Unit number/ manufacturer number	Material of image detector	The percentage of total numbers of exposures with given combination anode / filter [%]	The percentage of exposures not exceeding acceptable level [%]	The percentage of exposures not exceeding achievable level [%]
Unit 1 / Manufacturer 1	amorphous selenium	100.0 (W/Rh)	99.0	89.0
Unit 2 / Manufacturer 2	amorphous selenium	84.0 (Mo/Mo) 16.0 (Mo/Rh)	49.0	32.0
Unit 3 / Manufacturer 2	amorphous selenium	7.5 (Mo/Mo) 92.5 (Mo/Rh)	80.5	47.0
Unit 4 / Manufacturer 3	amorphous selenium	100.0 (W/Rh)	92.0	85.5
Unit 5 / Manufacturer 4	amorphous silicon	1.0 (Mo/Mo) 15.0 (Mo/Rh) 84.0 (Rh/Rh)	80.0	52.5
Unit 6 / Manufacturer 2	amorphous selenium	50.5 (Mo/Mo) 49.5 (Mo/Rh)	76.5	57.0
Unit 7 / Manufacturer 1	amorphous selenium	100.0 (W/Rh)	99.5	97.0
Unit 8 / Manufacturer 2	amorphous selenium	64.5 (Mo/Mo) 35.5 (Mo/Rh)	97.5	92.05
Unit 9 / Manufacturer 3	amorphous selenium	100.0 (W/Rh)	100.0	100.0
Unit 10 / Manufacturer 3	amorphous selenium	100.0 (W/Rh)	100.0	99.0

Table 3. Material of image detector, the percentage of exposures performed with given anode/filter combination, the percentage of exposures for which the clinical breast doses did not exceed the acceptable and achievable limits for 10 DR systems.

The results of clinical breast dose calculated for 10 mammography units equipped with DR systems are presented in Fig. 1. in a form of a histogram in grey. These dose values range from 0.12 mGy to 5.80 mGy with the mean value of 1.78 mGy. They do not exceed the limit values for typical breasts at the acceptable level in 87.4% of cases and at the achievable level in 65.2% of cases. For comparison, in Fig. 1 a histogram, in black, of clinical breast doses calculated for 50 women examined with the use of one SFM unit is presented. This mammography unit was installed in the Coordination Centre of the Screening Program in Poland in 2007. The mammography unit and the accessories (film processor, viewing box, amplifying screens and films) were of good quality. They were systematically controlled and fulfilled all quality criteria given in „European guidelines for quality assurance in breast cancer screening and diagnosis Fourth edition". The clinical breast dose values determined for the SFM unit ranged from 0.40 mGy to 4.22 mGy with the mean value of 1.68 mGy. They did not exceed the limit values for typical breasts at the acceptable level in 98% of cases and at the achievable level in 95% of cases.

The comparison of two histograms in Fig. 1 shows that the frequently cited opinion that the women examined with the use of DR mammography systems receive smaller doses of radiation than the women examined with SFM systems is not generally true. Furthermore, the SFM system presented here generated small clinical breast doses with simultaneous fulfilling the quality requirements formulated by the „European guidelines for quality assurance in breast cancer screening and diagnosis Fourth edition".

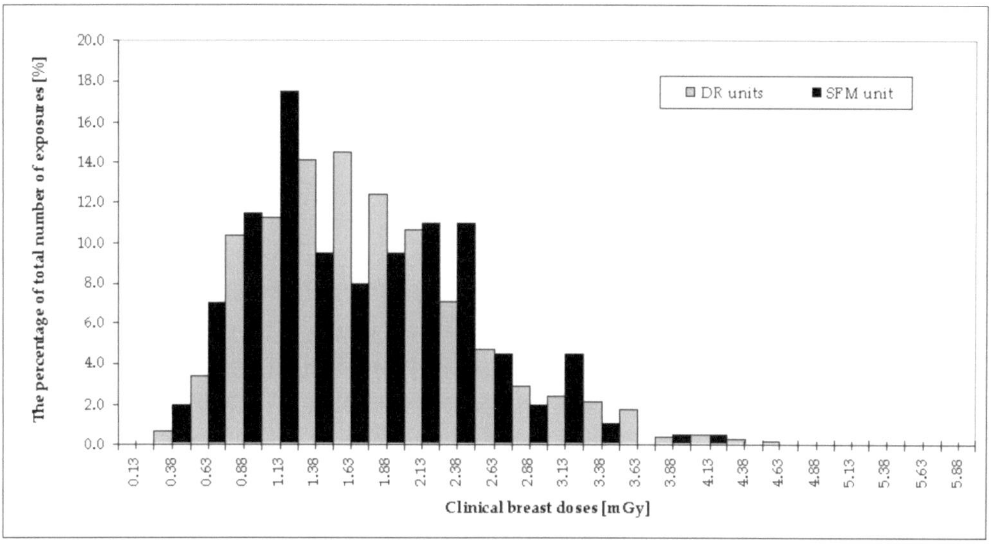

Fig. 1. The histograms of the clinical breast doses received by the women examined with the use of ten mammography units equipped with DR systems (in grey) and received by the women examined with the use of one SFM unit (in black).

2.4 The modifications in DR systems and the clinical breast doses

During the exploitation of the DR systems the manufacturer service upgrades the software of mammography unit, performs the calibration of the image detector and, in particular situations, replaces the image detector. Upgrade of the mammography unit software means changes of AEC area setting, exposure parameters setting and calibration setting. The replacement of the image detector is associated with the calibration of new image detector. All these activities should not influence the dose received by the examined women. However, the authors of this chapter noticed that the service actions in this area result in the increase of the clinical breast doses. For three mammography units (units 2, 3 and 4 are the same as in Table 3) the manufacturer service performed alterations of the image detector and the mammography system software. For the mammography units 2 and 3 the clinical breast doses were recalculated three times: directly after the installation of mammography unit, after the replacement of the image detector and the upgrade of the software, and for the mammography unit 4 twice: after the installation of mammography unit and before the calibration of the image detector. The data concerning the minimum, maximum and mean values for established clinical breast doses and the percentage of exposures meeting the acceptable and achievable limits are presented in Table 4.

The data analysis indicate that the mean values of clinical breast doses for the mammography unit 3 after the replacement of the image detector and after the upgrade of the software increased by about 44% and 50% in the relation to the mean value of clinical breast doses determined after installation of mammography unit. At the same time the number of exposures meeting the acceptable limit diminished from 22% to 1% and those meeting the achievable limit from 1% to 0%. In the case of the mammography unit 2 the mean clinical breast dose value after the upgrade of the software decreased by about 4% as compared to the mean value of clinical breast dose determined after the installation of the unit. On the other hand, after the replacement of the image detector mean value of the clinical breast dose increased by 8% in relation to the mean value of clinical breast doses calculated after the installation of the unit. The percentage values of exposures fulfilling the acceptable limits decreased after consecutive changes from 66% to 38% and 23% and for the achievable limits from 41% to 13% and 12%. For mammography unit 4 the mean value of clinical breast doses before the calibration of the image detector increased by about 9% in relation to clinical breast doses established just after the installation of the mammography unit and the small decrease of the number of exposures meeting the acceptable and achievable limits was observed.

Taking into account the three DR systems, two from the same manufacturer, it is possible to conclude that during the upgrade of the software, calibration and exchange of the image detector (made by the manufacturer services) changes are introducing which, as a consequence, induce increase of the doses received by the women during examinations (which was observed in the case of the mammography unit 3). The manufacturer service staff claimed that they were carefully following the manufacturer indications. It might suggest that these were minimal indications, which leave a lot of freedom in service activities. Therefore, it is reasonable to determine the clinical breast doses values after every manufacturer service intervention into the software and the image detector in order to be able, in case of increased doses, to optimize the exposure parameters.

Monitoring of the doses received by the women during mammography examinations, especially during screening, is necessary in order to protect potentially healthy population against additional irradiation. The values of AGD, calculated by the DR systems after every exposure and displayed on every mammography image would help the task. The accuracy of these values was tested during the clinical breast dose determination for the cases described above. For every exposure, the displayed AGD values were compared with clinical breast doses values calculated on the basis of exposure parameters. The percentage of the cases when the displayed AGD value agreeded with calculated one was established. As the criterion of the agreement between displayed and calculated values it was adopted that differences between these values could not be bigger than ±14% of calculated clinical breast doses values (i.e. the uncertainty of clinical breast dose value determination). The results of the comparisons are presented in Table 4. They indicate the discrepancies between the displayed and calculated values. The best agreement, for 71%exposures, was for mammography unit 2 just after its installation. The actions of manufacturer service resulted

Unit	Calculation of clinical breast doses	Clinical breast doses [mGy]			The percentage of exposures not exceeding		The compliance between the calculated and the displayed dose [%]	The percentage of exposures for which the displayed value is lower than the calculated value [%]
		minimum value	maximum value	mean value	acceptable level [%]	achievable level [%]		
2	After installation	1.41	3.92	2.36	66	41	71	100
	After the upgrade of the software	1.55	4.98	2.27	38	13	4	100
	After the replacement of the image detector	1.81	4.28	2.54	23	12	0	100
3	After installation	1.30	4.98	2.60	22	1	0	100
	After the replacement of the image detector	2.46	7.79	3.75	1	0	0	100
	After the upgrade of the software	2.45	7.71	3.89	1	0	0	100
4	After installation	0.67	4.13	1.72	100	97	65	92
	Before the calibration of the image detector	0.55	5.46	1.87	92	85.5	50.5	48.5

Table 4. The values of clinical breast doses (minimal, maximal and mean), percentage of exposures fulfilling acceptable and achievable limits of doses, percentage of calculated clinical breast doses values complied with AGD values displayed after exposure and percentage of exposures for which displayed values were lower than calculated values, after consecutive alterations introduced by the manufacturer service in three DR mammography systems (units 2, 3 and 4 are the same as in Table 3).

in diminishing of this agreement in every case. Additionally, in the majority of cases the displayed doses were lower than the calculated ones. It was not possible to establish the reason of such discrepancies between the displayed values and the values calculated according to recommendations of the „European guidelines for quality assurance in breast cancer screening and diagnosis Fourth edition". In any case, the displayed values could not be used for the evaluation of the radiation doses received by the examined women.

3. Optimization of exposure parameters

The significant increase of clinical breast dose values after the intervention of manufacturer service in mammography unit 3 (Table 4) forced the authors of this chapter into the attempt of exposure parameters optimization in order to reduce the doses received by the examined women. However, such dose reduction should not affect the image quality and the functioning of the automatic exposure control (AEC) system. The main parameter of image quality is the visibility of very small objects at the contrast threshold level. The functioning of AEC system is evaluated by a parameter linked to contrast handling by the system. This parameter is called the contrast to noise ratio (CNR) calculated for the objects of various thicknesses simulating typical breasts.

3.1 Contrast threshold level of the image

In mammography it is important to visualize and distinguish objects of low contrast and small dimensions on the image. The threshold contrast visibility is determined for circular objects of diameters from 0.1 mm to 2.0 mm placed in the homogenous PMMA plates of 4.5 cm total thickness. The small objects are made of gold, and the radiation contrast variability is attained by their various thicknesses. One of the phantoms suitable for contrast threshold determination is the CDMAM phantom manufactured by Artinis (Fig. 2). This phantom is composed of an aluminium plate type Al 1050 (99.5% purity) of 0.5 mm thickness with embedded golden discs (Au 99.9999 purity) of various thicknesses (from 0.03 μm to 2.00 μm) and various diameters (from 0.06 mm to 2.00 mm). The golden discs are placed in a matrix of 16 lines and 16 columns which is turned by 45° in relation to the phantom longer side (in order to minimize the so called heel-effect[1] on the image quality). Every matrix element contains two identical discs, one in the middle of the element and the other one in one of the corners of the element. The reason of the placement of the second disc in an arbitrarily selected corner is to not allow the observer analysing the images to memorize the disc positions. The aluminium plate is placed in the homogenous PMMA plate of 0.5 cm thickness. In the phantom set there are additional four PMMA plates (each 1.0 cm thick). The phantom dimensions are adapted to the dimensions of the standard mammography films (18 cm x 24 cm).

According to the recommendations of the manufacturer of the CDMAM phantom ("Manual Contrast Detail Phantom CDMAM 3.4. & CDMAM Analyser software V1.2.") the evaluation of objects visibility should be done on the basis of the analysis of the unprocessed (by mammography system software) image. On this kind of image (Fig. 3a) the observer is not able to detect any object, even the largest discs of 2.0 mm diameter. For comparison, in

[1] Heel - effect: The non-uniform distribution of air kerma rate and of the beam hardness in an X-ray beam in planes perpendicular to the beam axis and in the direction cathode to anode (according to "Dosimetry in Diagnostic Radiology: An International Code of Practice" by International Atomic Energy Agency).

Fig. 3b the processed (by mammography system software) CDMAM phantom image is presented.

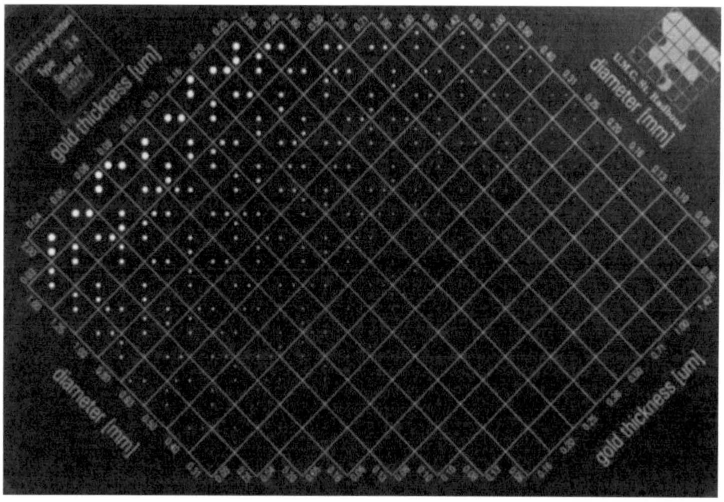

Fig. 2. CDMAM phantom manufactured by Artinis.

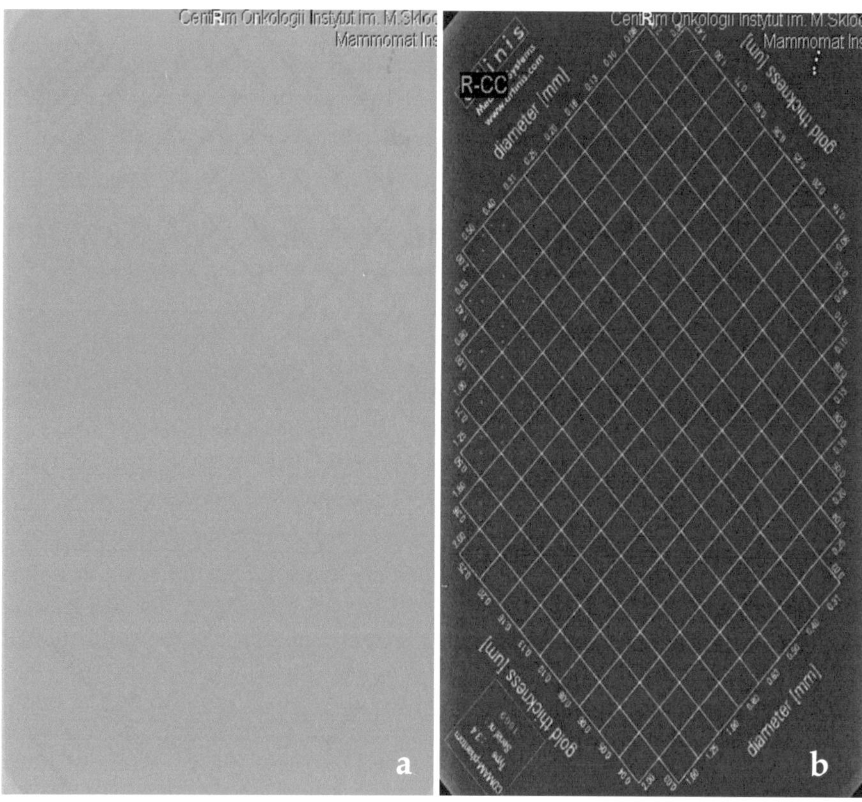

Fig. 3. Unprocessed image (a) and processed image (b) of CDMAM phantom for mammography unit 10 (unit 10 is the same as in Table 3).

The unprocessed image is transferred from workstation of mammography unit to the separate computer software provided by the manufacturer of the CDMAM phantom (i.e. CDMAM Analyser software) in order to analyse this image. Thicknesses of the objects of worst visibility for every object diameter are the final result of the computer analysis. As an example, in Table 5 the results of the image computer analysis for one of the DR systems are presented. Diameters of the objects are given in mm and thicknesses of the objects are given in μm.

Diameter:	0.060	0.080	0.100	0.130	0.160	0.200	0.250	0.310	0.400	0.500	0.630	0.800	1.000	1.250	1.600	2.000
Thickness:	2.500	0.992	0.525	0.429	0.334	0.152	0.125	0.079	0.067	0.068	0.038	0.030	0.030	0.030	0.030	0.040

Table 5. The results of the image analysis with CDMAM Analyser software V1.2.

In order to get reliable results at least eight images should be analysed. In Fig. 4 the Contrast Detail Curves for a single image and for eight images are presented. It may be easily notice that the curves differ considerably, especially for discs of 0.13 mm and of 1.00 m diameter. The analysis of larger number of images is necessary to avoid random errors.

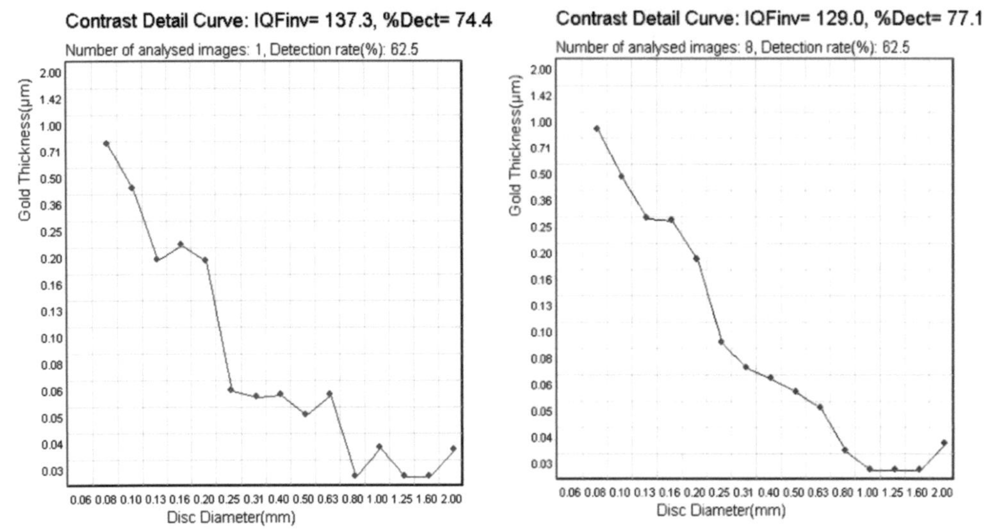

Fig. 4. Contrast Detail Curves for a single image (left) and for eight images of the same series (right) for mammography unit 2 (unit 2 is the same as in Table 3).

The CDMAM Analyser software does not provide the contrast values for structures contained in the CDMAM phantom. Therefore the next step after the plotting of the Contrast Detail Curve is to determine the threshold contrast on the basis of determined object thicknesses. The threshold contrast values of the object for several selected thicknesses are given in the "European guidelines for quality assurance in breast cancer screening and diagnosis Fourth edition". These values were calculated for X-ray spectrum of 28 kV, molybdenum anode and additional filtration of 0.03 mm Mo on the basis of the data from the „Catalogue of diagnostic X - ray spectra & other data" (IPEM report 78) published by the British Institute of Physics and Engineering in Medicine. In digital mammography various anode/filter combinations are employed, different from Mo/Mo, for example W/Rh (Table 3), and therefore the X-ray spectra differ considerably (for example the HVL) from the Mo/Mo spectrum at 28 kV. In theory, the data contained in the „Catalogue of diagnostic X - ray spectra & other data" may be used for calculation of contrasts for different spectra. The software included in the catalogue allows for the generation of pre-attenuated spectra with additional filtration, and for calculation of tube output for such spectra (expressed as air kerma value per tube load value at 75 cm distance from the focal spot). The CDMAM phantom, with 4.0 cm of PMMA added, can be here treated as an additional filter consisting of 4.3 cm of PMMA, 0.5 mm aluminium, and 0.03-2.00 μm of gold. Only the phantom is taken into account, attenuation caused by elements of the mammography unit (compression plate, breast support table, anti scatter grid, etc) is omitted. The radiation contrast can be defined as the percentage difference between the intensity of the beam passing through the phantom with a structure and beam passing through the phantom without the structure. However, the „Catalogue of diagnostic X - ray spectra & other data" contains only a limited range of spectra. The spectra for molybdenum and rhodium targets are available for tube voltage values from 25 kV to 32 kV, and spectra for a tungsten target are only available for tube voltage values from 30 kV to 150 kV, while in mammography the tube voltage values beyond these ranges are also used. Beam spectra for all target materials and wider range of tube voltage values (18 kV to 40 kV) can be generated using polynomial models ("Molybdenum, rhodium, and tungsten anode spectral models using interpolating polynomials with application to mammography"). An Excel spreadsheet was written that generates such spectra, calculates their attenuation by filter material (e.g., Mo or Rh) and by the CDMAM phantom (similarly as in the software included with IPEM report 78), and calculates radiation contrast of the structures. Linear attenuation coefficients and photon to kerma-in-air conversion factors taken from „Catalogue of diagnostic X - ray spectra & other data" are used in the calculations. The spreadsheet allows the user to calculate radiation contrast for virtually any beam quality used in digital mammography.

In Table 6, the values of threshold contrast in the case of the exposures at W/Rh combination of the CDMAM phantom for mammography units 4 and 10 are presented. The contrast values for the phantom structures were calculated following two methods. In the first one the catalogue of spectra from IPEM report 78 was used and adopted the same spectrum (Mo/0.03 mm Mo, 28 kV) as per „European guidelines for quality assurance in breast cancer screening and diagnosis Fourth edition". In the second one the contrast was calculated for the actual spectrum, in this case the W/0.05 mm Rh and 28 kV with the use of the above described spreadsheet. For both mammography units the contrast values determined for beam Mo/0.03 mm Mo, 28 kV are higher than to the contrast values for the actual beam. It shows that the differences of 26% - 27% in calculation of threshold contrast exist for both methods for all diameters and thicknesses values. It must be taken into account during the evaluation of quality control tests and all kinds of comparisons. It may be expected that the differences of threshold contrast values may be larger if the tube voltage value of the actual spectrum differs from 28 kV.

The values of the threshold contrast cannot exceed the limits given in the „European guidelines for quality assurance in breast cancer screening and diagnosis Fourth edition". For every object diameter two limits were set up (acceptable and achievable) expressed by the thickness of the object and by the corresponding threshold contrast (Table 7). These limits were established with the use of the CDMAM phantom placed between two PMMA plates of 2.0 cm thick and for typical X-ray spectrum for tube voltage value 28 kV, molybdenum target material and 30 μm thick molybdenum filter.

Diameter of detail [mm]	Gold thickness [µm]	Unit no 4			Diameter of detail [mm]	Gold thickness [µm]	Unit no 10		
		Threshold contrast [%]					Threshold contrast [%]		
		Typical spectrum (28 kV Mo/Mo)	Actual spectrum (28 kV W/Rh)	Difference [%]			Typical spectrum (28 kV Mo/Mo)	Actual spectrum (28 kV W/Rh)	Difference [%]
0.1	0.567	9.69	7.70	26	0.1	0.716	12.06	9.60	26
0.25	0.108	1.93	1.53	26	0.25	0.125	2.23	1.76	26
0.5	0.055	0.99	0.78	27	0.5	0.060	1.08	0.85	27
1.0	0.036	0.65	0.51	27	1.0	0.030	0.54	0.43	26
2.0	0.040	0.72	0.57	26	2.0	0.040	0.72	0.57	26

Table 6. Values of the threshold contrast for the exposures at the W/Rh combination of the CDMAM phantom, determined with two methods for mammography unit 4 and 10 (units 4 and 10 are the same as in Table 3).

Diameter of detail [mm]	Acceptable value		Achievable value	
	gold thickness [μm]	threshold contrast [%]	gold thickness [μm]	threshold contrast [%]
0.10	1.68	23.00	1.10	15.80
0.25	0.352	5.45	0.244	3.80
0.50	0.150	2.35	0.103	1.60
1.00	0.091	1.40	0.056	0.85
2.00	0.069	1.05	0.038	0.55

Table 7. Limiting values (acceptable and achievable levels) of the thickness of gold objects and corresponding value of threshold contrast for discs diameters from 0.10 mm to 2.00 mm according to the „European guidelines for quality assurance in breast cancer screening and diagnosis Fourth edition".

In Table 8 the examples of the image quality evaluation for four DR mammography units are presented. For the structures of the largest diameter (2.00 mm) on all images the structures of the same thicknesses were visible. The largest differences between the mammography units were seen for the low contrast objects of the smallest dimensions. While comparing the results of the analysis with the criteria given in the „European guidelines for quality assurance in breast cancer screening and diagnosis Fourth edition" (Table 7) one should consider mainly the visibility of the objects of specified thickness and not the specified contrast. The radiation contrast depends on the radiation quality used and does not characterize specifically the actual structure but the structure imaged with a given radiation beam. On the other hand the size of the structures visible on the phantom image is directly linked to the size of structures visible on the breast image.

Unit number	Parameter	Diameter of detail [mm]				
		0.10	0.25	0.50	1.00	2.00
2	Gold thickness [μm]	0.522	0.097	0.060	0.030	0.040
	Threshold contrast [%]	8.74	1.69	1.05	0.53	0.70
3	Gold thickness [μm]	0.806	0.143	0.056	0.036	0.040
	Threshold contrast [%]	11.93	2.24	0.88	0.57	0.63
4	Gold thickness [μm]	0.567	0.108	0.055	0.036	0.040
	Threshold contrast [%]	7.36	1.43	0.75	0.49	0.62
10	Gold thickness [μm]	0.716	0.125	0.060	0.030	0.040
	Threshold contrast [%]	9.17	1.69	0.82	0.41	0.55

Table 8. The example of the golden objects thicknesses for particular diameters and corresponding values of threshold contrast values for unprocessed images for mammography units 2, 3, 4 and 10 (units 2, 3, 4 and 10 are the same as in Table 3).

3.2 Contrast to noise ratio

The contrast to noise ratio (CNR) is used for the evaluation of the functioning of the AEC systems (so called object thickness and tube voltage compensation) for a given mammography unit. The functioning of the AEC systems should be controlled by exposures of PMMA plates of the thicknesses between 20 mm and 70 mm (10 mm step) with clinical settings of the AEC (tube voltage, target, filter, mode and exposure control step). During these exposures the compression paddle should be maximally pressed against the top surface of the plates. On the PMMA plates an aluminium object of 0.2 mm thickness should be placed. The dimensions of the object should be large enough to be able to mark on the image an area of 4 cm^2 as a region-of-interest (ROI). The PMMA plates have to cover the whole image detector. In Fig. 5 the positioning of the aluminium object on the PMMA plates and the position of the ROI (for which the mean pixel value and standard deviation are calculated) is indicated.

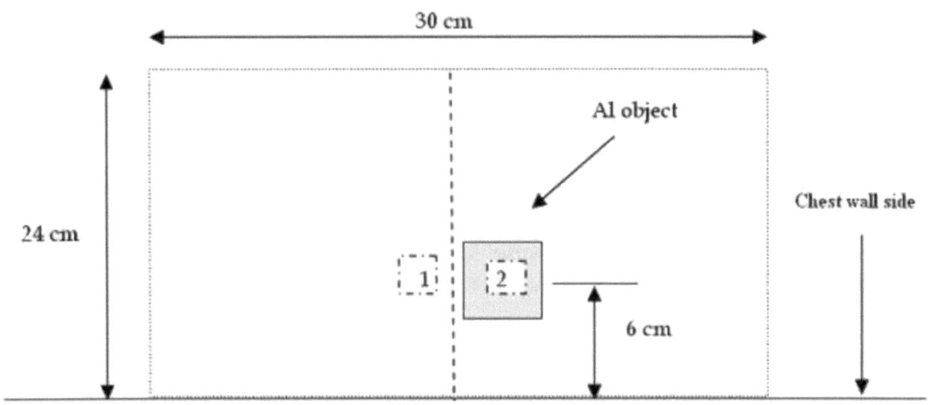

Fig. 5. The positioning of the aluminium object on PMMA plates and the ROI delineation for the CNR measurement.

The contrast to noise ratio (CNR) parameter should be calculated for a particular object according to the below presented formula from the „European guidelines for quality assurance in breast cancer screening and diagnosis Fourth edition":

$$CNR = \frac{mean\ pixel\ value(signal) - mean\ pixel\ value\ (background)}{\sqrt{\frac{Standard\ deviation\ (signal)^2 + Standard\ deviation\ (background)^2}{2}}} \quad (5)$$

where:

mean pixel value (signal) - mean pixel value for the ROI in position 2;
mean pixel value (background) - mean pixel value for ROI in position 1;
standard deviation (signal) – standard deviation for ROI in position 2;
standard deviation (background) – standard deviation for ROI in position 1.

On the basis of these data the CNR should be calculated according to the formula (5) for every PMMA plate from 20 mm to 70 mm thickness. The calculated CNR values should be referred to the limiting value ($CNR_{limiting\ value}$) calculated according to the formula (6) below:

$$CNR_{i/5cm} = \frac{CNR_i}{CNR_{limiting\ value}} \cdot 100\% \quad (6)$$

where:

$CNR_{i/5\,cm}$ - CNR value for PMMA plates of 20 mm, 30 mm, 40 mm, 45 mm, 50 mm, 60 mm and 70 mm thicknesses referred to the CNR value for PMMA phantom of 50 mm thickness;
CNR_i - CNR value determined for PMMA plates of 20 mm, 30 mm, 40 mm, 45 mm, 50 mm, 60 mm and 70 mm thickness;
$CNR_{limiting\ value}$ - the value calculated according to the formula (7) below;

$$CNR_{limiting\,value} = \frac{Treshold\,contrast_{measured} \cdot CNR_{measured}}{Treshold\ contrast_{limiting\,value}} \tag{7}$$

where:

Threshold $contrast_{measured}$ - the value of the threshold contrast determined for the golden object of 0.1 mm diameter placed in PMMA 50 mm thick (determined according to the methodology presented in 3.1);
$CNR_{measured}$ - CNR value determined for 50 mm PMMA;
Threshold $contrast_{limiting\ value}$ - limiting value of threshold contrast for a golden object of 0.1 mm diameter, equal to 23%.

According to the „European guidelines for quality assurance in breast cancer screening and diagnosis Fourth edition" the CNR values relative to the CNR for 50 mm PMMA must be determined during every control of the AEC system, at least every six month. The exemplary results for three mammography DR systems are presented in Table 9. In Table 9 in the second column the limiting values are listed. All results met the tolerance limits. The CNR values established for 70 mm PMMA thicknesses relative to the CNR for 50 mm PMMA were about 2 times higher (for every system) than the limiting value. In the case of 20 mm PMMA it was larger than the limiting value by about 3 to 4 times (depending on the system). This means that the AEC system setting by the manufacturer service is done to meet the minimum manufacturer requirements without trying to reach maximum values. This leads to the increased exposure of the image detector without taking into account the fact that even with the lower exposure the CNR limiting requirements would be met.

PMMA thickness [mm]	$CNR_{limiting\ value}$	Unit 2 / Manufacturer 2	Unit 3 / Manufacturer 2	Unit 4/ Manufacturer 3
	CNR relative to CNR for 50 mm PMMA [%]			
20	> 115	420	467	305
30	> 110	388	415	266
40	> 105	322	345	249
45	> 103	298	308	252
50	> 100	259	270	238
60	> 95	192	214	225
70	> 90	178	194	209

Table 9. The limiting values of the CNR relative to the CNR value for 50 mm PMMA for the objects of different thicknesses („European guidelines for quality assurance in breast cancer screening and diagnosis Fourth edition") and the exemplary results of CNR values relative to CNR for 50 mm PMMA for mammography units 2, 3 and 4 (units 2, 3 and 4 are the same as in Table 3).

3.3 Optimization

The user of the mammography system 3 did not agree to make exposures at the AEC system setting other than Auto-filter mode. The only way to introduce changes in exposure parameters setting was selecting different (than these which were used at that moment) service settings of the unit. For this particular unit the manufacturer service could select one of the available AEC system modes named in the mammography unit documentation as "Table 0", "Table 1", "Table 2" and "Table 3" (Table 10). The manufacturer described the way in which the AEC system adapts the tube voltage value to the breast thickness after compression. Before the optimization attempt the "Table 0" mode was set, for which the clinical breast doses did not fulfil the acceptance criteria. It was necessary to find out for which setting the clinical breast doses could be lowered to the acceptance limits without affecting the threshold contrast and CNR for various PMMA plates thicknesses.

For each AEC mode:

- AGD values were calculated for typical breasts (described in 2.2 above);
- evaluation of threshold contrast for discs of various diameters was performed (described in 3.1 above);
- CNR values were determined for exposures of the PMMA plates of the thickness in the range from 20 mm to 70 mm (10 mm step) and for 45 mm (described in. 3.2 above).

All these activities were carried out with the exposure control step set to "0", in Auto-filter mode and with the main region of detector of the AEC system manually set closest to the chest wall. The results are presented in Table 11 and Table 12. In Table 11, the values of tube voltage, tube load and anode/filter combination selected by the AEC system for various thicknesses of PMMA plates, CNR relative to CNR for 50 mm PMMA and the AGD values calculated for typical breasts for four possible settings of the mammography unit 3, are given. In Table 12, the thicknesses of golden objects of various diameters and corresponding values of threshold contrast for four settings of the mammography unit 3, are presented. When comparing the values in Tables 11 and 12 with limiting levels given in Tables 2, 7 and 9 one can see that quality criteria at the acceptable levels concerning all parameters (AGD, threshold contrast and CNR) are met for modes "Table 1", "Table 2" and "Table 3" with the lowest clinical breast doses for mode "Table 3". For this particular mammography unit all routine mammography examinations, before the optimization of exposure parameters, were performed with the "Table 0". For this mode the clinical breast doses were the highest and for PMMA plates of 4.0 cm and 4.5 cm thickness the AGD values exceed slightly the acceptable level, but the image quality was the best of the four modes. For the "Table 2" mode the image quality was the worst. Out of remaining two modes, "Table 1" and "Table 3", the "Table 3" mode was selected because of the lower clinical breast doses.

With the AEC setting in mode "Table 3" the mammography examinations were performed and the quality of the images was accepted by the radiologists. The "Table 3" mode was set by the manufacturer service as the permanent option not to be changed. The exposure control step ("0") wasn't changed. At these settings of the mammography unit the examinations of women have been started. For the examined women the clinical breast doses were calculated according to the methodology given in 2.3 above. In Table 13, the minimum, maximum and mean values of clinical breast doses calculated for the women examined with the use of the mammography unit 3 before and after the optimization of

Step #	Thickness (cm)	kV for "Table 0"	kV for "Table 1"	kV for "Table 2"	kV for "Table 3"
02	1.0	24	24	27	25
03	1.5	24	24	27	25
04	2.0	24	24	27	25
05	2.5	24	24	27	26
06	3.0	25	25	27	27
07	3.5	26	25	28	28
08	4.0	27	25	28	28
09	4.5	28	26	28	29
10	5.0	29	27	30	30
11	5.5	30	28	31	30
12	6.0	31	29	32	31
13	6.5	32	29	32	31
14	7.0	32	30	32	32
15	7.5	32	31	33	32
16	8.0	33	32	33	33
17	8.5	33	33	33	33
18	9.0	34	34	34	34
19	9.5	34	34	35	34
20	10.0	35	35	36	35
21	10.5	35	35	37	36
22	11.0	37	37	38	37
23	11.5	38	38	39	38
24	12.0	39	39	39	39
25	12.5	39	39	39	39
26	13.0	39	39	39	39
27	13.5	39	39	39	39
28	14.0	39	39	39	39
29	14.5	39	39	39	39
30	15.0	39	39	39	39
31	15.5	39	39	39	39

Table 10. Tube voltage selection scheme by the AEC system according to the breast thickness after compression - from technical documentation of the mammography unit 3.

Setting of AEC system	Parameter	PMMA thickness [cm]						
		2.0	3.0	4.0	4.5	5.0	6.0	7.0
"Table 0"	Tube voltage [kV]	24	26	28	29	30	32	32
	Tube load [mAs]	40.9	56.0	72.9	85.0	91.7	94.3	147.2
	Target/filter	Mo/Mo	Mo/Mo	Mo/Mo	Mo/Mo	Mo/Mo	Mo/Rh	Mo/Rh
	CNR relative to CNR for 50 mm PMMA [%]	467	415	345	308	270	214	194
	AGD [mGy]	0.92	1.36	2.04	2.51	2.93	3.12	4.42
"Table 1"	Tube voltage [kV]	24	26	28	29	30	32	32
	Tube load [mAs]	35.2	48.2	61.9	72.8	78.6	80.9	124.7
	Target/filter	Mo/Mo	Mo/Mo	Mo/Mo	Mo/Mo	Mo/Mo	Mo/Rh	Mo/Rh
	CNR relative to CNR for 50 mm PMMA [%]	444	396	329	289	259	212	191
	AGD [mGy]	0.79	1.17	1.73	2.14	2.51	2.66	3.74
"Table 2"	Tube voltage [kV]	27	28	28	30	31	32	33
	Tube load [mAs]	16.3	27.2	60.0	59.0	57.0	80.0	101.3
	Target/filter	Mo/Mo	Mo/Mo	Mo/Mo	Mo/Mo	Mo/Rh	Mo/Rh	Mo/Rh
	CNR relative to CNR for 50 mm PMMA [%]	328	289	270	226	198	172	144
	AGD [mGy]	0.61	0.90	1.68	1.98	1.80	2.64	3.36
"Table 3"	Tube voltage [kV]	26	28	27	30	30	31	32
	Tube load [mAs]	22.7	27.2	58.1	47.0	60.9	88.1	127.7
	Target/filter	Mo/Mo	Mo/Mo	Mo/Rh	Mo/Rh	Mo/Rh	Mo/Rh	Mo/Rh
	CNR relative to CNR for 50 mm PMMA [%]	336	278	238	207	201	171	148
	AGD [mGy]	0.72	0.90	1.20	1.41	1.73	2.59	3.77

Table 11. Tube voltage, tube load and anode/filter combination selected by the AEC system for PMMA plates of various thicknesses, CNR values relative to 5.0 cm PMMA and AGD values calculated for typical breasts for four operation modes of the AEC system for mammography unit 3.

Setting of AEC system	Parameter	Diameter of detail [mm]				
		0.10	0.25	0.50	1.00	2.00
"Table 0"	Gold thickness [μm]	0.525	0.125	0.068	0.030	0.040
	Threshold contrast [%]	8.758	2.173	1.189	0.526	0.701
"Table 1"	Gold thickness [μm]	0.547	0.134	0.060	0.030	0.040
	Threshold contrast [%]	9.134	2.327	1.049	0.526	0.701
"Table 2"	Gold thickness [μm]	0.753	0.138	0.081	0.037	0.040
	Threshold contrast [%]	12.333	2.396	1.414	0.649	0.701
"Table 3"	Gold thickness [μm]	0.806	0.143	0.056	0.036	0.040
	Threshold contrast [%]	11.925	2.239	0.883	0.569	0.632

Table 12. The thicknesses of golden objects of various diameters and corresponding values of threshold contrast for four settings of the AEC system for the mammography unit no 3.

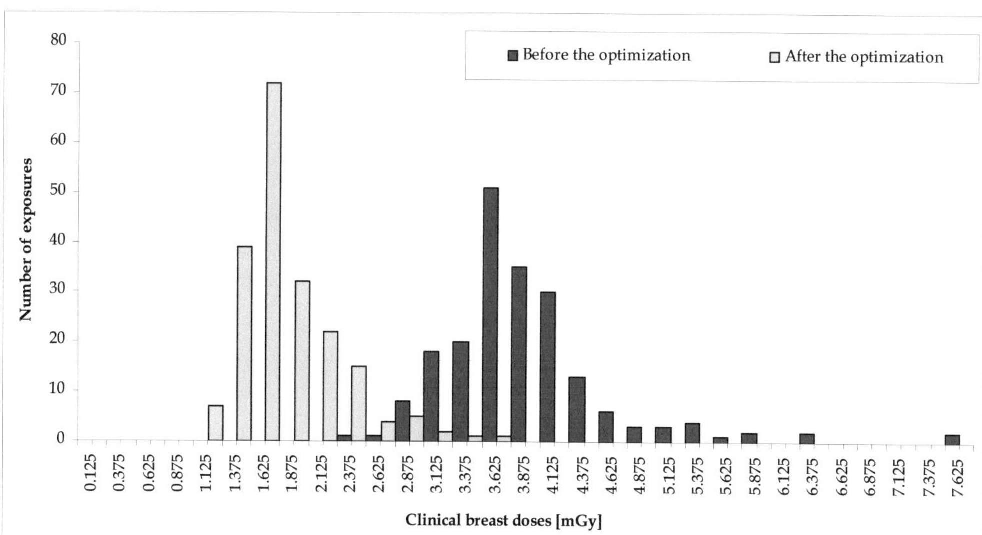

Fig. 6. Clinical breast doses calculated for two groups of women examined with the mammography unit 3: before the optimization of exposure parameters (in black) and after the optimization (in grey).

Calculation of clinical breast doses	Clinical breast doses [mGy]			The percentage of exposures not exceeding	
	minimum value	maximum value	mean value	acceptable level	achievable level
Before the optimization	2.45	7.71	3.89	1 %	0 %
After the optimization	1.16	3.64	1.80	80.5 %	47 %

Table 13. Minimum, maximum and mean values of clinical breast doses calculated and the percentage of exposures, for which the clinical breast doses were below the acceptable and achievable level, before and after the optimization of exposure parameters for the mammography unit 3.

exposure parameters, are presented. The percentage of exposures, for which the clinical breast dose values do not exceed the limiting values at the acceptable and achievable levels, are also given. The maximum, minimum and mean values of clinical breast doses after the optimization of exposure parameters were lower than these values before the optimization by about 53%. The values of clinical breast doses after the optimization of exposure parameters were below the acceptable level in 80.5% of cases and below the achievable level in 47% of cases.

The decrease of the clinical breast dose values after setting the "Table 3" AEC mode on the mammography unit 3 is better presented in Fig. 6. Two histograms of clinical breast dose values, before the optimization of exposure parameters (in black) and after the optimization (in grey) are presented. They are clearly separated which means that the efforts to optimize the exposure parameters brought about a significant reduction of the clinical breast doses received by the women during examination. It should be noted that it was achieved at the cost of slight reduction of the visibility of the objects at the threshold contrast level, but it was accepted by the radiologists involved in image analysis in the mammography screening program.

4. Conclusion

The optimization procedure presented in this chapter is only a proposal of actions which could lead to the reduction of the doses received by the women during mammography examinations, especially in case of screening programs when probably healthy women are irradiated. The proposed approach has an advantage of not resigning of the system settings allowing for fully automatic of tube voltage and filter selection. Evidently, mammography units of various types and from different manufacturers have different capabilities but every capability should be first used for the optimization of exposure parameters and clinical breast doses reduction during mammography examinations.

5. References

Boone, J.M.; Fewell, T.R. & Jennings, R.J. Molybdenum, rhodium, and tungsten anode spectral models using interpolating polynomials with application to mammography. *Medical Physics*, 24, 12, (December 1997), pp. 1863-1874, ISSN 0094-2405

Chevalier, M.; Morán, P.; Ten, J.I.; Soto, J.M.F.; Cepeda, T. & Vañó, E. Patient dose in digital mammography. *Medical Physics*, 31, 9, (September 2004), pp. 2471-2479, ISSN 0094-2405.

Cranley, K.; Gilmore, B.J.; Fogarty, G.W.A. & Desponds, L. (1997) *Catalogue of diagnostic X – ray spectra & other data*, Institute of Physics and Engineering in Medicine, ISBN 090418188X, York, UK

Dance, D. R.; Skinner, C.L.; Young, K.C.; Beckett, J.R. & Kotre, C.J. Additional factors for the estimation of mean glandular breast dose using the UK mammography dosimetry protocol, *Physics in Medicine and Biology*, 45, (November 2000), pp. 3225-3240, ISSN 0031-9155

Dosimetry in Diagnostic Radiology: An International Code of Practice, International Atomic Energy Agency, (September 2007), ISBN 92-0-115406-2, Vienna, Austria

Fischmann, A.; Siegmann, K.C.; Wersebe, A.; Claussen, C.D. & Müller - Schimpfle, M. Comparison of full-field digital mammography and film-screen mammography: image quality and lesion detection, *British Journal of Radiology*, 78, (April 2005), pp. 312–315, ISSN 0007-1285

Gennaro, G. & di Magio, C. Dose comparison between screen/film and full-field digital mammography, *European Radiology*, 16, (November 2006), pp. 2559–2566, ISSN 1432-1084

Gennaro, G.; Baldelli, P.; Taibi, A.; di Magio, C. & Gambaccini, M. Patient dose in full-field digital mammography: an Italian survey, *European Radiology*, 14, (April 2004), pp. 645-652, ISSN 1432-1084

Gosch, D.; Jendrass, S.; Scholz, M. & Kahn, T. Radiation exposure in full-field digital mammography with a selenium flat-panel detector, *RoFo Fortschritte auf dem Gebiete der Rontgenstrahlen und der Nuklearme*, 178, (July 2006), pp. 693-697, ISSN 1438-9029

Hermann, K.P.; Obenauer, S.; Marten, K.; Kehbel, S.; Fischer, U. & Grabbe, E. Average glandular dose with amorphous silicon full-field digital mammography - Clinical results," *RoFo Fortschritte auf dem Gebiete der Rontgenstrahlen und der Nuklearme*, 174, (June 2002), pp. 696-699, ISSN 1438-9029

Lawinski, C.P.; Cole, J.A.; Emerton, D.P.; Clinch, P.J. & Mackenzie, A. (July 2008). Buyer's guide Digital mammography, Available from: <http://nhscep.useconnect.co.uk/CEPProducts/Catalogue.aspx?ReportType=Buyers%27+guide>

Perry, N.; Broeders, M.; de Wolf, C.; Törnberg, S.; Holland, R. & von Karsa, L. (2006) *European guidelines for quality assurance in breast cancer screening and diagnosis Fourth edition*, European Commission, ISBN 92-79-01258-4, Belgium

Van der Burght, R.; Thijssen, M. & Bijkerk, R. (2010). *Manual Contrast Detail Phantom CDMAM 3.4. & CDMAM Analyser software V1.2.*, Artinis Medical systems BV, Zetten, Netherlands

7

An Analysis of Application of Mean Glandular Dose and Factors on Which It Depends to Patients of Various Age Groups

Suad Kunosic[1,2]
[1]*Department of Physics, Faculty of Natural Sciences and Mathematics, University of Tuzla*
[2]*Department of Biophysics, Medical Faculty, University of Tuzla*
Bosnia and Herzegovina

1. Introduction

Breast cancer is the most frequently diagnosed type of cancer nowadays and it is the leading cause of death caused by cancer in women (Jemal et al., 2011). It has become one of the main health problems both in developed and in developing countries. More than a million new cases of breast cancer are diagnosed every year all over the world (Ferlay et al., 2004). According to researches of the American Cancer Society (American Cancer Society, 2002), since 2002 breast cancer has been the second largest cause of death caused by cancer in women. According to a research conducted in 2007 in Korea, breast cancer was the second most frequently detected type of cancer in women (Kyu-Won et al., 2010). In 2008 there were 3, 2 million (Ferlay et al., 2010) new cases of cancer in Europe out of which 421, 000 (13,1%) (Ferlay et al., 2010) cases were breast cancers. According to the mentioned research, after colorectal cancer (436, 000 cases) breast cancer is the second most frequently registered cancer in Europe (Ferlay et al., 2010). In Bosnia and Herzegovina 1600 new cases of breast cancer are registered every year (Saric, 2009). Nowadays, mammography represents the best diagnostic way for detection of breast cancer. This diagnostic medical discipline applies a specially designed roentgen apparatus for breast examination. A good topographic position and a high degree of mobility of the breast (Fajdic, 2001) enable a great number of early diagnosed breast cancers detected with mammography. Ultrasound breast diagnostic is often used as an additional method to classic mammography for breast cancer detection, especially identification of cysts in the breast (Fajdic, 2001). Nowadays there are classic (film-screen) and digital mammography. While digital mammography enables a superior contrast resolution, its spatial resolution is somewhat lower in regard to the standard technique (Kuzmiak et al., 2005). Advantages and disadvantages of these two types of mammography were compared in more than ten studies (Rosselli Del Turco et al., 2007; Skaane, 2009). One of the main arguments for giving priority to digital mammography in regard to classic mammography was the fact that digital systems cause less radiation during an examination (Hermann et al., 2002; Moran et al., 2005). The newest study shows that digital mammography cannot guarantee significantly lower patient doses in regard to classic mammography (Hauge et al., 2011). The objective of most studies about mammography is to define benefits and risks caused by application of radiation in mammography. The size which best describes amount of risk for glandular tissue caused by application of radiation in mammography is called mean glandular dose (MGD). There are two critical age groups of patients in mammography: patients 40 to 49 years of age and patients 50 to 64 years of age. Naturally, patient doses have to be defined for all other patients who undergo mammographic diagnostic but do not belong to the mentioned age groups. Advantages of a routine mammography in timely diagnosing of breast diseases are great. Mammographic screening reduces mortality caused by breast cancer for women 39 to 69 years of age (Heidi D. Nelson et al., 2009). This study aims to define patient doses and factors which influence them for all critical groups of patients in routine mammography. Since a mammographic examination of each breast consists of mediolateral and craniocaudal projection, it was necessary to define patient doses for individual projections and for the complete mammographic examination.

2. Materials and methods

2.1 A procedure for measuring of measurable parameters in mammography

Like any other study in diagnostic radiology, this one also aimed to first collect all measurable parameters during a routine mammography. It was necessary to collect not only physical but also technical, diagnostic and medical parameters.

During mammographic diagnostic, it is necessary to note physical and technical parameters, and after completion of mammography also diagnostic and medical parameters which can be offered by a radiologist. On a basis of collected data about a patient (age, mass, height) and with an established body mass index (BMI), one can examine its relation with patient doses in mammography (Schubauer-Berigan et al., 2002; Jamal et al., 2003) and a frequency of patient's going for a regular mammographic examination (Zhu et al., 2006). All experimental measuring of doses during diagnostic mammographic examinations was performed at the Department of Mammography of Public Health Institution Health Center Tuzla. For diagnostic examinations of patients we used a GE Healthcare Alpha ST (Mo/Mo) mammographic apparatus. In classic mammography (film-screen), Mo/Mo dominates as one of the most frequently used meta/filter combinations (Hauge et al., 2011), and many mammographic systems, such as Alpha ST, have a Mo/Mo meta/filter combination as their only choice. The measuring was done in the period from May 2008 to January 2011 and it involved 329 female patients between 40 and 64 years of age.

The following data were recorded during a diagnostic examination:

a. patient's age,
b. applied clinical spectrum (meta/filter combination),
c. CBT (compressed breast thickness) and type of projection (CC, MLO) for each breast,
d. exposition factors: charge I·t (mAs) and voltage (kVp),
e. size of applied film (18 x 24 or 24 x 32),
f. number of previous mammographic examinations underwent by every patient,
g. type of diagnostic examination: routine control examination, post-operative control examination; an enlarged additional image of a certain projection is necessary; a repeated image because of insufficient sharpness.
h. possible ultrasound control.

The mentioned data were used for calculation of strength of kerma in the air, filter half-values and conversion factors for age groups. Mean glandular dose (MGD) for the breast was defined according to these parameters. MGD doses were defined for every individual projection and for the complete mammographic examination. A statistical dependency (correlation) between compressed breast thickness and MGD dose was defined for every age group and for mediolateral and craniocaudal projection of every age group.

A correlation between ultrasound and mammographic breast examination was found and it was confirmed that these two diagnostic disciplines complement each other excellently in early breast cancer prevention (Harlow et al., 1999; Kuhl et al., 2005). A combination of mammography and ultrasound with a possible ultrasound cytological puncture offers a basis for a reliable diagnosis of the smallest malignant formations in breasts (Mainiero, 2010). A number of underwent mammographic examinations in a correlation with patient's age gave an answer to many questions, such as: a level of information about breast cancer available to patients, need for a routine mammography in breast cancer prevention, importance of self-examination for women and differences in psychological behavior of patients during the first and after several mammographic examinations. A type of diagnostic examination on a mammography unit and a way of its performance showed the importance of a role of a radiology technician and his/her direct communication with a patient during the process for obtaining a good quality of image in mammographic diagnostics.

2.2 Quality control

Quality control (Geise et al., 1988; Hendrick et al., 2002) in mammography contains a set of tests (Perry et al., 2006) which can be divided according to priority and a level of training of personnel who perform them. Some tests require usage of special equipment or special work conditions. That is why sometimes in some institutions there is a possibility of failure to implement a complete quality control of a mammography system. Regular quality controls of mammography units in some countries contributed to decreasing of patient doses and improvement of quality of mammographic images (Maccia et al., 1995; Zdesar, 2000; Vassileva et al., 2005; Ciraj-Bjelac et al., 2011) and improvement of functioning of a mammography unit (Zoetelief et al., 1992). The tests can be grouped in the following way:

- Tests for mammographic device,
- Tests for films, foil and processor,
- Tests for quality of images,
- Calculation of breast dose

Quality control in mammography was regularly performed during a three-year period of data collection and its long-term strategy was to support reduction of mortality rate caused by breast cancer. A special attention was dedicated to tests for mammographic devices. Anode voltage value, dose reproducibility and filter half-value (HVL) without returnable radiation were measured for different settings of kVp and meta filter combination (a controlled mammography unit had only one meta filter combination Mo/Mo) following recommendations of the quality control protocol (Perry et al., 2006), which defines measuring methodology and frequency. When measuring half filter value (HVL) one used aluminium filters of extremely high purity (99,9%). First, measuring was done several times without a filter in order to obtain an initial exposition value. Afterwards, sets of aluminium filters of various thicknesses were settled between the focus and detectors. Roentgen tube voltage ranged from 22 to 32 kVp and every voltage value was measured several times in order to obtain half the dose in regard to the initial dose value on the detector. Possible HVL values in mammography range from 0,25 to 0,45 mmAl. All tests for mammographic device were done with Barracuda instrument.

2.3 Dosimetry

For every mammogram MGD was defined on a basis of conversion factors calculated by Dance et. al. (Dance et al., 2000) and a calculated *K* (entering air kerma measured freely in air without backscatter), using the following relation:

$$\mathrm{MGD} = \mathrm{K\,g\,c\,s}$$

For every individual exposition *K* was calculated from post - exposure mAs (I · t) and output data for the x - ray set in μGy mAs^{-1} used in an exposition field. Conversion factors were calculated by Dance for a different clinical spectrum (target/filter combination), HVL, compressed breast thickness and breast glandularity. *G* and *c* are conversion factors to account for both X-ray beam characteristics and breast composition i.e., various percentages of fat and glandular tissue. Factor *s* includes a correction for applied type of the clinical spectrum and all screens were made using the same clinical spectra Mo/Mo.

2.4 Statistical analysis

The data were statistically processed in SPSS 17.0 and they were shown as standard deviation and confidence interval. Pearson´s coefficient was used for statistical significance of correlation between MGD and CBT. A value of $p<0.05$ was considered as indicative of significance.

3. Results and discussion

3.1 Age and compressed breast thickness

Age of examined patients varied from 40 to 64. The average age of the first group (40 - 49) was 45, 27 years (SD: 2,76) and of the second age group (50 - 64) it was 55,90 years (SD: 4,20). The average age of all of the patients was 51,63 (SD: 6,39). Distribution of compressed breast thickness in mammography was symmetrical to patient's age and it varied from 20 to 100 mm. Errors in defining compressed breast thickness varied in the range of ± 1 mm. There was a good correlation between patient's age and compressed breast thickness. A similar symmetry was noted in other works (Beckett & Kotre, 2000; Kunosic et al., 2010; Kunosic et al., 2011). Mean value of compressed breast thickness of the complete sample was 42,24 mm (SD : 14,86). It is known that compressed breast thickness value shows a certain tendency of growth in younger patients and a tendency of decline in older patients (Law et al., 1994), which proved as true in our examined sample. Mean value of compressed breast thickness in mediolateral projection was 20 to 23 % higher than in craniocaudal projection. This information is very important for understanding of results and explanation of obtained glandular doses for the breast from Tables 4. and 5.

3.2 Quality control

Accuracy of measured voltage in roentgen tube (maximum deviation) was ± 0,89 kVp for voltage ranging from 22 to 32 kVp. Outgoing radiation (mGy/mAs) was measured several times during this study and it was within the range of ± 4 % from the initial value. The most frequently used voltage during performance of diagnostic examinations was 25 kVp (45,08 %). This voltage was applied in cases when compressed breast thickness varied from 20 to 28 mm, and sometimes with higher values of compressed breast thickness depending on age group to which a patient belongs.

Voltage of 26 kVp (19,18 %) was applied in most cases when compressed breast thickness was 28 to 34 mm while voltage of 27 kVp (13,69 %) was mainly applied when compressed breast thickness varied from 35 to 45 mm. Percentage of utilization voltage of 25, 26 and 27 kVp leads us to a conclusion that the greatest number of patients who underwent a routine mammography in this study had compressed breast thickness from 20 to 45 mm, if we assess utilization voltage. A significant percent of utilization was ascribed to voltage of 28 kVp (10,57 %) and 29 kVp (8,03 %) when compresses breast thickness varied from 40 to 53 mm and 54 to 63 mm, respectively. Voltage of 30 kVp (1,97 %) and 31 kVp (0,82 %) was applied for compressed breast thickness from 64 to 80 mm to make a compromise between mentioned values and obtain an image of better quality. Voltage of 32 (0,49 %) and 33 (0,16 %) kVp was used for extremely great values of compressed breast thickness from 81 to 100 mm.

Age group (years)	Number of images	Voltage								
		25 (kVp)	26 (kVp)	27 (kVp)	28 (kVp)	29 (kVp)	30 (kVp)	31 (kVp)	32 (kVp)	33 (kVp)
40 - 49	493	200	99	93	66	35	0	0	0	0
	(%)	40,57	20,08	18,86	13,39	7,10	0,00	0,00	0,00	0,00
50 - 64	727	350	135	74	63	63	24	10	6	2
	(%)	48,14	18,57	10,18	8,67	8,67	3,30	1,38	0,83	0,28
Total	1220	550	234	167	129	98	24	10	6	2
	(%)	45,08	19,18	13,69	10,57	8,03	1,97	0,82	0,49	0,16

Table 1. Statistical illustration of applied voltage per age groups for complete sample during mammographic diagnostics.

When we analyze percentage of representation of voltage applied during diagnostic examinations per age groups we draw similar conclusions like for the complete sample, with a slight deviation. What is interesting to note here is that voltage of 30 - 33 kVp was not applied for the age group 40 - 49. Voltage of 25 kVp was mostly applied for this group while the difference in application of voltage of 26 and 27 kVp was insignificant. These three voltages were applied for about 80 % diagnostic examinations (Table 1.) of this age group. It is important to note that absence of application of extremely high voltage was compensated with significant application of voltage of 28 and 29 kVp, which representation is greater in this age group in regard to the other age group (Table 1.).

A tendency of application of voltage of 25 kVp and voltage of 26 kVp was retained in the age group 50 to 64 years of age (Table 1). The difference in regard to the age group 40 - 49 reflects in significantly less application of voltage of 27 and 28 kVp (Table 1.) and greater utilization of voltage ranging from 30 to 33 kVp. This wide spectrum of voltage applied in the age group 50 - 64 was caused by a wide spectrum of compressed breast thickness.

3.3 X – ray technique

The greatest number of images taken during mammographic diagnostic was two for MLO and two for CC projection. The total number of images used for a complete diagnostic examination was 4. The same clinical spectrum (meta/filter) Mo/Mo was applied for all diagnostic examinations. 1220 images were taken to examine 329 patients (Table 2.), out of which 1172 images were taken for the complete mammographic examination of 293 (89,06 %) patients (two images for each projection). In this way both breasts were completely diagnostically processed (Hackshaw et al., 2000). 24 images were used for a routine control examination of one breast after a surgery or additional controls because of a certain doubt (one for each projection) to examine 12 (3,65 %) patients.

Remaining 24 (7,29 %) patients were examined with application of 24 images mainly because of a need for an improved image (of better quality) for some of projections.

Age group (years)	Number of patients	Number of images taken per a patient during mammography			Type of film applied per a patient	
		4 images	2 images	1 images	18 x 24	24 x 32
	132	119	4	9	71	61
40 - 49	(%)	90,15	3,03	6,82	53,79	46,21
	197	174	8	15	97	100
50 - 64	(%)	88,32	4,06	7,61	49,24	50,76
	329	293	12	24	168	161
Total	(%)	89,06	3,65	7,29	51,06	48,94

Table 2. Statistical illustration of number of images taken and types of films applied for all age groups and complete sample during mammographic diagnostic.

Percentage of patients for whom taking two images was necessary for examination of one breast was 3,65 %, and it indicates a need for a routine mammographic control because it represents a percentage of patients in whom a timely routine control detected breast cancer. It is in common in all of developed countries of the world which have a developed program for early breast cancer detection to examine all patients with application of 4 images (two images for each projection) with a desire to obtain a complete clinical picture (Nelson et al., 2002; Miller, 2005).

Such approach is a result of routine mammography which is compulsory every third year in developed countries. As a result, there is a great number of patients with early detected breast cancer (Greenlee et al., 2000), which automatically influences a decrease of mortality caused by breast cancer (Tabar et al., 2003; Gøtzsche & Nielsen, 2006; Gøtzsche, 2011; D'Orsi & Newell, 2011).

Age group (years)	Number of images	Mammographic image 18 x 24 (cassette)			Mammographic image 24 x 32 (cassette)		
		4 images	2 images	1 image	4 images	2 images	1 image
	493	63	3	5	56	1	4
40 - 49	(%)	88,73	4,23	7,04	91,80	1,64	6,56
	727	88	4	5	86	4	10
50 - 64	(%)	90,72	4,12	5,15	86,00	4,00	10,00
	1220	151	7	10	142	5	14
Total	(%)	89,88	4,17	5,95	88,20	3,11	8,70

Table 3. Statistical illustration of number of images taken depending on size of film applied for all age groups.

An analysis of applied mammographic images per age categories (Table 3.) revealed new interesting information. Over 90% of complete mammographic examinations were performed in the first age group where belong younger patients (40 to 49 years of age). As expected, number of 18 x 24 images is greater because this is the population where the breast (Kopans et al., 2003), as a very dynamic organ, passes through a set of dynamic changes during its growth and development. Mammographic images 24 x 32 are mainly used for patients between 46 and 49. A percentage of control examinations after a surgery of one breast is small, not greater than 3,1 %. It is expected for this age category to have a lot of blur and unclearness in mammographic images, which sometimes cause repetition of one of diagnostic projections (1 image, CC or MLO). Percentage of repeated images is a bit smaller than 7 % (Table 3.), which is quite satisfactory for such huge population and adequate for a radiologist to obtain a clear clinical picture and to define a final diagnosis on a basis of an additional image. A complete mammographic examination was conducted in 44, 67 cases from the second age group (50 - 64) with 18 x 24 film and in 43,65 % cases with 24 x 32 films. With this population, there is a tendency of increasing of a number of control examinations for 50% in regard to the younger age group. This is a confirmation of the tendency of growth of early breast cancer detection in women who frequently undergo routine controls and self-examinations. Percentage trend of 7,62 % of repeated images in one projection is retained, although a number of diagnostically treated patients increased for 33% in regard to the previous group. A slight advantage for the benefit of usage of smaller 18 x 24 images in regard to bigger 24 x 32 images in a complete diagnostic examination corresponds to the average compressed breast thickness of diagnostically processed population (Table 5.). The mentioned data leads us to the conclusion that the average compressed breast thickness of the examined population with such great sample must be less than 50 mm, in comparison with other study (Kunosic et al., 2010).

3.4 Patient's doses

The most frequently used procedure in a routine mammography includes 2 images of every breast, craniocaudal and mediolateral. Even if there is a visible anomaly at one breast, it is necessary to perform a diagnostic mammographic examination of both breasts. Such procedure enables us to compare both breasts and to detect possible anomalies into details (Hackshaw et al., 2000). In the last 20 years a set of studies has been conducted in Europe with the objective to define MGD (Wall & Roberts, 1992; Faulkner et al., 1995; Klein et al., 1997; Beckett & Kotre, 2000; Adlien et al., 2005; Assiamah et al., 2005; Tsapaki et al., 2008; Kunosic et al., 2010; Ciraj-Bijelac et al., 2010). Similar researches were conducted on Thailand (Sookpeng & Ketted, 2006), in Iran (Bouzarjomehri et al., 2006), in the USA(Gentry & De Werd, 1996), Malaysia (Jamal et al., 2003), Australia (Heggie, 1996), Korea (Oh et al., 2003) and many other countries all over the world. Table 10.4. illustrates results regarding MGD for every individual projection and for the complete diagnostic examination of all patients during MLO and CC diagnostic examinations.

	Number of images	Voltage	CBT (mm)	I t (mAs)	MGD (mGy)	
		kVp ± SD	Mean ± SD	Mean ± SD	MGD ± CI	Third quartile
Total	1220	26,31 ± 1,56	42,24 ± 14,86	40,71 ± 12,73	0,90 ± 0,01	0,99
CC	613	25,75 ± 1,09	36,88 ± 11,95	35,88 ± 10,27	0,83 ± 0,01	0,91
MLO	607	26,87 ± 1,75	47,76 ± 15,54	45,58 ± 13,12	0,96 ± 0,02	1,09

Table 4. Complete statistical illustration of voltage, compressed breast thickness,MGD for all patients and two different projections (CC, MLO). (MLO - Mediolateral oblique view; CC - Craniocaudal view; SD - Standard deviation, CI - Confidence interval for the mean of 95 %; CBT - Compressed breast thickness)

Values of MGD and compressed breast thickness (CBT) were defined for a sample of 1220 images (613 CC and 607 MLO projections). Mean value of a patient dose for the complete CC projection was 1,66 mGy and for MLO projection 1,92 mGy. A significant difference (Table 4.) between the mentioned doses (according to calculated values) was caused by compressed breast thickness and it was 13,54 %. Similar results were noted in works of other authors (Gentry & De Werd, 1996; Heggie, 1996; Young, 2000; Jamal et al., 2003; Oh et al., 2003; Bouzarjomehri et al., 2006; Sookpeng & Ketted, 2006; Tsapaki et al., 2008; Kunosic et al., 2010). A sample of a significant increase of doses in MLO in regard to CC projection can be explained with the fact that pectoral muscle (Helvie et al., 1994; Young, 2000) is involved in MLO projection which causes an increase of thickness of compressed tissue and requires greater exposition for an image of a better quality. The total dose for a complete mammographic examination was 3,58 mGy, which is much less than 4 mGy which is the ceiling for mammography. In comparison with other studies (based on a principle of a great sample) the obtained patient dose is less in regard to a study conducted in Sweden (Eklund et al., 1993) which involved a sample of 1350 patients and in regard to a study conducted on 490 patients in Australia (Heggie, 1996), and it correlates well with results of studies from Korea (Oh et al., 2003) and Greece (Tsapaki et al., 2008). A study conducted in Iran included 246 patients (Bouzarjomehri et al., 2006) and showed that an obtained MGD dose for a complete mammographic examination in that country was 5,57 mGy, which is significantly more in regard to this study and which, most probably, is a consequence of a quality control system which was established late and differences in compressed breast thickness. The mentioned studies did not use conversion factors according to Dance (which are used in this study), but in Austra, Korea and Malaysia one used conversion factors according to Wu (Wu et al., 1991), in Sweden according to Rosenstein and in Iran according to Sobol (Sobol & Wu, 1997). Values of MGD dose for a complete mammographic examination in Bosnia and Herzegovina are 5,0 % higher in regard to results obtained from 300 patients in Malaysia (Jamal et al., 2003) and 7,8 % higher in regard to the most complete study (Young & Burch, 2000) conducted in the Great Britain which included 8745 patients. More than 70 % of all of mammographic diagnostic examinations was done with doses less than 3,2 mGy. According to a correlation analysis (Picture 10.2.), there was a considerable significance (Fig. 1.) between MGD and CBT ($r = 0,689$, $p<0,01$).

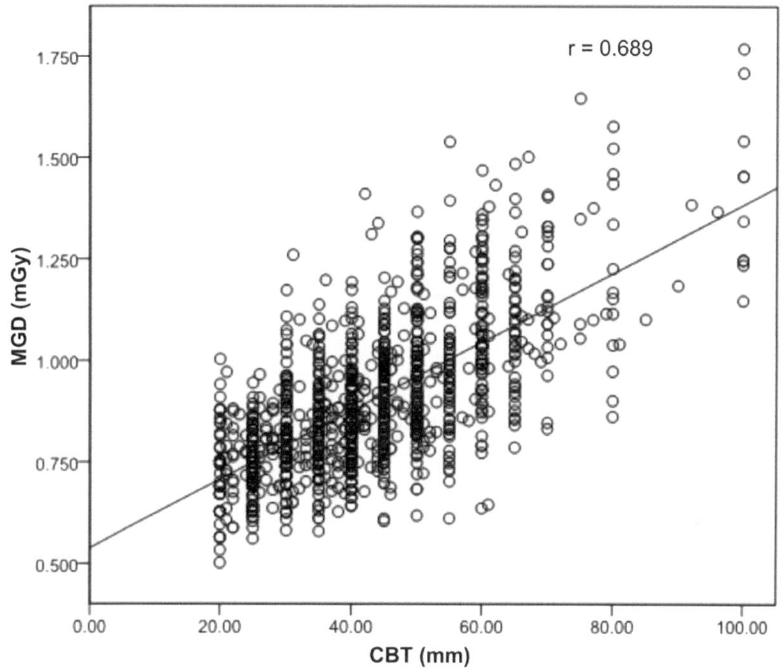

Fig. 1. Correlation between MGD and CBT.

A similar positive correlation between MGD and CBT was noted on a much smaller sample of Bosnian patients (Kunosic et al., 2010). An influence of CBT on patient doses during mammographic diagnostic examinations was confirmed by other authors in their researches (Wall & Roberts, 1992; Gentry & De Werd, 1996; Dance et al, 2000; Kruger et al, 2001; Oh et al., 2003; Bouzarjomehri et al., 2006; Sookpeng & Ketted, 2006; Bor et al, 2008; Robinson & Kotre, 2008) and some authors used this dependency to predict patient doses through training of artificial neural networks (Ceke et al., 2009). The number of previously conducted mammographic examinations for the complete group was 1,80 (SD: 0,66) while more than 75 % of patients underwent at least 2 mammographic examinations in their lives. All patients underwent an ultrasound breast examination.

3.5 Patient's doses for two different age groups

It is extremely important to examine a relation between projections (craniocaudal and mediolateral projection) during a mammographic diagnostic, compressed breast thickness and mean glandular dose received by a patient during one exposition and during the complete examination for two different age groups (Wall & Roberts, 1992; Gentry & De Werd, 1996; Heggie, 1996; Klein et al., 1997; Young, 2000; Young & Burch, 2000; Oh et al., 2003; Jamal et al., 2003; Sookpeng & Ketted, 2006; Bouzarjomehri et al., 2006; Tsapaki et al., 2008; Ciraj-Bijelac et al., 2010; Kunosic et al., 2010). Patients are divided into a group of younger patients (40 - 49) and a group of older patients (50 - 64), according to the European Protocol for Dosimetry in Mammography (Perry, et al., 2006). Table 5. illustrates results regarding MGD doses for every individual projection (MLO and CC) and for the complete mammographic examination of the mentioned projections. The first age group (40 – 49) consisted of 132 patients for whose examination 493 mammographic images were taken. Mean value of compressed breast thickness was 41,15 mm (SD: 15,06).

Age group (years)		Number of images	Voltage	CBT (mm)	I t (mAs)	MGD per exposure(mGy)	
			kVp ± SD	Mean ± SD	Mean ± SD	MGDs ± CI	Third quartile
	Total	493	26,26 ± 1,30	41,15 ± 15,06	40,46 ± 12,87	0,88 ± 0,01	0,96
40 - 49	CC	246	25,76 ± 0,99	36,18 ± 12,53	35,72 ± 10,81	0,82 ± 0,01	0,88
	MLO	247	26,74 ± 1,38	46,11 ± 15,74	45,18 ± 13,05	0,94 ± 0,02	1,05
	Total	727	26,34 ± 1,72	42,98 ± 14,69	40,87 ± 12,64	0,90 ± 0,01	1,00
50 - 64	CC	367	25,74 ± 1,16	37,35 ± 11,54	35,98 ± 9,90	0,83 ± 0,01	0,91
	MLO	360	26,95 ± 1,96	48,73 ± 15,34	45,86 ± 13,18	0,98 ± 0,02	1,12

Table 5. Complete statistical illustration for voltage, compressed breast thickness, MGD for three different age groups and two different projections (CC, MLO). (MLO - Mediolateral oblique view; CC - Craniocaudal view; SD - Standard deviation, CI - Confidence interval for the mean of 95 %; CBT - Compressed breast thickness).

A slight tendency of increasing of compressed breast thickness with aging was noted with this age group (Klein et al., 1997; Moore et al., 2005). Compressed breast thickness in MLO projection was 21,53 % higher than the one noted in CC projection. Doses in MLO and CC projection were 1,88 mGy and 1,64 mGy, respectively. The mentioned values of doses are within the frame of results promoted by K.C.Young (Young, 2000) for the age group 40 to 48. A considerable significance was noted between MGD and CBT (Fig. 2.) with this age group ($r = 0,689$; $p < 0,01$). More than 75 % of doses for individual (one) image in CC projection was less than 0,88 mGy while more than 75% of individual images in MLO projection was below 1,05 mGy. Doses received in an individual MLO projection were for about 12,76 % higher than in CC projection, which is mostly contributed by a difference in compressed breast thickness in the mentioned projections. The number of performed mammographic examinations for this age group as of now is 1,68 (SD: 0,60) while more than 75 % of patients underwent at least 2 mammographic examinations in their lives, which is a good average considering the fact that this is the youngest group and bearing in mind a very bad economic status of the country.

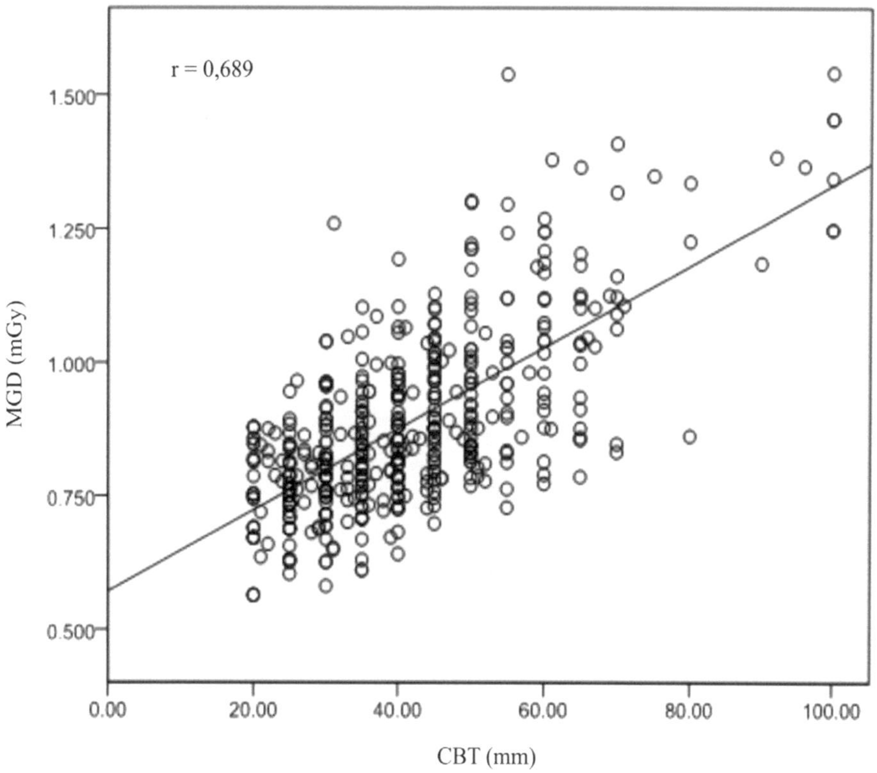

Fig. 2. Correlation between MGD and CBT for age group 40 - 49.

The second age group, 50 - 64 years of age, involved 197 patients for whose mammographic examination one made 727 images (Table 10.9.). Mean compressed breast thickness was 42,98 mm (SD: 14,69). Compressed breast thickness in MLO projection was 23,35 % higher than in CC projection. Patient doses for the complete MLO and CC image were 1,96 mGy and 1,66 mGy, respectively. These results comply well with results from the work of Burch and Goodman (Burch & Goodman, 1998). A patient dose in CC projection is something higher in regard to a study conducted in the USA (Gentry & De Werd, 1996) where one measured mean compressed breast thickness of 4,5 cm and MGD of 1,5 mGy for the mentioned projection. What is interesting is that values of doses decreased with an increase of patients' age in this group (Beckett & Kotre, 2000; Bouzarjomehri et al., 2006), probably because of a change (decrease) of breast glandularity (Eklund et al., 1993; Heggie, 1996). More than 75 % of doses for an individual (one) image in CC projection was less than 0,91 mGy while more than 75% of individual images in MLO projection was below 1,12 mGy. Doses received during an individual MLO projection were for 15,31 % higher than in CC projection, which is mostly contributed by a difference in compressed breast thickness in the mentioned projections. A correlation analysis of this age group showed a considerable significance between MGD and CBT ($r = 0,692$; $p < 0,01$). The number of performed mammographic examinations for this age group as of now is 1,88 (SD: 0,69) and more than 75 % of patients underwent less than 2 mammographic examinations in their lives. This information is discouraging since the number of examinations performed as of now in comparison with the number in developed countries should be much greater. Possible causes would be an insufficient number of mammographic apparatuses, lack of information, poor social status of this age category and lack of a program and measures for prevention and detection of breast cancer at the state level.

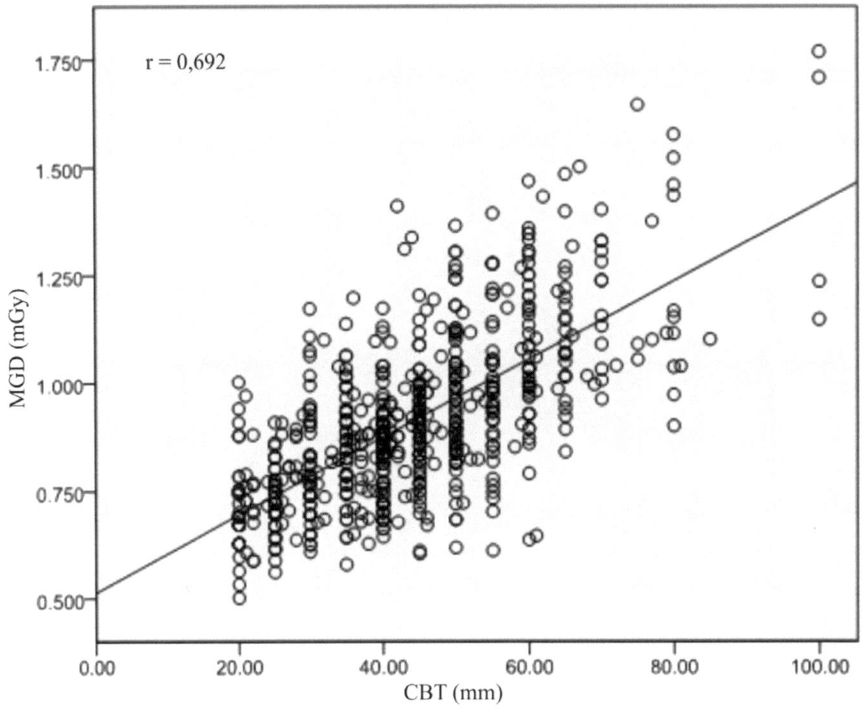

Fig. 3. Correlation between MGD and CBT for age group 50 - 64.

4. Conclusion

This work analyzes application of patient doses for various age groups of patients during a routine mammographic examination. One examined and analyzed factors on which patients doses depend. A correlation between patient doses and a complete spectrum of technical, physical, clinical and diagnostic parameters on which mammographic examination depends was established. The total dose for a complete mammographic examination was 3,58 mGy, which is significantly less than 4 mGy which is the ceiling for mammography. A slight tendency of compressed breast thickness increasing with age was noted for the age group 40 - 49. In the second age group, 50 - 64, it was noted that values of doses decreased with an increase of patients' age. It was defined that mean glandular dose depended on compressed breast thickness and that there was a positive correlation between these two sizes. More than 75 % of treated patients underwent at least 2 mammographic examinations in their lives. All patients underwent an ultrasound breast examination.

5. Acknowledgment

This study was supported by Public Health Institution "Health Centre Tuzla", Department of Medical Diagnostics / Radiology.

6. References

Adlien, D., Adlys, G., Cerapaite, R., Jonaitiene, E. & Cibulskaite, I. (2005) Optimisation of X - ray examinations in Lithuania: start of implementation in Mammography. *Radiat Prot Dosimetry*, 114, 399 - 402.

American Cancer Society. Facts and figures. (2002) Atlanta: American Cancer Society.

Assiamah, M., Nam, T.L. & Keddy, R.J. (2005) Comparison of mammography radiation dose values obtained from direct incident air kerma measurements with values from measured X - ray spectral data. *Appl Radiat Isot*, 62, 551-560.

Beckett, J.R. & Kotre, C.J. (2000) Dosimetric implications of age related glandular chnages in screening mammography. *Phys Med Biol*, 45, 801 - 813.

Bor, D., Tukel, S., Olgar, T., Toklu, T., Aydin, E. & Akyol, O. (2008) Investigation of mean glandular dose versus compressed breast thickness relationship for mammography. *Radiat Prot Dosimetry*, 129(1-3), 160-164.

Bouzarjomehri, F., Mostaar, A., Ghasemi, A., Ehramposh, M.H. & Khosravi, H. (2006) The study of mean glandular dose in mammography in Yazd and the factors affecting it. *Iran J Radiol*, 4(1), 29 - 35.

Burch, A. & Goodman, D.A. (1998) A pilot survey of radiation doses received in the United Kingdom breast screening program. *Br J Radiol*, 71, 517 - 527.

Ceke, D., Kunosic, S., Kopric, M. & Lincender, L. (2009) Using Neural Network Algorithms in Prediction of Mean Glandular Dose Based on the Measurable Parameters in Mammography. *Acta Informatica Medica*, 17 (4), 194-197.

Ciraj-Bijelac, O., Beciric, S., Arandjic, D., Kosutic, D. & Kovacevic, M. (2010) Mammography radiation dose: initial results from Serbia based on mean glandular dose assessment for phantoms and patients. *Radiat Prot Dosimetry*, 140(1), 75-80.

Ciraj-Bjelac, Olivera., Simona, Avramova-Cholakova., Adnan, Beganovic., Sotirios, Economides., Dario, Faj., Vesna, Gershan., Edward, Grupetta., Kharita, M.H. , Milomir, Milakovic., Constantin, Milu., Wilbroad, E. Muhogora., Pirunthavany, Muthuvelu., Samuel, Oola., Saeid, Setayeshi., Cyril, Schandorf., Ion, Ursulean., Ivan, R. Videnovic., Areesha, Zaman., Julius, Ziliukas. & Madan M Rehani. (2011) Image quality and dose in mammography in 17 countries in Africa, Asia and Eastern Europe: Results from IAEA projects. *Eur J Radiol*, doi:10.1016/j.ejrad.2011.05.026

Dance, D.R., Skinner, C.L., Young, K.C., Beckett, J.R. & Kotre, C.J. (2000) Additional factors for the estimation of mean glandular breast dose using the UK mammography dosimetry protocol. *Phys Med Biol*, 45, 3225 - 3240.

D'Orsi, C.J. & Newell, M.S. (2011) On the frontline of screening for breast cancer. *Semin Oncol*, 38(1), 119-127.

Eklund, S., Thilander, A., Leitz, W. & Mattsson, S. (1993) The impact of anatomic variations of absorbed radiation doses in mammography. *Radiat Prot Dosimetry*, 49, 167–170.

Fajdic, Josip. (2001) Suvremena dijagnostika bolesti dojke, Medicinska naklada, Zagreb.

Faulkner, K., Law, J. & Robson, K. J. (1995) Assessment of mean glandular dose in mammography. *Br J Radiol*, 75, 877 - 881.

Ferlay, J., Bray, F., Pisani, P., et al. (2004) GLOBOCAN 2002: Cancer Incidence, Mortality and Prevalence Worldwide. IARC CancerBase No. 5. Version 2.0, IARC Press, Lyon.

Ferlay, J., Parkin, D.M. & Steliarova-Foucher, E. (2010) Estimates of cancer incidence and mortality in Europe in 2008. *European Journal of Cancer*, 46 (4), 765-781.

Geise, R.A., Morin, R.L. & Wasserman, N.F. (1988) Routine quality control tests for film-screen mammographic systems with automatic exposure control. *Med Phys*, 15(6), 904-8.

Gentry, J.R. & De Werd, L.A. (1996) TLD measurements of in vivo mammographic exposures and the calculated mean glandular dose across the United States. *Med Phys*, 23, 899–903.

Gøtzsche, P.C. & Nielsen, M. (2006) Screening for breast cancer with mammography. *Cochrane Database Syst Rev*, 4, CD001877.

Gøtzsche, P.C. (2011) Relation between breast cancer mortality and screening effectiveness: systematic review of the mammography trials. *Dan Med Bull*, 58(3), A4246.

Greenlee, R.T., Murray, T., Bolden, S. & Wingo, P.A. (2000) Cancer statistics. *CA Cancer J Clin*, 50,7-33.

Hackshaw, A.K., Wald, N.J. & Michell, M.J. (2000) An investigation into why two - view mammography is better than one - view in breast cancer screening. *Clin Radiol*, 55, 454 - 458.

Harlow, S.P., Krag, D.N., Ames, S.E. & Weaver, D.L. (1999) Intraoperative ultrasound localization to guide surgical excision of nonpalpable breast carcinoma. *J Am Coll Surg*, 189(3), 241-246.

Hauge, I.H.R., Pedersen, K., Sanderud, A., Hofvind, S. & Olerud, H. M. (2011) Patient doses from screen-film and full-field digital mammography in a population-based screening programme. *Radiat Prot Dosimetry*, (2011) first published online February 17, 2011 doi:10.1093/rpd/ncq598.

Heggie, J.C.P. (1996) Survey of dose in screening mammography. *Australas Phys Eng Sci Med*, 19, 207–216.

Heidi, D. Nelson., Kari, Tyne., Arpana, Naik., Christina, Bougatsos., Benjamin, K. Chan. & Linda, Humphrey. (2009) Screening for Breast Cancer: An Update for the U.S. Preventive Services Task Force. *Annals of Internal Medicine*, 151(10), 727-737.

Helvie, M.A., Chan, H.P., Adler, D.D. & Boyd, P.G. (1994) Breast thickness in routine mammograms: effect on image quality and radiation dose. *AJR Am J Roentgenol*, 163(6), 1371-4.

Hendrick, R.E., Klabunde, C., Grivegnee, A. at al. (2002) Technical quality control practices in mammography screening programs in 22 countries. *Int J Qual Health Care*, 14 (3), 219-226.

Hermann, K.P. et al. (2002) Average glandular dose with amorphous silicon full-field digital mammography—clinical results. *Rofo*, 174(6), 696–699.

Jamal, N., Ng, K.H. & Mclean, D. (2003) A study of mean glandular dose during diagnostic mammography in Malaysia and some of the factors affecting it. *Brit J Radiol*, 76, 238-245.

Jemal, A., Bray, F., Center, M. M., Ferlay, J., Ward, E. & Forman, D. (2011) Global cancer statistics. *CA: A Cancer Journal for Clinicians*, 61, 69–90.

Klein, R., Aichinger, H. & Dierker, J. (1997) Determination of average glandular dose with modern Mammography units for two large groups of patients. *Phys Med Biol*, 42, 651 - 671.

Kopans, D.B., Rafferty, E., Georgian-Smith, D., et al. (2003) A simple model of breast cancer growth may provide explanations for observations of apparently complex phenomena. *Cancer*, 97, 2951 - 2955.

Kruger, R.L. & Schueler, B.A. (2001) A survey of clinical factors and patient dose in mammography. *Med Phys*, 28(7), 1449-54.

Kuhl, C.K., Schrading, S., Leutner, C.C., Morakkabati-Spitz, N., Wardelmann, E., Fimmers, R., Kuhn, W. & Schild, H.H. (2005) Mammography, breast ultrasound, and magnetic resonance imaging for surveillance of women at high familial risk for breast cancer. *J Clin Oncol*, 23(33), 8469-8476.

Kunosic, S., Ceke, D., Kopric, M. & Lincender, L. (2010) Determination of mean glandular dose from routine mammography for two age groups of patients. *HealthMED*, 4(1), 125-131.

Kunosic, S., Ceke, D., Beganovic, A. & Basic, B. (2011) Effects of dispersed radiation on the thyroid and the gonads during mammography. *HealthMED*, 5(6), 1774-1781.

Kuzmiak, C.M., Pisano, E.D., Cole E.B., Zeng, D., Burns, C.B., Roberto, C., Pavic, D., Lee, Y., Seo, B.K., Koomen, M. & Washburn, D. (2005) Comparison of full-field digital mammography to screen-film mammography with respect to contrast and spatial resolution in tissue equivalent breast phantoms. *Med Phys*, 32(10), 3144-50.

Kyu-Won, Jung., Sohee, Park., Hyun-Joo, Kong.,Young-Joo, Won.,You-Kyung, Boo., Hai-Rim, Shin., Eun-Cheol, Park., & Jin-Soo, Lee. (2010) Cancer Statistics in Korea: Incidence, Mortality and Survival in 2006-2007. *J Korean Med Sci*, 25(8), 1113–1121.

Law, J., Dance, D.R., Faulkner, K., Fitzgerald, M.C., Ramsdale, M.L. & Robinson, A. (1994). The commissioning and routine testing of mammographic X-ray systems. *IPSM report No 59*, Second Edition, IPSM, York.

Mainiero, M.B. (2010) Regional lymph node staging in breast cancer: the increasing role of imaging and ultrasound-guided axillary lymph node fine needle aspiration. *Radiol Clin North Am*, 48(5), 989-997.

Maccia, C., Nadeau, X., Renaud, R., et al. (1995) Quality control inmammography: the pilot campaign of breast screening inthe Bas-Rhin region. *Rad Prot Dosim*, 57, 323-328.

Miller, A. B.(2005) Screening for breast cancer - is there an alternative to mammography? *Asian Cancer Prev*, 6, 83 - 86.

Moore, A.C., Dance, D.R., Evans, D.S., Lawinski, C.P., Pitcher, E.M., Rust, A. & Young, K.C. (2005) The commissioning and routine testing of mammographic X-ray systems. *IPEM report No 89*, Third Edition, IPEM, York.

Moran, P. et al. (2005) A survey of patient dose and clinical factors in a full-field digital mammography system. *Radiat Prot Dosimetry*, 114(1-3), 375–379.

Nelson, D.E., Bland, S., Powell-Griner, E., et al. (2002) State trends in health risk factors and receipt of clinical preventive services among US adults during the 1990s. *JAMA*, 287(20), 2659-2667.

Oh, K.K., Hur, J., Kim, E.K. & Choo, S.S. (2003) Dosimetric evaluation of the mean glandular dose for mammography in Korean women: a preliminary report. *Yonsei Med J*, 44(5), 863-868.

Perry, N. et al. (2006) European guidelines for quality assurance in breast cancer screening and diagnosis. Fourth editions, European Communities, Luxembourg.

Robinson, M. & Kotre, C. J. (2008) Trends in compressed breast thickness and radiation dose in breast screening mammography. *Br J Radiol*, 81, 214-218.

Rosselli Del Turco, Marco., Paola, Mantellini., Stefano, Ciatto., Rita, Bonardi., Francesca, Martinelli., Barbara, Lazzari. & Nehmat, Houssami. (2007) Full-Field Digital Versus

Screen-Film Mammography: Comparative Accuracy in Concurrent Screening Cohorts. *Am J Roentgenol*, 189(4), 860-866.
Saric Sabina. (2009) Breast cancer patient`s quality of life compared to correctible risik factors of life style. *HealthMED*, 3 (3), 267-272.
Schubauer-Berigan, M.K., Frey, G.D., Baron, L. & Hoel, D.G. (2002) Mammography dose in relation to body mass index, race, and menopausal status. *Radiat Prot Dosimetry*, 98(4), 425-432.
Skaane, P. (2009) Studies comparing screen-film mammography and full-field digital mammography in breast cancer screening: updated review. *Acta Radiol*, 50(1), 3-14.
Sobol, W.T. & Wu, X. (1997) Parametrization of mammography normalized average glandular dose tables. *Med Phys*, 24(4), 574-54.
Sookpeng, S. & Ketted, P. (2006) Mean glandular dose from routine mammography. *NU Journal*. 14, 19-26.
Tabar, L., Yen, M.F., Vitak, B., Chen, H.H., Smith, R.A. & Duffy, S.W. (2003) Mammography service screening and mortality in breast cancer patients: 20-year follow-up before and after introduction of screening. *Lancet*, 361(9367), 1405-1410.
Tsapaki, V., Tsalafoutas, I.A., Poga, V., Louizi, A., Kottou, S. & Koulentianos, E. (2008) Investigation of breast dose in five screening mammography centres in Greece. *J Radiol Prot*, 28(3), 1405-1410.
Vassileva, J., Avramova-Cholakova, S., Dimov, A. & Lichev, A. (2005) Implemantation of the European Protocol for QualityControl of the Technical Aspects of Mammography Screening in Bulgaria. *Radiat Prot Dosimetry*, 114, 403-405.
Wall, M.A. & Roberts, P.J. (1992) Radiation dose in relation to compressed breast thickness for screening mammography. *Radiat Prot Dosimetry*, 43, 253 - 255.
Wu, X., Barnes, G.T. & Tucker, D.M. (1991) Spectral Dependences of Glandular Tissue Dose in Screen Film Mammography. *Radiology*, 179, 143-148.
Young, K.C. & Burch, A. (2000) Radiation dose received in the UK Breast Screening Program in 1997 and 1998. *Br J Radiol*, 73,278–287.
Young, K.C. (2000) Radiation doses in the UK trial of breast screening in women aged 40-48 years. *Br J Radiol*, 75, 362 - 370.
Zdesar, U. (2000) Simple optimisation method in mammography. *Radiat Prot Dosimetry*, 90, 221-223.
Zhu, K., Wu, H., Jatoi, I., Potter, J. & Shriver, C. (2006) Body mass index and use of mammography screening in the United States. *Prev Med*, 42(5), 381-385.
Zoetelief, J., Broerse, J. & Thijssen, M. (1992) A Dutch protocol for quality control in mammography screening: dosimetric aspects. *Radiat Prot Dosimetry*, 43(1-4), 261-264.

8

Assessment of AGD in UAE Hospital

Najlaa Almazrouei
Dubai Health Authority (DHA)–Medical Physics Section
United Arab Emirates

1. Introduction

X-ray mammography is the most reliable method of detecting breast cancer. It is the method of choice for the Breast Screening Program in a variety of developed countries In order to obtain high quality mammograms at an acceptable breast dose, it is essential to use the correct equipment.

In the United Arab Emirates (UAE), the number of mammography examinations has been rising steadily the past few years due to the rapid economic growth of the country and the increasing use of computed and digital radiography systems, as film based mammography systems are being abandoned progressively.

At present, there is a growing concern about the radiation doses incurred by patients when undergoing breast examinations. For this reason, the UAE has decided to join the IAEA Task4 project to undertake a survey of patient exposure in digital mammography in several Hospitals.

The objectives of this work are

- Achieve consistently high quality mammograms.
- Limit radiation dose by determine the Average Glandular Dose (DG) resulting cranio-caudal - projections.
- IAEA guidance was used for measuring the Entrance Surface Air Kerma (Ka,e) and EUREF - guidelines DG calculations.
- Minimize the number of supplementary and repeat examinations.
- Minimize the number of unnecessary invasive procedures.
- The main objective of this work was to evaluate the Average Glandular Dose (DG) resulting from exposure to mammographic X-rays while the ultimate aim of the project remains the establishment of Dose Reference Levels (DRL) in the UAE.

It is worth noting that the quantities and symbols used in this presentation are those suggested by the International Commission on radiation Units and Measurements (ICRU) in its publication 74.

The Total numbers of mammography system in Dubai are 26 facilities both in Governmental and Privet sector, the Average number of patients per year were 528, the number of CR system 18, the DR system 5 and the screen film 3.

There are some factors affecting the visibility of the objects:

Size, Contrast & Noise (from different sources)

Also the following Exposure parameters:

Anode (Mo, Rh, W...) => contrast, (resolution)

Filter (Mo, Rh, Al...) => contrast

Tube voltage (kV) => contrast

Dose or tube loading (mAs) => noise

Radiation dose to the breast is affected by the following parameter

- The breast composition and thickness
- The photon energy
- The sensitivity of the image receptor
- The breast composition has a significant influence on the dose
- The area of the compressed breast has a small influence on the dose
- Majority of the interactions are photoelectric

A Quality Control program should ensure:

- The best image quality
- With the minimum dose to the breast
- Hence regular check of important parameters

2. Methodology, equipment and tools used to perform the study

For tube quality

- Victoreen NERO mAx 8000 multimeter + Fluke Biomedical Detector
- Gamex test tool
- Unfors kit (as a substitute when Victoreen was not available)

For checking image quality

- ToRMAX-316 (Leeds Test Object) for Detailed Image (total thickness 7 cm)
- ACR phantom for general image

For measuring the Contrast-to-Noise-Ratio (CNR)

- ToRMAX-316 (Leeds Test Object)
- 2 cm x 2 cm piece of aluminum of thickness 0.2 mm
- ACR phantom

For the measurement of ESAK

- Victoreen NeroMax 8000 multimeter + Victoreen cylindrical Ion chamber 3.3 cc or
- Unfors kit (as a substitute when Victoreen was not available)

2.1 Quality control of the mammography machines

All parameters relevant to X-ray beam (mainly kVp, HVL & light field collimation) should be checked.

2.1.1 KVp accuracy

Method:

- Turn on the Victoreen NERO Max 8000 and select the Mammography option then press enter.
- Place the Victoreen NERO mAx 8000 Detector on the table.
- Insert 22-35 filters to the detector.
- Give exposure and write down the effective KVp and Dose.
- Action Limit: If the measured kVp differs more than ±5% of the set kVp then seeks service correction

2.1.2 Reproducibility

Method:

- Turn on the Victoreen NERO Max 8000 and select the Mammography option then press enter.
- Place the Victoreen NERO mAx 8000 Detector on the table.
- Insert 22-35 filters to the detector.
- Give exposure and fill down the table.
- Action Limit: if the coefficient of variation exceeds 0.02, then seek service correction.
- Formula used for calculation:

$$SD = \sqrt{[n \sum x^2 - (\sum x)^2 / n (n - 1)]} \quad (1)$$

$$CV = SD / Mean \quad (2)$$

2.1.3 Beam quality test (HVL)

Method:

1. Raise the compression paddle to its highest position. Mount the 6000-529 ionization chamber on a ring stand so there is approximately 5 cm of space between the bottom of the chamber and table. The chamber should be centered in the beam laterally, and approximately 4 cm from the chest wall.
2. Collimate the beam, using the light field, so that the entire chamber is included in the beam. The field should be approximately 6 cm x 6 cm. If necessary, relocate the chamber such that it is centered in the field.
3. Set the kVp selector at a kVp setting that is frequently used for making mammograms.
4. Connect the chamber to the Nero Max8000 device.
5. Make an exposure. Note the reading and label it X0.
6. Place a sheet of aluminum 0.2 mm thick on the compression paddle. Using the collimator light, be sure the entire ionization chamber is in the shadow of the aluminum sheet. Make an exposure. Record the reading and label it X1; also record the thickness of aluminum used to make the exposure. Label it t1.
7. Place an additional 0.01 mm of aluminum on top of the aluminum absorbers) already in place. Make an exposure. Record the reading, labeling it with sequential indices. Also, record the total thickness of aluminum used in making the measurement, labeling it as

tN where N is the total number of filtered exposures taken so far. If XN is less than one half of X0 proceed to step 7, otherwise, repeat step

8. It is now assumed that you have compiled a list of data pairs, labeled "ti" and "Xi"- If N is the total number of filtered exposures, then the half-value layer may then be calculated using the following formula:

$$HVL = \frac{{}^{t}N^{1n}\{2XN - 1 / x_0\} \ -{}^{t}N - 1^{1n}\{2XN / x_0\}}{1n\ \{XN - 1 / XN\}} \quad (3)$$

2.2 Image quality

For general image, we use the ACR mammography phantom contains test objects that are similar to microcalcifications, fibers, and masses

- Image quality tests were performed at clinical settings to ensure that the X-ray machines were functioning properly, in accordance to the manufacturer's specifications.
- Place the phantom on the image receptor surface in the same position as a breast. The nipple indent marker should be positioned away from the chest wall, just as the nipple of the patient's breast would be positioned.
- Position the x-ray tube and compression device as you would for a craniocaudal examination of a patient's breast.
- Choose the kVp and mAs factors as you would use for an average 4.5 cm breast and make an exposure.
- The image will represent the imaging abilities of your machine using these clinical factors.
- If the image is over or under exposed, make a suitable adjustment in your factors and repeat the exposure.
- This is an indication that adjustments may be necessary for patient imaging of these compressed breast thicknesses and should be checked.

Use the ToRMAX-316 (Leeds Test Object) for Detailed Image (total thickness 7 cm) and repeat the pervious step for each breast thickness.

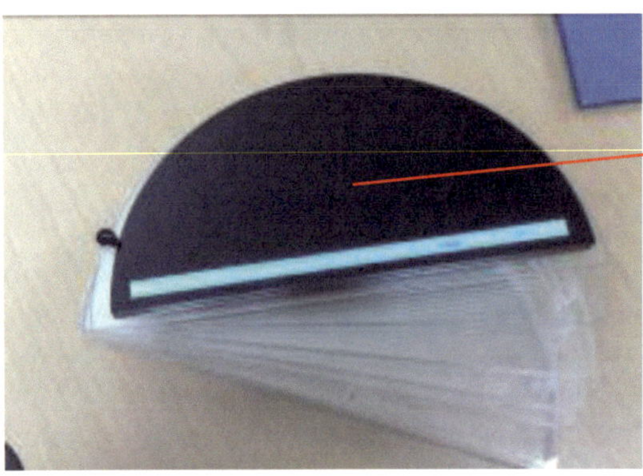

Image 1. ToRMAX-316 (Leeds Test Object).

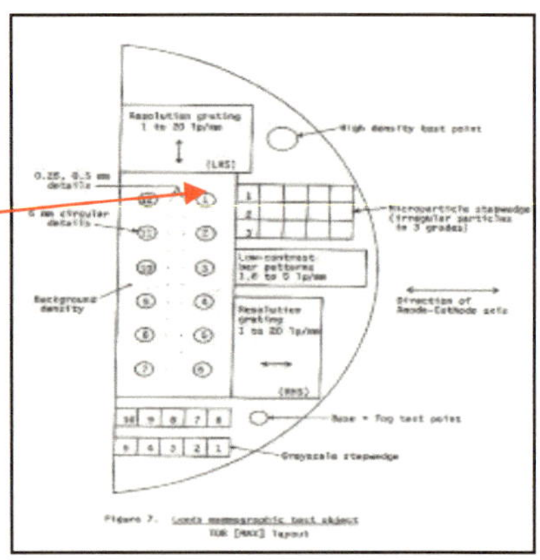

Image.2

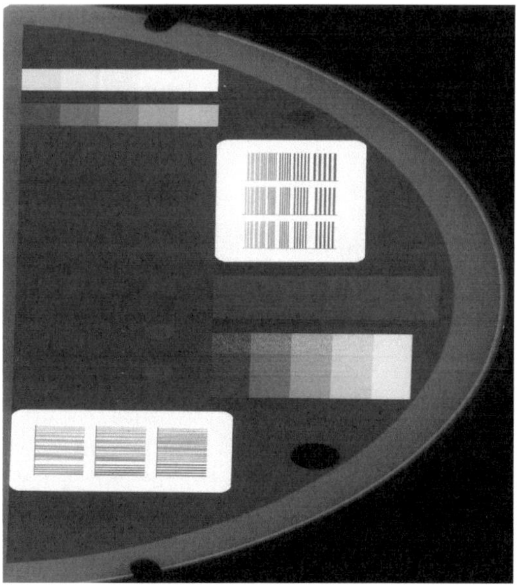

Image 3. this image reflect the image that we got from the phantom after exposure.

2.3 Contrast-to-Noise Ratio (CNR)

- The Contrast-to-Noise Ratio (CNR) was determined by placing a square-shaped 2 cm x 2 cm piece of aluminum of thickness 0.2 mm on the PMMA phantom, 6 cm from the edge of the phantom and table, in the centre of the phantom.
- Two ROIs of 4 cm2 were selected in the saved image to calculate the mean (S) and the standard deviation (σ).

The Contrast-to-Noise Ratio (CNR) is obtained using the equation:

$$CNR = \frac{S_{AL} - S}{\sqrt{\sigma_{AL}^{2} + \sigma^{2}}} \tag{4}$$

2.4 Average Glandular Dose, DG

The AGD cannot be measured directly but it is derived from measurements with the standard phantom for the actual technique set-up of the mammographic equipment.

The measurements of the Entrance Surface Air Kerma Ka,e were performed in two steps,

First

1. Set up the x-ray machine for a typical mammographic technique. Place a loaded cassette in the cassette holder, of the size and type consistent with the examination being simulated. Set the machine in the AEC mode and set the density control to the position most commonly used for the examination.
2. Place a mammographic LTO phantom on the cassette holder assembly at the position normally occupied by the breast. Be sure the phantom completely covers the AEC sensor.

3. The LTO phantom was exposed to X-ray beams using automatic mode to get the kVp, mAs, and target/filter combination used.
4. Then, remove the phantom and a similar exposure will perform in manual mode with no phantom.

Second

1. Now, place the Model 6000-529 ionization chamber in the center of the phantom.
2. Lower the compression paddle until it contacts the chamber. Take care not to put any mechanical stress on the chamber.
3. Connect the chamber cable to an NERO max8000; Follow the instructions accompanying the instrument for details of instrument operation.
4. Make an exposure. Record the reading from the electrometer. Apply whatever corrections are necessary to yield an accurate exposure reading.
5. Repeat step 4 three more times. Average all four results. The final result is the breast entrance exposure. You should now repeat the procedure for all other clinically used techniques. The value of Ka, e, the Entrance Surface Air Kerma (ESAK) is deduced

$$Ka, e = Od\ PIt\ (dsd\ /\ (dsd - T))\ 2 \tag{5}$$

Od = Tube output at level of detector
Pit= Tube current exposure time product (mAs)
dsd= Source to detector distance
T= Thickness of compressed breast (CBT)

Conversion factors from incident air kerma to average glandular dose have been obtained using Monte Carlo transport calculations in simple breast models e.g. Dance et al (2000)

The Average Glandular Dose DG is calculated as:

$$DG = Ka,e\ .\ g.\ c.\ s \tag{6}$$

- Where ***Ka,e*** is the entrance surface air kerma (without backscatter) calculated at the upper surface of the PMMA.
- The factor g, corresponds to a glandularity of 50%, and is derived from the values calculated by Dance et al 2000 and is shown in table.1 for a range of HVL.
- The c-factor corrects for the difference in composition of typical breasts from 50% glandularity [Dance et al 2000] and is given here for typical breasts in the age range 50 to 64 in table.2.
- Typical values of HVL for various spectra are given in table.3. The factor **s** shown in table 4 corrects for differences due to the choice of X-ray spectrum (Dance et al 2000).

Note that the c and g-factors applied are those for the corresponding thickness of typical breast rather than the thickness of PMMA block used. Where necessary interpolation may be made for different values of HVL.

The dose should be determined using the usual clinically selected exposure factors including any automatic selection of kV and target/filter combination.

PMMA Breast Thickness (mm)	Equivalent Breast Thickness (mm)	g-factors (mGy/mGy) HVL (mmAl)							
		0.25	0.30	0.35	0.40	0.45	0.50	0.55	0.60
20	21	0.329	0.378	0.421	0.460	0.496	0.529	0.559	0.585
30	32	0.222	0.261	0.294	0.326	0.357	0.388	0.419	0.448
40	45	0.155	0.183	0.208	0.232	0.258	0.285	0.311	0.339
45	53	0.130	0.155	0.177	0.198	0.220	0.245	0.272	0.295
50	60	0.112	0.135	0.154	0.172	0.192	0.214	0.236	0.261
60	75	0.088	0.106	0.121	0.136	0.152	0.166	0.189	0.210
70	90		0.086	0.098	0.111	0.123	0.136	0.154	0.172
80	103		0.074	0.085	0.096	0.106	0.117	0.133	0.149

Table.1. g-factors for breast simulated with PMMA.

PMMA Breast Thickness (mm)	Equivelant Breast Thickness (mm)	Glandularity of Equivelant Breast	c-factors (mGy/mGy) HVL (mmAl)						
			0.30	0.35	0.40	0.45	0.50	0.55	0.60
20	21	97	0.889	0.895	0.903	0.908	0.912	0.917	0.921
30	32	67	0.940	0.943	0.945	0.946	0.949	0.952	0.953
40	45	41	1.043	1.041	1.040	1.039	1.037	1.035	1.034
45	53	29	1.109	1.105	1.102	1.099	1.096	1.091	1.088
50	60	20	1.164	1.160	1.151	1.150	1.144	1.139	1.134
60	75	9	1.254	1.245	1.235	1.231	1.225	1.217	1.207
70	90	4	1.299	1.292	1.282	1.275	1.270	1.260	1.249
80	103	3	1.307	1.299	1.292	1.287	1.283	1.273	1.262

Table 2. c-factors for breast simulated with PMMA.

HVL (mm Al) for target filter combination					
Kv	Mo + 30 μm Mo	Mo +25 μm Rh	Rh +25 μm Rh	W +50 μm Rh	W +0.45 μm Al[22]
25	0.33 ± .02	0.40 ± .02	0.38 ± .02	0.52 ± .03	0.31 ± .03
28	0.36 ± .02	0.42 ± .02	0.43 ± .02	0.54 ± .03	0.37 ± .03
31	0.39 ± .02	0.44 ± .02	0.48 ± .02	0.56 ± .03	0.42 ± .03
34		0.47 ± .02		0.59 ± .03	0.47 ± .03
37		0.50 ± .02			0.51 ± .03
* Some compression paddles are made of Lexan, the HVL values with this type of compression plate are 0.01 mm Al lower compared with the values in the table.					

Table 3. Typical HVL measurements for different tube voltage and target filter combinations. (Data includes the effect on measured HVL of attenuation by a PMMA compression plate*.)

Spectrum	s-factor
Mo/Mo	1.000
Mo/Rh	1.017
Rh/Rh	1.061
Rh/Al	1.044
W/Rh	1.042
W/Al	1.05*

*This value is not given in the paper of Dance et al. The value in the table has been estimated using the S-values of other spectra.

Table 4. s-factors for clinically used spectra [Dance et al. 2000].

The recommended achievable and limiting dose values in the European guidelines for the same PMMA thickness (van Engen et al 2006) are 0.6, 1, 1.6, 2, 2.4, 3.6, 5.1 mGy and 1, 1.5, 2, 2.5, 3, 4.5, 6.5 mGy respectively for 2, 3, 4, 4.5, 5, 6 and 7 cm of PMMA.

In our survey we use the limiting dose values to compare our date with it, as it will be shown in the next figures.

PMMA thickness (cm)	European Guild lines for the Limits AGD (mGy)
2	1
3	1.5
4	2
4.5	2.5
5	3
6	4.5
7	6.5

Table.5. European guild line for limit AGD (mGy) for at different PMMA thickness (cm).

3. Discussion

The Results of the measured Average Glandular Dose (AGD) were performed on different breast thickness, we chose 2cm breast thickens, 4.5 cm breast thickens which simulate the standard breast thickens and the third thickens was 7 cm, so in our survey we were covered the small, medium and large breast thickness.

We inspected (21 facilities), and 4 of them have a DR mammography, 13 CR mammography and 3 screen film mammography.

Results of the DR Mammography system

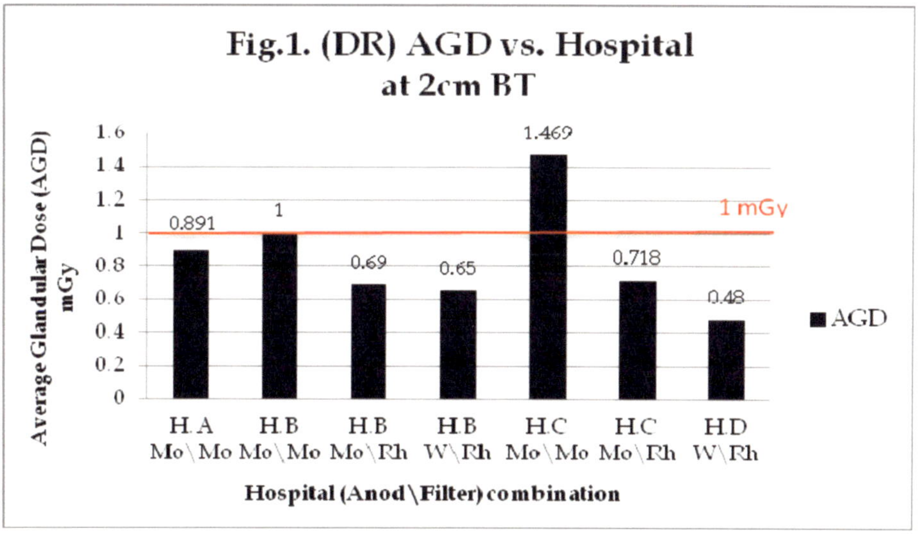

Fig. 1. ((DR) AGD vs. Hospital at 2cm BT), shows that one hospital (H.C Mo\Mo) is exceeding the acceptable limits, it was a test to observe the differences between the different Anode\Filter combinations that their machine have, and they are using the automatic mode (Auto-Kv mode) to acquire their images.

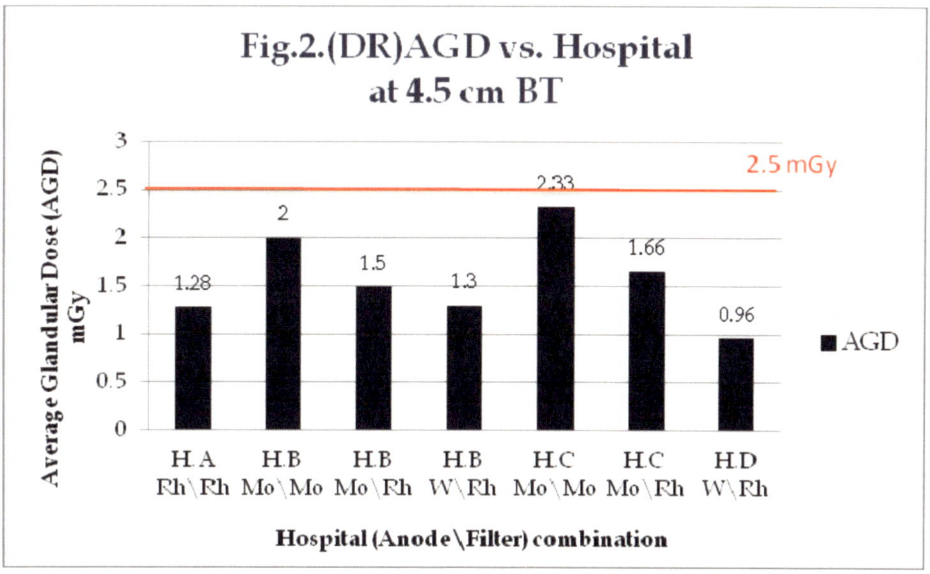

Fig. 2. ((DR) AGD vs. Hospital at 4.5cm BT), we observe that all hospital were within the AGD acceptable limit, all theses hospital are using the automatic mode to acquire their images, Except hospital A & B, the technician control the Kv parameter depending on the breast thickness.

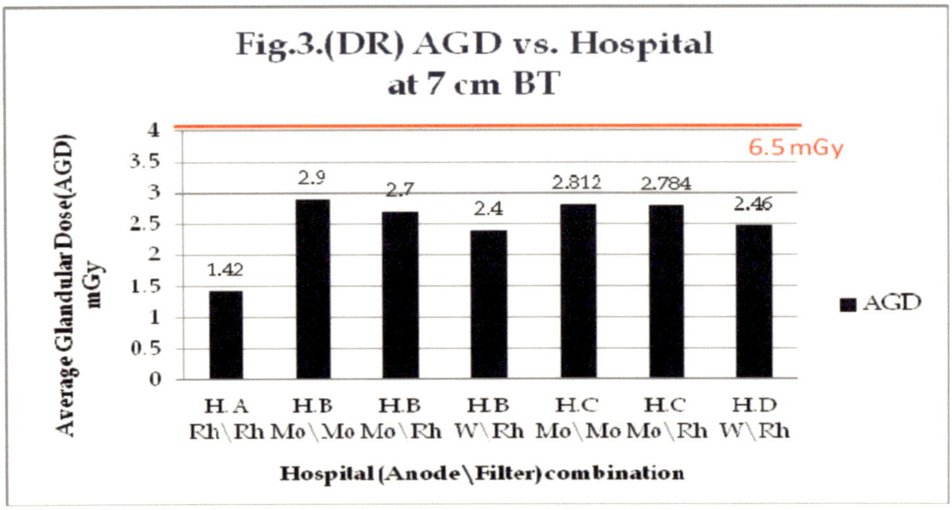

Fig. 3. ((DR) AGD vs. Hospital at 7cm BT), shows that all hospitals are below the AGD acceptable limit, all theses hospital are using the automatic setting to acquire their images, Except hospital A & B, the technician use the manual setting for the Kv parameter depending on the breast thickness.

Result of 13 Computed Mammography machine

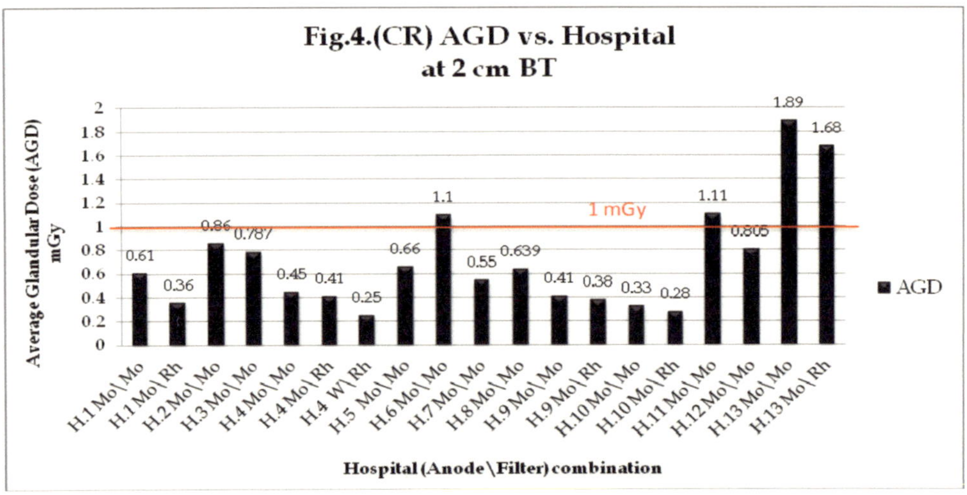

Fig. 4. ((CR) AGD vs. Hospital at 2cm BT), we observe from this figure that there are 3 hospitals were exceeding the AGD acceptable limit, which they are H6, H11&H13 with different anode\filter combination. H6: they are using the automatic mode, H11: they only have one Anode\Filter combination they use manual setting for Kv and automatic setting for mAs they were advice to change their setting to reduce the dose. H13: the technician were use the manual mode for acquiring their images , they were advised to fix call the service to fix their machine on the same time their cassette also were old and it was need to be changed. Regarding the other hospitals the most of them were fully automatic and the other have manual Kv settings.

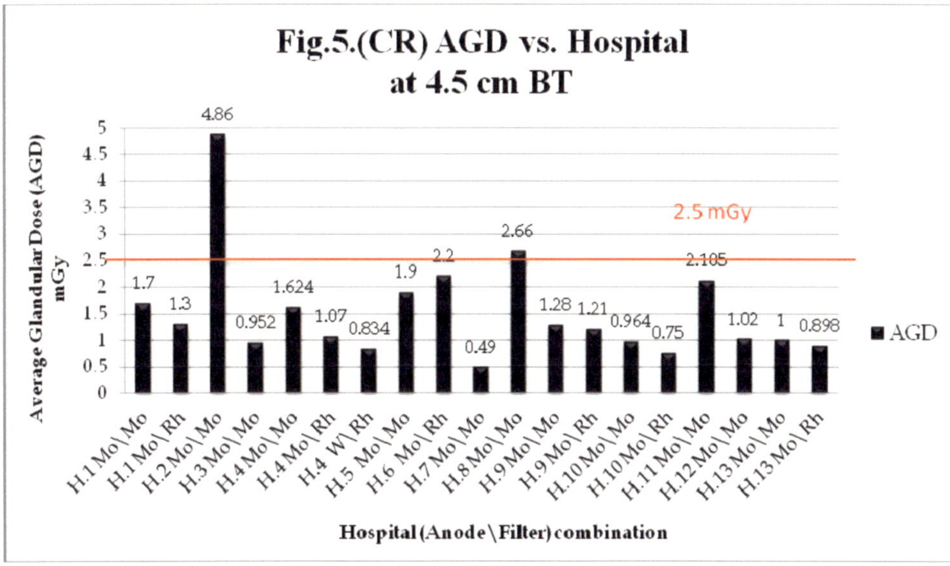

Fig. 5. ((CR) AGD vs. Hospital at 4.5 cm BT), shows that there was one hospital exceeding the acceptable dose limit (H2 Mo\Mo), the technician was use manual setting, they advise to call service to fix their machine. On the other hand we observe that (H7 Mo\Mo) have the lowest radiation dose to the patient, the technician were use manual setting for both KV & mAs.

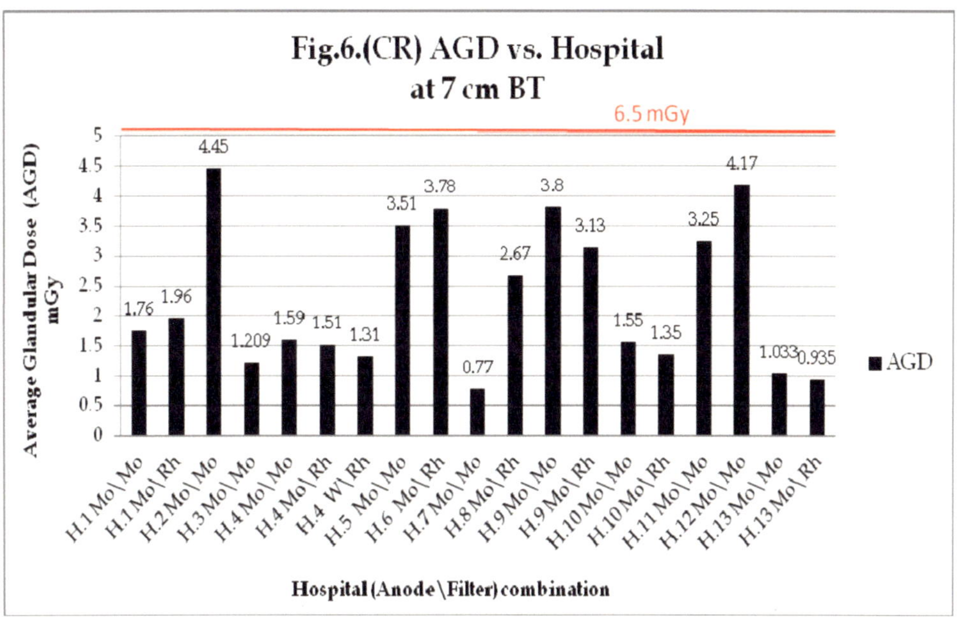

Fig. 6.((CR) AGD vs. Hospital at 7 cm BT),we observe that all hospital were below the AGD acceptable limit. As I explain before most of the hospital were using the manual settings for the Kv parameter. H7 Mo\Mo has the lowest radiation dose, the parameter that their use were so small Kv=27 & mAs= 50 the image quality was acceptable to their physician.

Results of the Three Screen Film Mammography machine

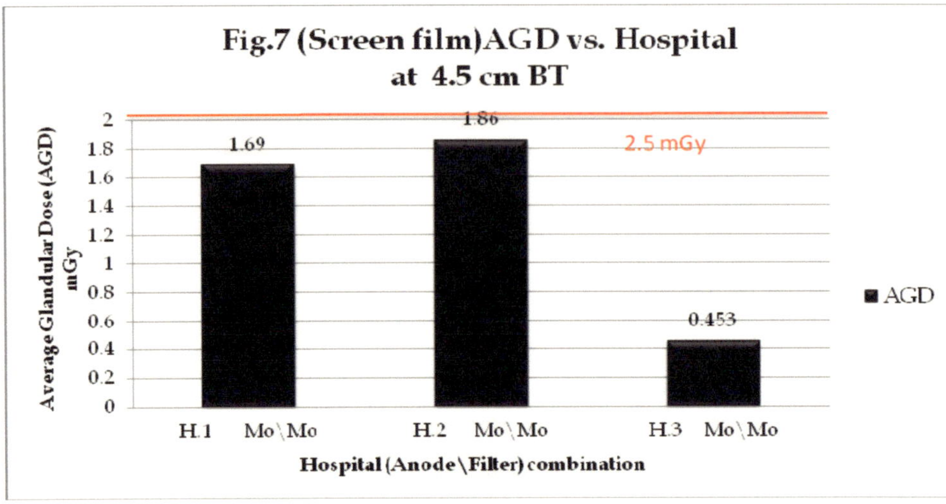

Fig. 7.((Screen film) AGD vs. Hospital at 4.5 cm BT), shows that all hospitals were below the AGD acceptable limit. All of these hospitals were using the manual setting for acquiring their images, their images were acceptable to their physician, for H3 the parameters used was Kv=28 & mAs=25.

Comparison between Calculated Average Glandular Dose (AGD) & System AGD

In most facilities, the difference between **AGD** values measured by the Physicist and those generated by the system were found acceptable, thus justifying a survey of patient doses on the basis of the AGD recorded by the system.

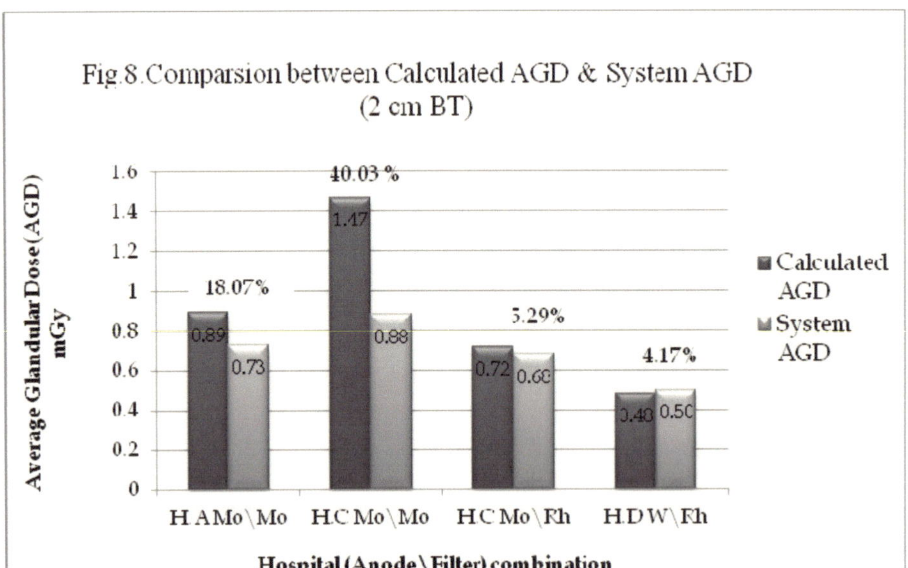

Fig. 8. Comparison between Calculated AGD & System AGD for 2 cm Breast Thickens.

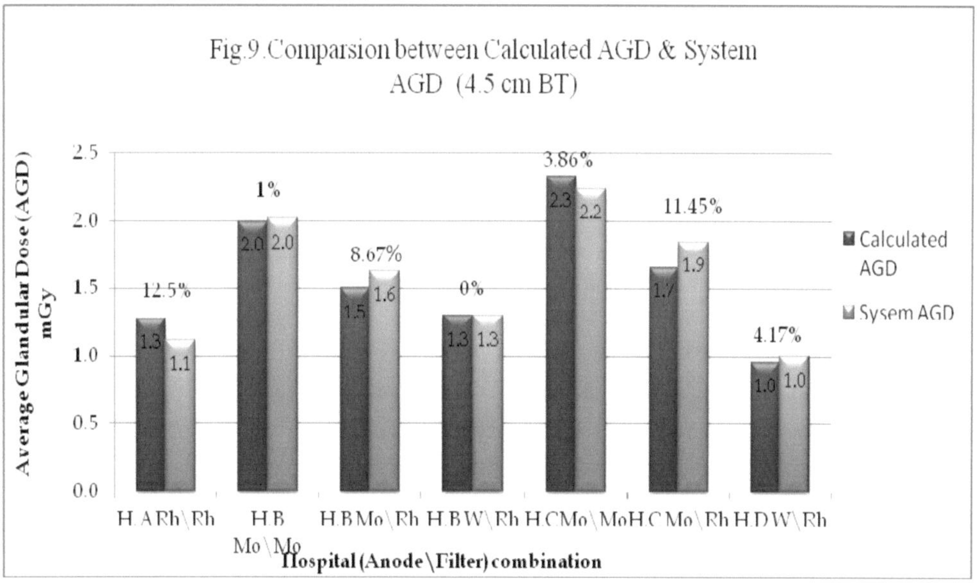

Fig. 9. Comparison between Calculated AGD & System AGD for 4.5 cm Breast Thickness.

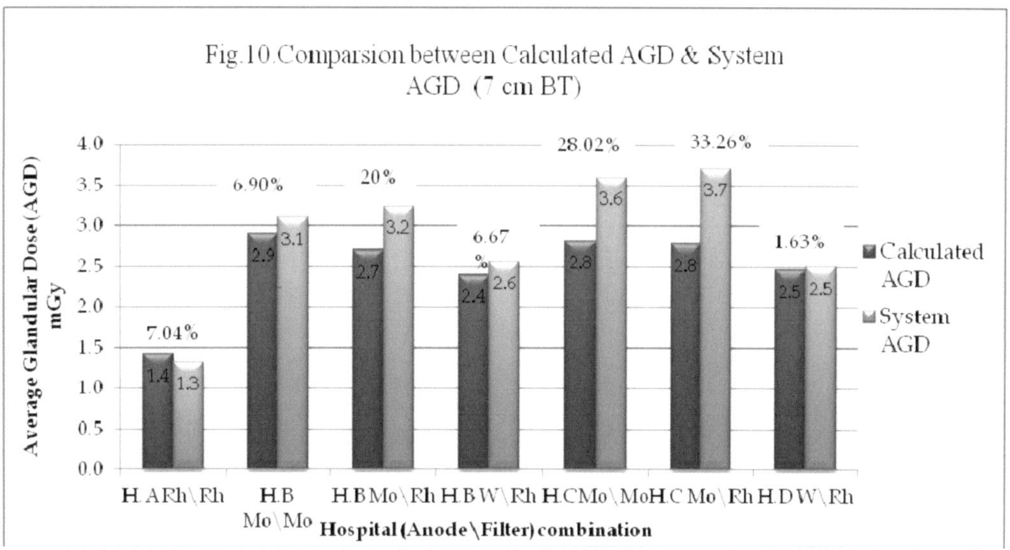

Fig. 10. Comparison between Calculated AGD & System AGD for 7 cm Breast Thickness.

Result of the Contrast to Noise Ratio results (CNR)

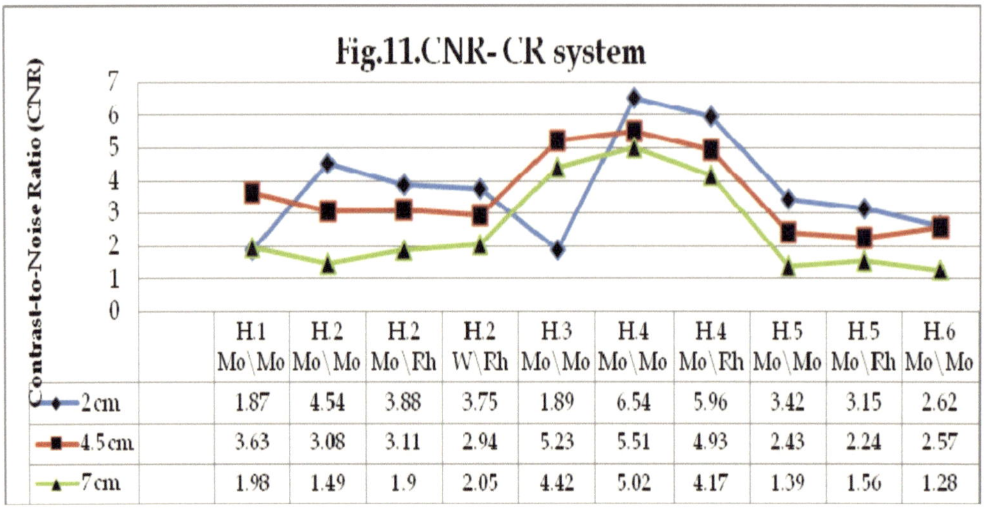

	H.1 Mo\Mo	H.2 Mo\Mo	H.2 Mo\Rh	H.2 W\Rh	H.3 Mo\Mo	H.4 Mo\Mo	H.4 Mo\Rh	H.5 Mo\Mo	H.5 Mo\Rh	H.6 Mo\Mo
2cm	1.87	4.54	3.88	3.75	1.89	6.54	5.96	3.42	3.15	2.62
4.5cm	3.63	3.08	3.11	2.94	5.23	5.51	4.93	2.43	2.24	2.57
7cm	1.98	1.49	1.9	2.05	4.42	5.02	4.17	1.39	1.56	1.28

Fig. 11. the Contrast to Noise Ratio (CNR) -CR system.

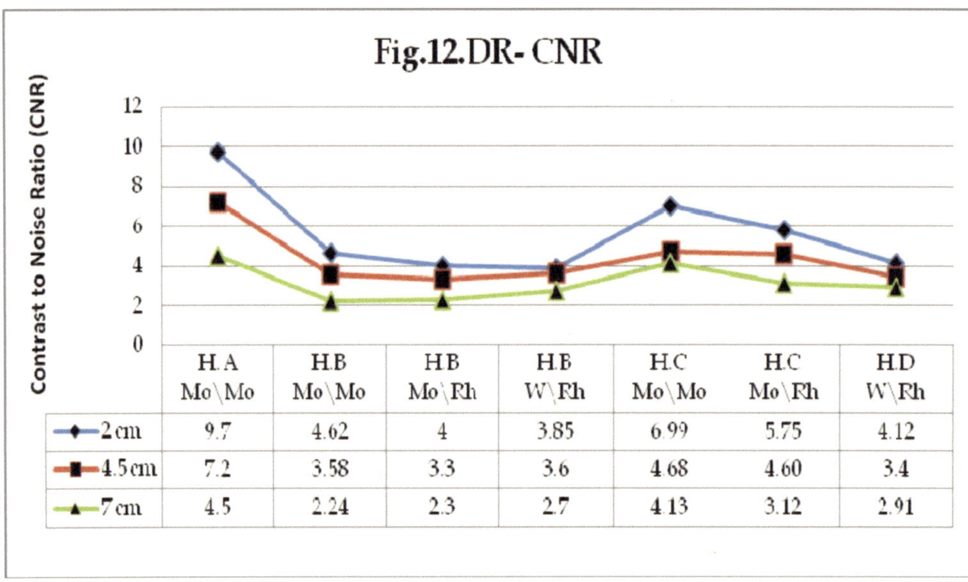

	H.A Mo\Mo	H.B Mo\Mo	H.B Mo\Rh	H.B W\Rh	H.C Mo\Mo	H.C Mo\Rh	H.D W\Rh
2cm	9.7	4.62	4	3.85	6.99	5.75	4.12
4.5cm	7.2	3.58	3.3	3.6	4.68	4.60	3.4
7cm	4.5	2.24	2.3	2.7	4.13	3.12	2.91

Fig. 12. the Contrast to Noise Ratio (CNR) -DR system.

4. Conclusion

This study on radiation exposure in mammography concerned number of facilities in Dubai region and will be extended to a larger number of facilities in the near future.

The results obtained show that quality control and patient Dosimetry are crucially needed in order to ensure a safe and efficient use of mammographic X-rays on patients whether for routine diagnosis or breast screening.

Also , we found that the value of the CNR is depend on the specification of the manufacture for each mammography machine , so we can't compare the value measured of the hospitals to each other because they are from different manufactures

5. Acknowledgment

- IAEA for initiating and supporting this project.
- Dubai Hospital Medical Physics Team.
- Dubai Health Authority (DHA)
- All hospitals participated in this project.

6. Appendix: The forms used to collect the data

Quality Control Findings – Mammography/ ------

Hospital: -- Done on: -----------------------

X-ray Tube	**Operation machine**
Manufacture: X-ray unit name: Model Number: Serial Number: Manufacture date:	Manufacture: Machine name: Serial Number: Manufacture date:

Exposure conditions

Radiographic projection:	Cranio-caudal/lateral/oblique			
Anode material:	Mo/W/Rh			
Inherent filtration material:				
Inherent filtration thickness:			mm	
Additional filtration material:				
Additional filtration thickness:			mm	
Focus to film distance:			cm	
Grid used:		Yes/No		
Automatic exposure control used:		Yes/No		
Tube potential:	kVp ;	Tube charge:	mAs	

Frequency: Acceptance, yearly and after tube or collimator repair/exchange.

6.1 Collimation assessment

Source to image receptor distance (SID) ---------- cm

Deviation between X-ray field and light field

Target material	Mo	Mo
Collimator (cm)	18x24	24x30
Left edge deviation		
Right edge deviation		
Sum of left and right edge deviations		
Sum as % of SID		
Anterior edge deviation		
Chest edge deviation		
Sum of anterior and chest edge deviations		
Sum as % of SID		

ACTION LIMIT: ACR/MQSA - If sum of left plus right edge deviations or anterior plus chest edge deviations exceeds 2% of SID, seek service adjustment.

Deviation between X-ray field and edges of the image receptor

Left edge deviation			
% of SID (retain sign)			
Right edge deviation			
% of SID (retain sign)			
Anterior edge deviation			
% of SID (retain sign)			
Chest edge deviation			
% of SID (retain sign)			

ACTION LIMIT: ACR/MQSA - If X-ray field exceeds image receptor at any side by more than 2% of SID or if X-ray field falls within image receptor on the chest wall side, seek service adjustment.

ACR - If X-ray field falls within image receptor by more than -2% on the left and right sides or by more than -4% on the anterior side, seek service adjustment.

Alignment of chest-wall edges of compression paddle and film

Difference between paddle edge and film					
Difference as % of SID					

ACTION LIMIT: ACR/MQSA -If chest-wall edge of compression paddle is within the image receptor or projects beyond the chest-wall edge of the image receptor by more than 1% of SID, seek service correction.

6.2 Kvp accuracy/reproducibility

KVp meter used-----------
Setting------/---------

	Set 1	Set 2	Set 3	Set 4
Nominal kVp setting				
Focal spot	L	L	L	L
Exposure time (sec)				
mA				
mAs	50	50	50	50

Measured kVp values

1					
2					
3					
4					
Mean kVp					
Standard deviation (SD)					
Mean kVp - Nominal kVp					
0.05 X Nominal kVp					
% Error					
Coefficient of variation					
Pass/Fail Results					
% Error Pass/Fail Criterion	5.00%	CV Pass/Fail Criterion			0.02

ACTION LIMIT: ACR/MQSA - If the mean kVp differs from the nominal by more than +5% of the nominal kVp, or if the coefficient of variation exceeds 0.02, then seek service correction.

6.3 Beam quality (HVL) measurement

Dosimetry system used-----------------

Nominal Kvp setting	30	30	30
Target material			
Filter			
mA			
Time			
mAs	50	50	50
No aluminum filtration, E(0a)			
0.2 mm of added aluminum, E(2)			
0.3 mm of added aluminum, E(3)			
0.4 mm of added aluminum, E(4)			
0.5 mm of added aluminum, E(5)			
0.6 mm of added aluminum, E(6)			
No aluminum filtration, E(0b)			
Average E(0)			
Average E(0)/2			
Calculated HVL (mm Al)			

MQSA X-Ray Tube Voltage and Minimum HVL	
Measured Voltage (kV)	Minimum HVL (mm Al)
20	0.2
25	0.25
30	0.3

6.4 Image quality

Using ACR Phantom:
Anode/Filter: ---------------------
The exposure factors were kV= mAs= ESAK= AGD=

NO.	**Region Materials**	**Visible**
1	1.56 mm nylon fiber	
2	1.12 mm nylon fiber	
3	0.89 mm nylon fiber	
4	0.75 mm nylon fiber	
5	0.54 mm nylon fiber	
6	0.40 mm nylon fiber	
7	0.54 mm simulated micro-calcification	
8	0.40 mm simulated micro-calcification	
9	0.32 mm simulated micro-calcification	
10	0.24 mm simulated micro-calcification	
11	0.16 mm simulated micro-calcification	
12	2.00 mm tumor-like mass	
13	1.00 mm tumor-like mass	
14	0.75 mm tumor-like mass	
15	0.50 mm tumor-like mass	
16	0.25 mm tumor-like mass	

6.5 Using TOR MAX phantom

Anode/Filter: ---------------------

BT = 2cm, Exposure factor: kV= mAs= ESAK= AGD=

BT = 4.5cm, Exposure factor: kV= mAs= ESAK= AGD=

BT =7cm, Exposure factor: kV= mAs= ESAK= AGD=

Unsharpness Measurements:

<table>
<tr><td rowspan="8">Resolution Limit</td><td rowspan="4">RHS Grating</td><td>BT</td><td>Groups</td><td>Line pairs/mm</td></tr>
<tr><td>2</td><td></td><td></td></tr>
<tr><td>5</td><td></td><td></td></tr>
<tr><td>7</td><td></td><td></td></tr>
<tr><td rowspan="4">LHS Grating</td><td>BT</td><td>Groups</td><td>Line pairs/mm</td></tr>
<tr><td>2</td><td></td><td></td></tr>
<tr><td>5</td><td></td><td></td></tr>
<tr><td>7</td><td></td><td></td></tr>
<tr><td colspan="2" rowspan="4">Low Contrast Bar Patterns</td><td>BT</td><td>Groups</td><td>Line pairs/mm</td></tr>
<tr><td>2</td><td></td><td></td></tr>
<tr><td>5</td><td></td><td></td></tr>
<tr><td>7</td><td></td><td></td></tr>
</table>

Low Contrast Sensitivity:

	BT	No. detected	Threshold Contrast
1.6 mm details:	2		
	5		
	7		

Small Detail Visibility:

	BT	No. detected	Threshold Contrast
0.5 mm details:	2		
	5		
	7		
0.25 mm details:	BT	No. detected	Threshold Contrast
	2		
	5		
	7		
Particle Stepwedage :	BT	Comment	
	2		
	5		
	7		

6.6 Contrast to noise ratio measurement

Exposure conditions

Radiographic projection:		Cranio-caudal
Anode material:	Mo/W/Rh	
Inherent filtration material:		
Inherent filtration thickness:		mm
Additional filtration material:		
Additional filtration thickness:		mm
Focus to film distance:		cm
Grid used:	Yes/No	
Automatic exposure control used: Yes/No		

$$CNR = \frac{S_{AL} - S}{\sqrt{(\sigma_{AL}{}^2 + \sigma^2)}}$$

PMMA (cm)	Anode /Filter	kV	mAs	AGD (mGy)	Under Al object S_{al}	SD_{al}	Side to Al object **S**	**SD**	CNR
2									
3									
4									
4.5									
5									
6									
7									
ACR Phantom									

6.7 Dose measurement

CBT = 2 cm

Exposure conditions

Focus-Chamber Distance (cm):
FBD Focus-Bucky Distance (cm):
${}_nK_i$ @FBD = K_i (FCD/FBD)^2 /mAs ${}_nK_e$=${}_nK_i$*BF

Note, BF=1.09; K_i should be correct for calibration factors, temperature and pressure

Anode/Filter	kV		mAs		Reading K_i (mGy)	${}_nK_i$/mAs @ FBD (mGy/mAs)	${}_nK_e$ (mGy/mAs)
	Auto	Manu	Auto	Manu			

ESAK calculation for clinical exposures
K_e=${}_nK_e$*mAs*(FBD/(FBD-BT))^2
Note: use proper ${}_nK_e$ for the used anode/filter combination

BT Breast thickness (cm)	Focus-Breast Distance (cm)	Anode/Filter	kV	mAs	Ke @FBD (mGy)	Ke (mGy/mAs)

7. References

AAPM Report No. 29, Equipment Requirements and Quality Control for Mammography, August 1990

IAEA Group Training on Radiation Protection dose assessment and dose management in Diagnostic and Interventional Radiology, 7-18 May 2008, Udine (Italy)

IAEA-TECDOC-1447, Optimization of the radiological protection of patients: Image quality and dose in mammography (coordinated research in Europe), May2005

Journal of the ICRU Vol. 5 No 2 (2005) Report 74- Oxford University Press, Chapter 3 - Quantities and Units for Measurement and Calculation in Medical X-Ray Imaging.

N.Perry, M. Broeders, C. de Wolf, S. Törnberg, R. Holland & L. von Karsa - 4th edition of the European Guidelines for Quality Assurance in Breast Cancer Screening and Diagnosis (EUREF) - Office for Official Publications of the European Communities, 2006

Nuclear Associates 18-220, Mammographic Accreditation Phantom, Instruction Manual© 2003 Cardinal Health, Inc. www.cardinal.com/rms

Priscilla F. Butler, M.S, Digital Mammography Quality Control and Accreditation, (July 1, 2006)

Part 3

Novel Diagnostic Approach by Mammography

9

Is Mammographic Density a Biomarker to Study the Molecular Causes of Breast Cancer?

Hanna Mirette and Diorio Caroline
Université Laval/Unité de Recherche en Santé des Populations
Canada

1. Introduction

Breast cancer is the most common cancer affecting females worldwide. It accounts for 31% of all new cancer cases diagnosed in females with 23% of cases diagnosed in women younger than 50 years old (Jemal et al., 2002; Smigal et al., 2006). Being the second cause of cancer deaths after lung cancer (Jemal et al., 2002), enormous scientific efforts have been done aiming to better understand, treat and prevent breast cancer. Despite these research efforts, breast cancer remains a major health problem.

Since their implementation, the mammographic screening programs have resulted in breast cancer detection at an earlier stage and consequently have contributed to a greater reduction in the breast cancer mortality rate (Lebovic et al., 2010). Routine screening mammograms usually target women aged from 50 to 69 years old (Bryant & Mai, 2011). However, many studies have identified 40 years old as an appropriate age to begin annual mammographic screening (Bryant & Mai, 2011; Lebovic et al., 2010). Besides being a screening and diagnostic device, the mammography is also used as a research tool.

Variations in the mammographic appearance of the breast referred to as "mammographic density", reveal histological changes in breast tissue composition. Nowadays, elevated mammographic density is proven to be one of the strongest risk factors for breast cancer. Whatever the method used to classify mammographic density, all have shown a substantial increased breast cancer risk associated with increased mammographic density (McCormack & dos Santos Silva, 2006). Mammographic density has been consistently associated with increased risk of hyperplasia, atypical hyperplasia and carcinoma *in situ* (Boyd et al., 2000). In addition, several recognized risk factors for breast cancer (such as number of full-term pregnancies, age at first full-term pregnancy, family history of breast cancer, personal history of breast biopsies and use of hormone replacement therapy) are also associated with mammographic density (Boyd et al., 2010; Heine & Malhotra, 2002). Mammographic density is related to levels of hormonal and growth factors involved in cellular proliferation, differentiation and apoptosis (Diorio et al., 2005b; Greendale et al., 2005; Howard & Gusterson, 2000) which have established roles in the etiology of breast cancer (Imagawa et al., 2002; Shekhar et al., 2003).

Mammographic density reflects the proportion of the breast occupied by epithelial and stromal tissues. Therefore, mammographic density is hypothesized to reflect the quantity of non-adipose breast tissue (Boyd et al., 2010; Li et al., 2005), representing the population of breast cells at risk of carcinogenic transformation (Trichopoulos et al., 2005). Breast cancer generally arises from epithelial cells (Russo et al., 1990), and an increase in the overall epithelial cell number is believed to increase the risk of breast cancer (Preston-Martin et al., 1990). However, there is also growing evidence that stroma plays an important role, not only in mammary gland development, but also in breast carcinogenesis (Imagawa et al., 2002; Shekhar et al., 2003; Woodward et al., 1998). Stroma is a major component of the breast (Imagawa et al., 2002; Page & Winfield, 1986; Shekhar et al., 2003) and variations in mammographic density may be more sensitive to changes in the stroma than to those in the epithelium (Warren & Lakhani, 2003). Knowledge of molecular markers (such as proteins and genes expression) in normal breast epithelium and stroma that are associated with mammographic density may provide important clues regarding breast cancer etiology. Studying the influence of such genes/proteins on mammographic density used as an end point in epidemiological studies may reduce the long term follow-up period needed to detect their effects on breast cancer incidence, thus providing an easier and more economic way to study the pathogenesis of breast cancer. A better understanding of molecular markers influencing mammographic density may also help to identify preventive targets.

In this review, we intend to shed light on the possibility of using mammographic density as an intermediate biomarker to study the molecular causes of breast cancer. We hypothesize that if breast cancer biomarkers ultimately exert their influence on mammographic density in the same direction as they influence breast cancer risk, then mammographic density could be considered as an intermediate biomarker for breast cancer rather than just a risk factor. An overview with emphasis on changes in genes and proteins expression in normal breast tissue and their relationship with mammographic density is provided.

2. Mammographic density

The breast is composed mainly of fibroglandular tissue and adipose tissue at different proportions. These constituents differ in their X-ray attenuation characteristics. Fibroglandular tissue, mainly composed of epithelial cells and supporting stroma, attenuates more X-rays and thus appears white on mammograms, while adipose tissue, which is radiolucent, appears dark on mammograms. Hence, variations in the radiological appearance of the breast on a mammogram reflect variations in breast tissue composition. Mammographic density represents the proportion of the breast occupied by radiologically dense tissue. Results from Li's study show that elevated mammographic density is associated with a greater nuclear area of both epithelial and non-epithelial cells, as well as with a greater proportion of collagen and a greater area of glandular structures (Li et al., 2005). It is believed that elevated mammographic density reflects the effects of mitogens and mutagens which influence cellular proliferation and genetic damage of these cells (Martin & Boyd, 2008). This provides a potential mechanism by which elevated mammographic density could influence the risk of breast cancer. Moreover, it has been suggested that mammographic density is more related to stromal changes rather than epithelial changes (Heine & Malhotra, 2002; Warren & Lakhani, 2003). This is consistent with Lin and colleagues findings who reported a higher number of stromal cells but not epithelial cells in high mammographic density regions when compared to low mammographic density regions within the same woman (p for trend < 0.01) (Lin et al., 2011).

3. Assessment and classifications of mammographic density

In 1976, Wolfe first described a method for classifying variations in the mammographic appearance of the breast into four categories based on the visual assessment of the extent of dense breast tissue on the mammogram as well as of characteristics of densities seen (prominent ducts and dysplasia). The four categories correlate with breast cancer risk, where breasts with the densest pattern were associated with the highest risk of developing breast cancer (Wolfe, 1976). Later, the Wolfe categories have been largely replaced by the American College of Radiology's Breast Imaging Reporting and Data System (BI-RADS). The BI-RADS, which is still frequently in use, also classifies mammographic density into four categories: 1 = almost entirely fatty breast, 2 = breast containing scattered densities, 3 = heterogeneously dense breast and 4 = extremely dense breast. Since then, several methods have been developed seeking to provide a quantitative and continuous measure of mammographic density. In 1995, Boyd proposed a six-category scale based on the visual estimation by a radiologist of the proportion of the breast occupied by radiologically dense tissue. The six categories are: 0%, < 10%, 10%-< 25%, 25%-< 50%, 50%-< 75%, ≥ 75% (Boyd et al., 1995). These previously mentioned methods depend on the visual assessment and are thus subjected to bias (Warren, 2004). Mammographic density is now often measured by a computer-assisted method on digitized images allowing the quantitative assessment of mammographic density. Results from such a method are expressed as absolute area of mammographic density in square centimeters or in percentage of mammographic density. The computer-assisted method is known to have a high degree of reliability and reproducibility for determining mammographic density (Boyd et al., 1995; Boyd et al., 2010). The limitation of this method is that it does not take into account the gradual transition from dense to non-dense breast tissue. Generally, the quantitative approaches have the advantage over the qualitative categorical approaches in providing a continuous measure of mammographic density. However, quantitative methods do not consider the breast volume; instead they take into account the breast area. Nonetheless, quantitative approaches give a more consistent estimate of the associated breast cancer risk and this risk persists after adjustment for other risk factors.

4. Mammographic density and breast cancer risk

The association between elevated mammographic density and increased breast cancer risk was investigated in many studies. In order to confirm this association, McCormak and dos Santos Silva conducted a systematic meta-analysis on 42 previously published studies (McCormack & dos Santos Silva, 2006). They included 14,000 women with breast cancer and 226,000 women without breast cancer. They concluded that elevated mammographic density, regardless of the type of assessment, was consistently positively associated with an increased risk of breast cancer. Women with the most dense breast (> 75%) have 3-5 fold greater risk of developing breast cancer compared to women with the least dense breast (< 5%). The authors also reported that the associations were stronger when mammographic density was measured in percent mammographic density rather than categorized according to Wolfe scale. Thus, it is well established that high mammographic density constitutes an independent risk factor for breast cancer and that it accounts for a large proportion of the disease incidence (Boyd et al., 2010). It has been recently shown that women who experienced a decrease in mammographic density of at least one BI-RADS category over a period of six years had a 28% lower breast cancer risk compared to women whose mammographic density was unchanged (Tanne, 2010).

5. Breast cancer risk factors associated to mammographic density

Mammographic density is not constant throughout life. It declines with increasing age reflecting the age-related changes in breast tissue composition. These age-related changes, referred to as involution, reveal the reduction of the epithelium and stroma within the breast and the simultaneous increase in fat. Premenopausal women have consistently been found to have more elevated mammographic density than postmenopausal women. It might be slightly confusing knowing that mammographic density, which constitutes a breast cancer risk factor, decreases with age while breast cancer incidence increases with advanced age. This apparent paradox can be resolved by the breast cancer incidence model proposed by Pike (Pike et al., 2004). Pike based his model on the concept that the relevant measure to describe the age-specific incidence of breast cancer is the cumulative breast tissue exposure rather than the chronological age. The breast tissue exposure reflects the cumulative exposure of mammary cells to hormones and growth factors and the accumulation of genetic damage. According to Pike's model, breast tissue exposure is at its peak at menarche, and then it decreases gradually during pregnancy, until it reaches its lowest values during the postmenopausal period. Thus, the incidence of breast cancer and the cumulative exposure of breast tissue both increase with age (Henson & Tarone, 1994; Pike et al., 2004).

Several known risk factors for breast cancer; hormonal, reproductive and anthropometric variables, are also associated with variations in mammographic density. The strongest associations are observed with body weight. Mammographic density is inversely associated with body mass index (Brisson et al., 1984; Diorio et al., 2005a). This is consistent with the inverse association between body mass index or weight and breast cancer risk among premenopausal, but inconsistent with the positive association among postmenopausal women (Hunter & Willett, 1993; Trentham-Dietz et al., 1997). Height, which is proven to be positively associated with an increased risk of breast cancer among pre- and postmenopausal women, is also positively associated with increased mammographic density (Brisson et al., 1984; Trentham-Dietz et al., 1997).

Moreover, hormonal-related breast cancer risk factors such as nulliparity, low number of live births, late age at first birth and combined hormone replacement therapy are positively associated with increased percent mammographic density (Boyd et al., 2010; El-Bastawissi et al., 2000). However, the association of circulating estrogen levels (known to be strongly positively associated with breast cancer risk) with mammographic density has so far been inconsistent (Boyd et al., 2002c; Greendale et al., 2005). It is believed that the exposure to endogenous and exogenous hormones accompanying reproductive and hormonal changes increases mammographic density by affecting the proliferative activity and the quantity of stroma and epithelium in breast tissue (Boyd et al., 2010). Furthermore, menopause was found to be associated with a reduction in dense areas accompanied by an increase in non-dense areas. These changes in mammographic density due to menopausal status are not fully explained by the effect of age on density (Boyd et al., 2002a).

However, all these epidemiological risk factors explain only about 20%-40% of the variability in percent mammographic density (Vachon et al., 2000). It seems that genetic factors (heritability) could be responsible for greater variations in mammographic density. Current evidence shows that mammographic density is highly heritable and is inherited as a quantitative trait (Boyd et al., 2002b; Ursin et al., 2009). Heritability accounts for 50%-60% of the variation in mammographic density. Heritability of mammographic density may explain, at least in part, the familial aggregation pattern of breast cancer. Women with elevated percent mammographic density are more likely to have a first-degree relative with a history of breast cancer (Ziv et al., 2003).

Recently, it has been demonstrated that tamoxifen, which reduces the extent of mammographic density, also decreases the burden of invasive breast cancer (Cuzick et al., 2011). In that trial, for the 46% of women in the tamoxifen arm whose density was reduced by 10% or more, the risk of breast cancer was reduced by 63% relative to the control group (odds ratio (OR) = 0.37, p = 0.002) while for the 54% of women whose density was reduced by less than 10%, there was no reduction in breast cancer risk (OR = 1.13, p = 0.60). The action of tamoxifen is mediated through its effects on several gene products including insulin-like growth factor-1 (IGF-1) (Pollak et al., 1990), a protein that is believed to play a role in mammographic density (Diorio et al., 2005b) and breast cancer development (Schernhammer et al., 2005). This action can therefore be schematized as follow:

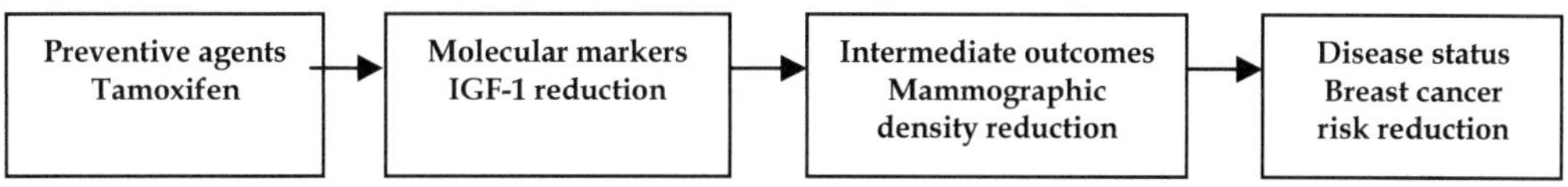

The number of proteins / genes that can be measured in breast tissue rather than in the circulation is rapidly increasing because of new molecular technologies. Given that some preventive agents can decrease mammographic density and consequently breast cancer risk through their modifying effects on several proteins and/or genes, it seems important to study proteins/genes that could influence mammographic density. These proteins/genes may be further used as preventive targets in future breast cancer intervention studies.

6. Proteins expression in breast tissue associated to mammographic density

6.1 Insulin-like growth factors

Knowing that mammographic density declines gradually with age and that circulating levels of IGF-1 also decrease with age and that both are related to an increased risk of breast cancer, it might be of great importance to study the relationship between the two. A pioneer study investigated the association between IGF-1 expression in breast tissue and mammographic density among women aged 45-55 years old who underwent breast biopsies with a final diagnosis of benign lesions (Guo et al., 2001). They used 92 formalin-fixed paraffin blocks of breast tissues surrounding benign lesions obtained from women with little (< 25%, n = 46) or extensive (> 50%, n = 46) mammographic density matched according to age at time of biopsy. In this study, tissue levels of IGF-1 from nuclear areas were analysed by immunohistochemistry and quantified using quantitative microscopy. Guo and colleagues found that breast tissue from subjects with extensive mammographic density had a greater IGF-1 staining when compared to subjects with little mammographic density (p = 0.02). After stratification by age, this association was significant only for subjects less than 50 years old. The IGF-1 staining was about three times greater in blocks obtained from women with high mammographic density compared to blocks from women with low mammographic density among subjects less than 50 years of age ($p = 0.0009$). A main pitfall of Guo's study was the lack of information regarding the menopausal status of the participants. Nonetheless, data from laboratory and epidemiological studies seem to support these findings.

The IGF-1 is a member of a superfamily of multifunctional peptides. The majority of circulating IGFs are produced by the liver in response to growth hormone, but many other tissues including the breast tissue can also express IGFs. IGF-1 plays a crucial role in regulating many cellular functions such as cell proliferation, differentiation and apoptosis. It is well known that IGF-1 is essential for normal mammary cells development (Marshman & Streuli, 2002). Strange and colleagues have demonstrated that IGF-1 increases the proliferative activity of cultured mammary cells and hence the risk of breast cancer. They added that IGF-1 is able to stimulate the growth of cultured human breast epithelial and stromal cells in a dose-dependent manner (Strange et al., 2002; Strange et al., 2004). Several epidemiological studies have provided evidence that elevated circulating levels of IGF-1 are associated with increased breast cancer risk in pre- but not postmenopausal women (Hankinson et al., 1998; Krajcik et al., 2002; Schernhammer et al., 2005; Toniolo et al., 2000). This is in line with the positive association between increased circulating levels of IGF-1 and percent mammographic density among pre- ($p = 0.02$) but not postmenopausal women ($p = 0.37$) that was observed in our large study specifically designed to confirm what other studies of smaller sample size had observed (Diorio et al., 2005b). More recently, we showed that single nucleotide polymorphisms (SNPs) located on IGF-1 gene were also associated with premenopausal mammographic density, and this association remained after adjustment for IGF-1 levels (Diorio et al., 2008). Although circulating levels of IGF-1, mainly produced in the liver, have been linked to breast morphogenesis and breast cancer risk, our results support the idea that IGF-1 at tissue levels are important in this respect, at least among premenopausal women. This association only found among premenopausal women may reflect a cross-talk between IGF-1 and steroid hormones. In fact, a previous study has observed a strong evidence of a cross-talk between IGF-1 and estrogen in breast tissue (Martin & Stoica, 2002). Estrogen induces IGF-1 expression through binding to estrogen receptor-α (ERα), and IGF-1, by binding to its receptor, initiates a cascade of phosphorylation that ends by activating ERα. This estrogen-IGF-1 cross-talk may induce mammary epithelial cells proliferation and possibly tumor development.

6.2 Hormone receptors

Since mammographic density reflects the cumulative effect of steroid hormones on breast tissue and blood estradiol level is a risk factor for breast cancer, then mammographic density is expected to be associated to hormone receptors in breast tissue. So far, two studies assessed the association between the two subtypes of ER, ERα and ERβ, separately and mammographic density (Lundstrom et al., 2006; Verheus et al., 2009), while two others assessed the association between ER, with no mention of the subtype, and mammographic density (Harvey et al., 2008; Yang et al., 2010). Among these, three groups also assessed the association between the progesterone receptor (PgR) and mammographic density (Harvey et al., 2008; Verheus et al., 2009; Yang et al., 2010).

Lundstrom and colleagues obtained normal tissue specimens from 28 postmenopausal women aged ≥ 52 years old undergoing surgery for breast cancer as first treatment.

Radiological examination was performed on tissue blocks, and pair-wise samples of dense and non-dense tissue were selected. They analysed semi-quantitatively ERα and ERβ in glandular epithelium by immunohistochemical staining intensity. They observed a higher ERα staining in glandular epithelium in mammographically dense compared to non-dense breast tissue (2.4 ± 0.2 versus 1.6 ± 0.2; $p < 0.01$). Conversely, there was no significant association between ERβ and mammographic density (2.2 ± 0.2 versus 1.9 ± 0.3; $p > 0.05$ for dense and non-dense tissue respectively) (Lundstrom et al., 2006). The major strengths of Lunstrom's study were the measurement of the two subtypes of ER separately and the usage of paired samples of dense and non-dense normal breast tissue at a distance of at least 2 cm from the tumor from each patient. The small sample size, the lack of premenopausal women included in the study sample and the usage of normal breast tissue obtained from breast cancer patients which may not be completely representative of normal breast tissue were the main limitations of this study.

In the study conducted by Verheus and colleagues, they assessed the epithelial expression of ERα, ERβ, and PgR in relation to mammographic density among 159 pre- and postmenopausal women having breast cancer, 60 years old on average, and of different ethnicities. They prepared tissue microarrays (TMAs) from benign breast tissue samples obtained from tumor blocks (mean = 1.7 specimens per woman). The TMAs were then immunostained for ERα, ERβ and PgR, which were measured by quantitative microscopy and categorized as < 10% or ≥ 10% of staining. Mammographic density from the craniocaudal views before breast cancer diagnosis was assessed using a computer-assisted method. None of the markers measured in breast tissue was significantly associated with percent or absolute mammographic density among the whole study population or among Japanese women. However, they observed a negative association between ERα expression and percent mammographic density ($p = 0.04$), a positive association between ERβ and percent mammographic density ($p = 0.05$) and a positive association between PgR and absolute mammographic density ($p = 0.03$) among Caucasian women (Verheus et al., 2009). Assessment of ERα and ERβ separately, the usage of TMA approach which allows the assessment of several markers expression in a large number of samples under the same staining conditions, the classification of mammographic density by a computer-assisted method and the adjustment for several potential confounders in the analysis were the main advantages of Verheus' study. However, the usage of benign breast tissue obtained from tumor blocks may not be fully representative of normal breast tissue and markers expression in benign tissue could have been influenced by potential paracrine effects of the adjacent tumors.

Harvey and colleagues included in their study 56 postmenopausal women aged from 45 to 85 years old having a surgical treatment for breast cancer. Mammographic density of the contralateral breast was assessed by a computer-assisted method. The ER and PgR content in ducts, lobules and fibrous stroma was measured by immunohistochemistry performed on tissue blocks free from cancer, and the intensity of staining, as negative or positive, was visually estimated. Contrary to what one might have expected, the authors did not find any significant association between ER or PgR and mammographic density after adjustment for hormonal replacement therapy use and age (Harvey et al., 2008). The small sample size, the lack of premenopausal women among the study population, the usage of tissue blocks from mastectomy specimens which might not be completely free from foci of carcinoma in addition to be sampled in densest areas of the breast and the lack of adjustment for potential confounding factors may explain the absence of association. The major strength of this study was the use of a computer-assisted method providing a continuous and reproducible measure of mammographic density.

For their study, Yang and colleagues identified 27 premenopausal women and 39 postmenopausal women (29-88 years old) who underwent surgery for breast cancer as first treatment. These women had low (BI-RADS 1 or 2, n = 28) or high (BI-RADS 3 or 4, n = 38) mammographic density. They analysed ER and PgR expression immunohistochemically in stroma and epithelium separately, from normal frozen breast tissue located at least 5 cm away from the tumor. The Allred scoring system was used by a breast pathologist to measure each marker. In this study, the authors did not find any significant positive association between ER or PgR and mammographic density in univariate models (Yang et al., 2010). Unfortunately, their small sample size did not allow analysis stratified by menopausal status. As in the above studies, they used normal breast tissue obtained from breast cancer patients which may not truly represent normal breast tissue.

Therefore, out of the studies that analysed the association between specified subtypes of ER expression in breast tissue and mammographic density, one study observed a positive association between epithelial ERα expression and mammographic density among postmenopausal women (Lundstrom et al., 2006), while another study observed an inverse association among pre- and postmenopausal Caucasian women (Verheus et al., 2009). In this latter population, a positive association of ERβ and PgR expression in breast tissue with mammographic density was also observed (Verheus et al., 2009). However, none of the other two studies that assessed PgR found any significant association among pre- and/or postmenopausal women (Harvey et al., 2008; Yang et al., 2010).

It is well known that ovarian steroid hormones play a critical role in normal mammary cell development, proliferation and differentiation (Graham & Clarke, 1997; Nilsson et al., 2001). While most of the studies agree that estrogen increases the risk of breast cancer, the effect of progesterone on this risk remains a subject of controversy (Hankinson & Eliassen, 2007). In fact, PgR could be considered a marker of both estrogen and progesterone actions in the mammary gland, since PgR expression is regulated by estrogen (Shyamala et al., 2002). Estrogen exerts its biological activity on mammary cells particularly through nuclear ERs. ERs are further subdivided into two subtypes; ERα and ERβ, having different expression levels in normal and malignant breast tissues. ERα and ERβ, encoded by different genes, exert different biological actions on breast tissue cells. Activation of ERα increases the rate of breast cells proliferation by up-regulating several genes involved in cellular proliferation such as cyclin D (Liu et al., 2002b), while down-regulating other genes known to inhibit proliferation such as transforming growth factor-β (TGF-β) (Chang et al., 2006). In a recent study, Woolcott and colleagues observed that ERα levels were higher in nonneoplastic epithelium obtained from breast cancer cases when compared to control biopsies obtained from women free from breast cancer (OR = 2.6; 95% CI 1.1-6.2). However, there was no significant difference between PgR expression in nonneoplastic epithelium obtained from breast cancer cases and that obtained from control women (OR = 0.7; 95% CI 0.4-1.3) (Woolcott et al., 2008). The ERα-induced breast cells proliferation is consistent with Lundstrom's finding (Lundstrom et al., 2006) of increased epithelial ERα expression in dense breast tissue compared to non-dense tissue. These results suggest that breast tissue could be influenced by increased ERα expression, leading to increased mammographic density and finally to increased breast cancer risk at least among postmenopausal women. On the other hand, the overexpression of ERβ decreases ERα transcriptional activity. ERβ has been found to modulate the expression of many ERα regulated genes involved in cell proliferation such as cyclin D and TGF-β genes (Chang et al., 2006; Liu et al., 2002b). Also, ERβ down-regulates the ERα protein level (Chang et al., 2006). Furthermore, ERβ staining was inversely correlated with the Ki67, marker of cellular proliferation, in normal breast tissue and preinvasive mammary tumor (Roger et al., 2001). This suggests that ERβ acts as a tumor suppressor (Bardin et al., 2004). Thus, it is evident that the ratio between both subtypes is the most important determinant of the overall response. The increased expression of ERα concomitant with decreased ERβ expression was found to take place in early breast cancer stages (Leygue et al., 1998a; Roger et al., 2001). Knowing that ER subtypes have opposite actions on breast tissue could provide further explanation regarding the opposite associations found in Verheus and colleagues study, who did not consider the ratio or the mutual adjustment of both subtypes in their analysis since both subtypes were associated to mammographic density.

6.3 Aromatase enzyme

A recent study assessed the association between breast tissue aromatase expression, a rate-limiting enzyme in the estrogen pathway, and mammographic density (Vachon et al., 2011). They looked for this association among 49 healthy Caucasian women aged from 40-82 years old. Mammographic density was visually assessed using the mammographic films and identifying areas of low and high mammographic density. They applied a fine-needle guided ultrasound to obtain tissue biopsies from dense and from non-dense breast areas for each woman. Biopsies were analysed by immunohistochemistry, and immunostaining for aromatase was scored visually in terms of extent and intensity of staining for each cell type (stroma, epithelium and adipocytes) using a modified H-score (Santen et al., 1994). They observed greater aromatase staining in dense breast tissue when compared to non-dense tissue ($p < 0.0003$). This result was consistent for pre- and postmenopausal women when assessed separately. The aromatase staining was higher in both stromal and epithelial cells from dense tissue compared to those from non-dense tissue (both $p < 0.01$). Conversely, it was lower in adipocytes from dense tissue versus non-dense tissue ($p < 0.01$). Concerning dense breast tissue, aromatase staining in stromal cells was threefold higher than that in epithelial cells. The major strengths of Vachon's study were the paired samples of dense and non-dense normal breast tissue taken from healthy subjects and the scoring of aromatase using both the extent and the intensity of staining. To our knowledge, this is the only study assessing the association between breast tissue aromatase level and mammographic density and therefore further larger studies are recommended to confirm these promising findings.

The aromatase enzyme catalyzes the conversion of androgens, androstenedione and testosterone to estrogen, estrone and estradiol. Thus, it is largely responsible for estrogen levels in breast tissue, especially after menopause, when the *in situ* production of estrogen in mammary adipose tissue takes the upper hand following the cessation of ovarian estrogen synthesis. Increased aromatase expression would result in higher estrogen levels and subsequently greater breast tissue exposure to estrogen. Irahara and colleagues observed an elevated level of aromatase mRNA in breast cancer cells when compared to normal breast tissue (Irahara et al., 2006). Furthermore, aromatase has been shown to stimulate the growth of breast cancer cells *in vitro* (Macaulay et al., 1994). The aromatase is the product of the CYP19 gene which is a member of the cytochrome P450 enzymes family. A comprehensive haplotype analysis of CYP19 and breast cancer risk reveals that a common specific long-range haplotype is associated with an increased risk of breast cancer (OR = 1.31; 95% CI 1.11-1.54) (Haiman et al., 2003). In contrast, no association has been observed in a recent comprehensive examination of CYP19 variants and mammographic density (Olson et al., 2007). However, the common long-range haplotype associated with breast cancer risk has not been assessed by Olson and colleagues. The identification of causal variants associated with the CYP19 long-range haplotype should be investigated.

6.4 Epidermal growth factors

Among the complete family of epidermal growth factor receptors and their ligands expressed in breast tissue, human epidermal growth factor receptor-2 (HER-2) and transforming growth factor-α (TGF-α) have been evaluated for their association with mammographic density.

In the study conducted by Verheus and colleagues described earlier (Verheus et al., 2009), the authors also measured the expression of HER-2 in breast tissue. They observed no association between HER-2 staining and mammographic density among the whole study population (p = 0.82 and p = 0.74 for percent and absolute mammographic density respectively), among Caucasian women (p = 0.38 and p = 0.99 for percent and absolute mammographic density respectively) or among Japanese women (p = 0.57 and p = 0.73 for percent and absolute mammographic density respectively). HER-2 belongs to the human epidermal growth factor receptor family which is involved in the regulation of normal breast growth and development. In fact, HER-2 is overexpressed in 20-30% of cases of breast cancer (Cho et al., 2008). When HER-2 is overexpressed, it sends signals to the nucleus to proliferate, resulting in increased cellular multiplication and consequently malignant growth (Yarden, 2001). A recent meta-analysis found that the functional SNP Ile655Val of HER-2 is associated to breast cancer risk among Asian women but not among Caucasian nor European women (Tao et al., 2009). Moreover, no association has been observed between HER-2 Ile655Val SNP and mammographic density among Australian women (Stone et al., 2007). The Ile655Val is believed to destabilize the active HER-2 reducing its activation (Fleishman et al., 2002).

In the study previously considered, Guo and colleagues also quantified TGF-α staining, and found no association with mammographic density before or after stratification for age (all p > 0.30) (Guo et al., 2001). The influence of TGF-α, a member of the epidermal growth factor family of peptides, on breast cancer incidence is not fully explored. However, a previous laboratory study has demonstrated that TGF-α enhances the growth of normal mouse mammary epithelial cell line (Casey et al., 2007). Furthermore, TGF-α can act as a mitogen and differentiation factor in mammary epithelium inducing multifocal hyperplastic and malignant lesions in an animal model (Smith et al., 1995).

Additional research will be needed to clarify the role of epidermal growth factor family in breast morphogenesis and breast cancer risk.

6.5 Matrix metalloproteinases

In a recent study, Steude and colleagues attempted to assess the association between matrix metalloproteinases (MMPs) 1, 3, 9, 12 and their inhibitor (TIMP-3) in breast tissue and mammographic density (Steude et al., 2009). Their study population was composed of 75 premenopausal and 202 postmenopausal breast cancer patients with mainly Caucasian and Japanese ancestry. To achieve their goal, they prepared TMAs with up to 4 cores from areas representing benign breast tissues (mean = 2.9 cores per woman). The expression of MMPs and TIMP-3 was immunohistochemically measured and visually classified in the stroma as no versus any stain (available for 169 women) and in the epithelium as no, weak or strong stain intensity (available for 259 women) separately. A computer-assisted method was applied for the evaluation of mammographic density from prediagnostic digitized mammograms from the craniocaudal views. Because the expression of MMP-3 and MMP-9 was observed in less than 20% of epithelial and less than 5% of stromal breast tissue, the authors did not examine their associations with percent mammographic density. Contrary to what was expected, MMP-1, MMP-12 and TIMP-3 analysed in stromal and in epithelial tissue were not significantly related to percent mammographic density after adjustment for confounders among the whole study population or across ethnic groups.

Although Guo and colleagues did not measure MMPs, they assayed TIMP-3 in addition to IGF-1 and TGF-α reported earlier (Guo et al., 2001). They found that TIMP-3 expression was higher in tissue from subjects with extensive mammographic density compared to age-matched subjects with little mammographic density (p = 0.08). Moreover, this association was statistically significant for women less than 50 years old (p = 0.004), but not for women 50 years old or more (p = 0.48). Guo and colleagues hypothesized that TIMP-3 may influence epithelial and stromal proliferation contributing to higher mammographic density and subsequently increased breast cancer risk. The discrepancy between Steude and Guo's studies could be due to different means used in classifying mammographic density, different immunostaining techniques applied, and different study population regarding their breast diseases, ethnicity and mean age. In particular, participants in Guo's study were younger (ranging from 45-55 years old) than those recruited in Steude's study (mean age = 60.2 ± 8.7 years old) suggesting that the association between TIMP-3 and breast density could be limited to young women. A further larger study, stratifying analyses according to menopausal status, will be needed to clarify these observations.

The MMPs are proteases responsible for cleaving proteins of the extracellular matrix. MMPs regulate a wide range of biological functions such as cell death, proliferation, differentiation, tumor associated angiogenesis and malignant conversion (Coussens et al., 2002). They can also induce tumor invasion and metastasis (Balduyck et al., 2000). MMPs have been found to be greatly expressed in malignant breast tissue when compared to the surrounding normal breast tissue (Bartsch et al., 2003; Garbett et al., 2000). However, their roles in breast cancer development are unclear. According to Shin and colleagues, none of the two common SNPs in the MMP-12 gene (A-82G in the promoter region and A1082G in the exon) was associated with breast cancer risk among pre- and postmenopausal Chinese women (Shin et al., 2005). A recently published meta-analysis, looked for the association between MMP-1 (rs1799750), MMP-2 (rs243865), MMP-3 (rs3025058) and MMP-9 (rs3918242) SNPs and breast cancer risk (Zhou et al., 2011). They selected 9 case-control studies including 2,597 cases and 2,618 controls, and found only an association between MMP-2 SNP and breast cancer risk. However, MMP-2 expression in breast tissue has not yet been examined in association with mammographic density.

TIMP-3 was found able to induce cellular apoptosis (Baker et al., 1999; Jiang et al., 2002). However, an increased TIMP-3 expression was observed in breast cancer (Byrne et al., 1995;

Uria et al., 1994). This is in line with Guo's observation who suggested that TIMP-3 might increase the risk of premenopausal breast cancer through its effect on epithelial and stromal cells proliferation. According to Peterson, who evaluated the association between 19 SNPs of TIMP-3 and breast cancer risk among 1,062 Chinese women with breast cancer and 1,069 without, women with the rs9609643 AA genotype had 60% lower risk of developing breast cancer when compared to women with GG genotype (OR = 0.4, 95% CI 0.2-1.0). Whereas, women with the rs8136803 TT genotype were 5 times more at risk of developing breast cancer when compared to women with the GG genotype (OR = 5.1, 95% CI 1.1-24.3) (Peterson et al., 2009). However, it is still unknown if these SNPs have a functional relevance. Lei and colleagues observed a moderately increased breast cancer risk for the C allele carriers of the TIMP-3 rs9619311 SNP (OR = 1.25, 95%CI 1.05-1.50) among Swedish women (Lei et al., 2007). A similar non-significant association was also observed in Peterson's study (OR = 1.2, 95%CI 0.9-1.5). Since TIMP-3 rs9619311 SNP is located in the promoter region, it is possible that it may affect transcription binding sites. Further studies will be needed to confirm if TIMP-3 is associated with mammographic density and breast cancer risk.

6.6 Proteoglycans

Two groups examined the association between the expression of some proteoglycans in breast tissue and mammographic density (Alowami et al., 2003; Lundstrom et al., 2006). In the study conducted by Alowami and colleagues, they assessed the association between the expression of small leucine-rich proteoglycans, lumican and decorin in breast tissue and percent mammographic density. In their study, they included 62 women aged 54-75 years old diagnosed with benign or preinvasive breast diseases. Immunohistochemical analysis of lumican and decorin was performed on tissue blocks obtained from resection margins distant from the lesion, and immunostainings were scored visually in terms of extent and intensity of staining. Following the localization of biopsies on previous screening mammograms, the authors assessed mammographic density of the surrounding breast tissue distant from the lesion using the six-category Boyd scale. For this study, they excluded all women whose mammographic density score ranged from 25%-50% and subdivided all remaining participants into low (< 25%, n = 35) and high (> 50%, n = 27) mammographic density subgroups. They observed that the expression of lumican and decorin was restricted to the stroma surrounding the epithelium. The median value of the expression of both lumican and decorin was 2-3 times higher in specimens from women with high mammographic density compared to those with low mammographic density (both with $p < 0.0001$). No adjustment for age has been made, but women in the categories of low and high mammographic density had similar range of age (54-74 and 54-75 years old, respectively). In their study, Alowami and colleagues included mainly postmenopausal women thus reducing the proportion of cases with high mammographic density and limiting the generalizability of their results.

The study considered earlier in the ERα-related section also compared the expression of syndecan-1, a cell surface heparan proteoglycan, in pair-wise samples of dense and non-dense normal breast tissue from 28 postmenopausal women undergoing surgery for breast cancer (Lundstrom et al., 2006). They performed an immunohistochemical staining to assess syndecan-1 intensity semi-quantitatively in stroma, stromal cells, ductal and lobular epithelium. They found that syndecan-1 expression was significantly higher in dense than non-dense normal breast tissue ($p = 0.004$, $p = 0.02$, $p = 0.008$ and $p = 0.02$ for stroma, stromal cells, ductal and lobular epithelium respectively). Moreover, syndecan-1 expression was higher in stroma than in epithelial tissue ($p < 0.01$). They concluded that the redistribution of syndecan-1 from epithelium to stroma maybe a key step in increased mammographic density.

The main proteoglycan synthesis inducer in breast tissue remains unknown. In addition, the role of proteoglycans in tumorigenesis has not been sufficiently explored. Previous studies have demonstrated an increased lumican expression in stroma from invasive breast carcinoma compared to stroma from adjacent normal breast tissue (Leygue et al., 1998b; Leygue et al., 2000). However, the exact mechanism by which lumican can induce cellular proliferation is not known. Contrary to lumican, decorin is believed to suppress cellular growth through epidermal growth factor receptor activation and p21 cell-cycle inhibitor induction (Moscatello et al., 1998; Santra et al., 1997). This is in line with Leygue's findings, who reported a decreased decorin expression in stroma from neoplastic breast tissue compared to stroma from normal adjacent breast tissue (Leygue et al., 2000). Kelemen and colleagues investigated the association between 14 common SNPs in the lumican (LUM) and decorin (DCN) genes among 1641 Caucasian women (798 breast cancer cases and 843 controls). Then, SNPs showing the strongest associations (one SNP per gene) were assessed among 4,470 breast cancer cases and 4,560 controls from England. The authors identified three SNPs in LUM (rs2268578, rs10859110 and rs17018765) and three SNPs in DCN (rs7441, rs516115 and rs3138165) which were each associated with increased breast cancer risk among their first study population. However, only LUM rs2268578 SNP was associated with increased breast cancer risk among pooled studies, but did not reach statistical significance among English women only (Kelemen et al., 2008). Since this SNP is located in an intron, more research will be needed to identify a functional SNP in LUM gene with an effect on mammographic density and breast cancer risk.

Proteoglycans are present either free in the extracellular compartment or attached to the cell surface as syndecans and glypicans (Liu et al., 2002a). The heparin sulphate proteoglycans (HSPG) play a crucial role in normal developmental processes, such as embryogenesis, as well as pathological conditions such as tumorigenesis (Liu et al., 2002a; Perrimon & Bernfield, 2000). In particular, syndecan-1 plays a critical role in the regulation of cellular adhesion, migration and proliferation. Syndecan-1 is expressed in stroma of breast cancer tissue as well as in normal epithelium but less in normal breast tissue stroma (Maeda et al., 2004). This suggests that syndecan-1 is redistributed in cancerous tissue (Lofgren et al., 2007). Syndecan-1 expression in stromal cells seems to promote growth of breast carcinoma cells in direct coculture by inducing cell proliferation rather than reducing its apoptosis. It is thought that the expression of syndecan-1 in stroma of tumors is a sort of oncofetal reaction of a regulatory pathway. Syndecan-1 exerts its biological action on the cell, through binding to various extracellular proteins, growth factors and cytokines via the heparan sulphate chain (Lofgren et al., 2007; Maeda et al., 2004). Syndecan-1 forms a complex with fibroblast growth factor (FGF-2), FGF-2/HSPG/FGF receptor-1, determining breast cancer cells response to FGFs *in vitro* (Mundhenke et al., 2002). Knowing that syndecan-1 is more abundantly expressed in stroma of malignant breast tissue and that it can promote cellular proliferation, one may hypothesize that syndecan-1 can affect mammographic density by promoting cellular proliferation and subsequently increasing the risk of breast cancer.

Recently, Menashe and colleagues conducted a pathway analysis of breast cancer genome-wide association study (Menashe et al., 2010). In their study, they included 69,525 SNPs representing 421 pathways and 3,962 genes, and performed the analysis on 1,145 postmenopausal women of European ancestry with invasive breast cancer and 1,142 controls. They observed that genetic alterations associated with three pathways, including the top ranked "syndecan-1 signaling", may contribute to breast cancer susceptibility. The pathway related to "syndecan-1 signaling" namely "FGF signaling" was ranked 10th in this study. The "syndecan-1 signaling" pathway contains 13 genes involved in different cellular processes mediated by syndecan-1. In this study, syndecan-1 rs7563245 SNP was moderately associated with increased breast cancer risk (p for trend = 0.019).

6.7 Cyclooxygenase-2

One study investigated the cyclooxygenase-2 (COX-2) enzyme expression in breast tissue from 66 women aged 29-88 years old with dense or non-dense breasts according to BI-RADS categories (Yang et al., 2010). In addition to hormone receptors previously described, they analysed COX-2 expression immunohistochemically in stroma and epithelium of normal breast tissue obtained from mastectomy specimens, and quantified immunostainings using the Allred scoring system. In their study, Yang and colleagues observed higher COX-2 expression in stroma ($p < 0.001$) and epithelium ($p < 0.02$) from dense breasts compared to non-dense breasts. However, after inclusion of all immunohistochemical factors in the model, only COX-2 expression in the stroma was statistically significant ($p < 0.01$).

The COX enzymes influence cellular proliferation by catalyzing the formation of prostaglandins (Soslow et al., 2000). Growing evidence supports the role of COX-2 in promoting tumorigenesis by catalyzing the synthesis of several prostaglandins, mainly prostaglandin E2, which in turn stimulates angiogenesis and inhibits the immune surveillance (Ben-Av et al., 1995; Soslow et al., 2000). By inducing prostaglandin E2 synthesis, COX-2 can also promote increased aromatase activity and mRNA production in the mammary gland and thereby augment estrogen production (Subbaramaiah et al., 2008; Zhao et al., 1996). Nevertheless, COX-2 has been shown to inhibit TGF-β which is known to reduce mammary epithelial cell proliferation (Studer & Chu, 2005; Yang et al., 2010). In support of this, COX-2 has been found to be up-regulated in 41% and 80% of invasive breast tumors and ductal carcinoma *in situ* respectively, which is significantly different from the negligible expression in nonneoplastic epithelium ($p < 0.0001$) (Soslow et al., 2000). In an effort to better assess the association between COX-2 and breast cancer risk, Yu and colleagues conducted a meta-analysis on the relationship between common SNPs in the COX-2 gene and breast cancer risk (Yu et al., 2010). In their meta-analysis, they found no clear association of rs5275, rs5277 or rs20417 SNPs with breast cancer risk in any model (codominant, dominant or recessive model). However, a novel SNP located in exon 2 (169 C > G) of the COX-2 gene has been recently associated to breast cancer risk (OR (GG vs. CC) = 1.76, 95% CI 1.20-3.05) (Li et al., 2009). Because of its location in an exon, the role of this SNP on the COX-2 expression should be investigated.

7. Genes expression in breast tissue associated to mammographic density

The hypothesis that specific genetic pathways could influence mammographic density was tested by two research groups (Haakensen et al., 2010; Yang et al., 2010). The first study, described above (Yang et al., 2010), used RNA isolated from frozen biopsy specimens from normal breast tissue containing at least 60% epithelial content and obtained at a distance of more than 5 cm from the primary tumor. The authors compared about 34,000 different genes expression in tissues from women with high (n = 28) and low (n = 38) mammographic densities. They identified 73 genes differentially expressed by ≥ 1.5 folds with a $p < 0.001$ (false discovery rate (FDR) < 0.10). Of those, 26 genes were up-regulated in dense breast tissue versus non-dense tissue, and 47 genes were down-regulated in dense tissue when compared to non-dense tissue. Consistent with the link between stroma and mammographic density, the biological functions analysis revealed that the differentially expressed genes were involved in tissue morphology, connective tissue development, function and disorders, developmental, skeletal and muscular disorders and tumor morphology. It was also found from both network and canonical pathways analysis that decreased TGF-β signaling was related to mammographic density, including the identification of the TGF-β receptor II (TGFBR2) as being lowly expressed in breast tissue of women with high compared to low mammographic density.

In addition to increased COX-2 enzyme expression (an inhibitor of TGF-β), Yang and colleagues observed a decreased signaling of TGF-β in dense versus non-dense breast tissue (Yang et al., 2010). Growing evidence suggests a dual action of TGF-β, shifting from tumor suppressor in early tumor initiation steps to tumor growth promoter in advanced malignant stages. The dual action of TGF-β is mediated through two opposing receptors, the antiangiogenic receptor ALK5 (TGFBR1) and the proangiogenic receptor ALK1. The balance between the two pathways determines the net result. TGF-β exerts its protective effect against breast cancer by inducing cell cycle arrest and promoting apoptosis of normal mammary epithelial cells (Casey et al., 2007). Data from 6,703 cases and 6,840 controls have been assessed in a recent meta-analysis performed by Scollen and colleagues in attempt to better understand the association between TGF-β and breast cancer risk (Scollen et al., 2011). The authors identified the most common variants in 17 genes comprising both arms of TGF-β signaling pathways. The minor G allele of SNP rs10512263 of the TGFBR1 gene and the G allele of SNP rs4522809 of the TGFBR2 gene had a protective effect (OR (G vs. A) = 0.87, 95% CI 0.81-0.95, $p = 0.001$ and OR (G vs. A) = 0.95, 95% CI 0.91-0.99, $p = 0.02$, respectively). The TGFBR1 rs10512263 SNP, located in intron 1, is either a causal variant of unknown function or marking the causal SNP, while rs4522809 SNP located in intron 2 of the TGFBR2 gene is most likely marking a putative causal variant. Conversely, for rs1982073 SNP located in TGFB1 gene, there was a dose-dependent association between the proline-encoding allele and increased breast cancer risk (OR (Pro vs. Leu) = 1.05, 95% CI 1.02-1.09, $p = 0.002$). The Pro allele induces TGFB1 secretion *in vitro* compared to the Leu allele. The authors observed no detectable effect of SNPs on genes that regulate the proangiogenic pathway.

The second study that examined genes differentially expressed in breast tissue according to mammographic density included 79 healthy women (Haakensen et al., 2010). They assessed percent mammographic density using a computer-assisted method from digitized craniocaudal mammograms of both breasts. In this study, they used RNA isolated from biopsies that were taken from areas with no visible pathology, but with some mammographic density in order to obtain sufficient RNA amount. They tested 9,767 different probes expression for their associations with percent mammographic density, and identified 25 probes representing 24 genes of decreased expression associated with increased mammographic density (FDR < 0.25). No particular biological function or pathway was found to be associated to this set of genes. Among identified genes, Haakensen and colleagues found that three uridine 5′-diphospho-glucuronosyltransferase genes (UGT2B7, UGT2B10 and UGT2B11) and the ERα gene were down-regulated in tissues with high mammographic density compared to those with low mammographic density. When the expressions of these genes were in models taking into account age and body mass index, only UGT2B10 expression among women younger than 50 years old and ERα expression among women 50 years or older remained statistically significant. Inclusion of healthy women was the major strength of this study.

The UGT genes encode enzymes responsible for the inactivation of several compounds, including sex hormones. They catalyse the glucuronidation of sex hormones to less active compounds (Guillemette et al., 2004). Like UGT2B7, UGT2B10 is capable of estrone conjugation. A study has demonstrated that the mRNA and activity of both UGT were down-regulated in cancerous breast tissue when compared to normal breast tissue (Starlard-Davenport et al., 2008). The mRNA expression of UGT2B7 and UGT2B10 were decreased by almost four folds and more than eight folds respectively in cancerous breast tissue biopsies compared to normal breast tissue (p = 0.01 and p = 0.04, respectively). Moreover, estrogen glucuronidation, which is considered as an index of UGT activity, was reduced by two folds in cancerous breast tissue compared to normal tissue. These results suggest that UGT2B7 and UGT2B10 have a protective role for breast tissue against estrogen metabolites and that decreased UGT2B7 and UGT2B10 expressions can promote breast carcinogenesis. This finding is consistent with that of Haakenssen and colleagues who observed decreased UGT2B7 and UGT2B10 expressions in mammographically dense breast tissue. The association between UGT variants or levels and breast cancer risk is not yet reported.

Contrary to what one would expect, Haakensen and colleagues found that the expression of ERα gene was significantly down-regulated in breasts with higher mammographic density among women 50 years or older. According to the authors, this decrease in ERα expression in dense breast tissue could be explained, at least in part, by the increased estrogen levels in postmenopausal breast tissue (Borras et al., 1994; Saceda et al., 1988). However, as stated previously, measurement of both ERα and ERβ expressions according to menopausal status may be required to evaluate the link between these receptors and mammographic density.

There was no overlap in lists of genes up-regulated or down-regulated according to mammographic density between both studies. The divergence between Yang and Haakensen results could be attributed to different means used to evaluate mammographic density (BI-RADS vs. computer-assisted method) and genes expression (Affymetrix U133Plus 2 Gene chip vs. Agilent Human Whole genome Oligo Microarrays G4110A platform), as well as the selection of normal breast tissue (≥ 60% epithelial content from breast cancer patient vs. mammographically dense tissue from healthy women). The main pitfall of both studies was the use of breast tissue specimens containing various proportions of types of cells (epithelial, stromal, adipocyte, etc.) We believe that it is important to distinguish tissue types, like epithelium from stroma, because it has been clearly determined that these two tissues exhibit distinct expression profiles (Finak et al., 2006). This is also in line with results from our previous sections.

8. Conclusion

In summary, some candidate proteins and genes in normal breast tissue such as IGF-1, TIMP3, TGF-β, UGT, stromal COX-2 and stromal and epithelial aromatase among pre- and postmenopausal women and epithelial ERα, stromal lumican and decorin, and epithelial and stromal syndecan-1 among postmenopausal women have been found to be associated with mammographic density. Among these, IGF-1, ERα, aromatase, TIMP3, lumican, syndecan-1, COX-2, TGF-β and UGT have also been related to breast cancer risk in the same direction of their association with mammographic density. However, the small number of studies that examined each protein/gene limited the conclusions that could be drawn.

Nonetheless, these data provide some support to the hypothesis that mammographic density could be used as an intermediate biomarker of breast cancer. Mammographic density promises a relatively quick exploration of the effect of several mitogens on breast tissue eliminating the long period of time elapsing between exposure to mitogen and the detection of their effect on breast tissue. Future investigations incorporating both pre- and postmenopausal women and examining the association of various molecular markers (proteins and genes expression) on epithelial and stromal breast tissue separately with mammographic density are therefore required to confirm the above findings and to identify new promising ones. The identification of molecular markers influencing mammographic density may provide important clues regarding the molecular causes of breast cancer.

9. Acknowledgments

This work was supported by the Canadian Breast Cancer Research Alliance (grant #20462). CD is a Junior Investigator of the Canadian Research Society (2011-700657).

10. References

Alowami, S.; Troup, S.; Al-Haddad, S.; Kirkpatrick, I. & Watson, P. H. (2003). Mammographic density is related to stroma and stromal proteoglycan expression. *Breast Cancer Res,* Vol.5, No.5, pp.R129-135, ISSN 1465-542

Baker, A. H.; George, S. J.; Zaltsman, A. B.; Murphy, G. & Newby, A. C. (1999). Inhibition of invasion and induction of apoptotic cell death of cancer cell lines by overexpression of TIMP-3. *Br J Cancer,* Vol.79, No.9-10, pp.1347-1355, ISSN 0007-0920

Balduyck, M.; Zerimech, F.; Gouyer, V.; Lemaire, R.; Hemon, B.; Grard, G.; Thiebaut, C.; Lemaire, V.; Dacquembronne, E.; Duhem, T.; Lebrun, A.; Dejonghe, M. J. & Huet, G. (2000). Specific expression of matrix metalloproteinases 1, 3, 9 and 13 associated with invasiveness of breast cancer cells in vitro. *Clin Exp Metastasis,* Vol.18, No.2, pp.171-178, ISSN 0262-0898

Bardin, A.; Boulle, N.; Lazennec, G.; Vignon, F. & Pujol, P. (2004). Loss of ERbeta expression as a common step in estrogen-dependent tumor progression. *Endocr Relat Cancer,* Vol.11, No.3, pp.537-551, ISSN 1351-0088

Bartsch, J. E.; Staren, E. D. & Appert, H. E. (2003). Matrix metalloproteinase expression in breast cancer. *J Surg Res,* Vol.110, No.2, pp.383-392, ISSN 0022-4804

Ben-Av, P.; Crofford, L. J.; Wilder, R. L. & Hla, T. (1995). Induction of vascular endothelial growth factor expression in synovial fibroblasts by prostaglandin E and interleukin-1: a potential mechanism for inflammatory angiogenesis. *FEBS Lett,* Vol.372, No.1, pp.83-87, ISSN 0014-5793

Borras, M.; Hardy, L.; Lempereur, F.; el Khissiin, A. H.; Legros, N.; Gol-Winkler, R. & Leclercq, G. (1994). Estradiol-induced down-regulation of estrogen receptor. Effect of various modulators of protein synthesis and expression. *J Steroid Biochem Mol Biol,* Vol.48, No.4, pp.325-336, ISSN 0960-0760

Boyd, N.; Martin, L.; Stone, J.; Little, L.; Minkin, S. & Yaffe, M. (2002a). A longitudinal study of the effects of menopause on mammographic features. *Cancer Epidemiol Biomarkers Prev,* Vol.11, No.10 Pt 1, pp.1048-1053, ISSN 1055-9965

Boyd, N. F.; Byng, J. W.; Jong, R. A.; Fishell, E. K.; Little, L. E.; Miller, A. B.; Lockwood, G. A.; Tritchler, D. L. & Yaffe, M. J. (1995). Quantitative classification of mammographic densities and breast cancer risk: results from the Canadian National Breast Screening Study. *J Natl Cancer Inst,* Vol.87, No.9, pp.670-675, ISSN 0027-8874

Boyd, N. F.; Jensen, H. M.; Cooke, G.; Han, H. L.; Lockwood, G. A. & Miller, A. B. (2000). Mammographic densities and the prevalence and incidence of histological types of benign breast disease. Reference Pathologists of the Canadian National Breast Screening Study. *Eur J Cancer Prev,* Vol.9, No.1, pp.15-24, ISSN 0959-8278

Boyd, N. F.; Dite, G. S.; Stone, J.; Gunasekara, A.; English, D. R.; McCredie, M. R.; Giles, G. G.; Tritchler, D.; Chiarelli, A.; Yaffe, M. J. & Hopper, J. L. (2002b). Heritability of mammographic density, a risk factor for breast cancer. *N Engl J Med,* Vol.347, No.12, pp.886-894, ISSN 1533-4406

Boyd, N. F.; Stone, J.; Martin, L. J.; Jong, R.; Fishell, E.; Yaffe, M.; Hammond, G. & Minkin, S. (2002c). The association of breast mitogens with mammographic densities. *Br J Cancer,* Vol.87, No.8, pp.876-882, ISSN 0007-0920

Boyd, N. F.; Martin, L. J.; Bronskill, M.; Yaffe, M. J.; Duric, N. & Minkin, S. (2010). Breast tissue composition and susceptibility to breast cancer. *J Natl Cancer Inst,* Vol.102, No.16, pp.1224-1237, ISSN 1460-2105

Brisson, J.; Morrison, A. S.; Kopans, D. B.; Sadowsky, N. L.; Kalisher, L.; Twaddle, J. A.; Meyer, J. E.; Henschke, C. I. & Cole, P. (1984). Height and weight, mammographic features of breast tissue, and breast cancer risk. *Am J Epidemiol,* Vol.119, No.3, pp.371-381, ISSN 0002-9262

Bryant, H. & Mai, V. (2011). Impact of age-specific recommendation changes on organized breast screening programs. *Prev Med,* ISSN 1096-0260

Byrne, J. A.; Tomasetto, C.; Rouyer, N.; Bellocq, J. P.; Rio, M. C. & Basset, P. (1995). The tissue inhibitor of metalloproteinases-3 gene in breast carcinoma: identification of multiple polyadenylation sites and a stromal pattern of expression. *Mol Med,* Vol.1, No.4, pp.418-427, ISSN 1076-1551

Casey, T. M.; Mulvey, T. M.; Patnode, T. A.; Dean, A.; Zakrzewska, E. & Plaut, K. (2007). Mammary epithelial cells treated concurrently with TGF-alpha and TGF-beta exhibit enhanced proliferation and death. *Exp Biol Med (Maywood),* Vol.232, No.8, pp.1027-1040, ISSN 1535-3702

Chang, E. C.; Frasor, J.; Komm, B. & Katzenellenbogen, B. S. (2006). Impact of estrogen receptor beta on gene networks regulated by estrogen receptor alpha in breast cancer cells. *Endocrinology,* Vol.147, No.10, pp.4831-4842, ISSN 0013-7227

Cho, E. Y.; Choi, Y. L.; Han, J. J.; Kim, K. M. & Oh, Y. L. (2008). Expression and amplification of Her2, EGFR and cyclin D1 in breast cancer: immunohistochemistry and chromogenic in situ hybridization. *Pathol Int,* Vol.58, No.1, pp.17-25, ISSN 1320-5463

Coussens, L. M.; Fingleton, B. & Matrisian, L. M. (2002). Matrix metalloproteinase inhibitors and cancer: trials and tribulations. *Science,* Vol.295, No.5564, pp.2387-2392, ISSN 1095-9203

Cuzick, J.; Warwick, J.; Pinney, E.; Duffy, S. W.; Cawthorn, S.; Howell, A.; Forbes, J. F. & Warren, R. M. (2011). Tamoxifen-induced reduction in mammographic density and breast cancer risk reduction: a nested case-control study. *J Natl Cancer Inst,* Vol.103, No.9, pp.744-752, ISSN 1460-2105

Diorio, C.; Pollak, M.; Byrne, C.; Masse, B.; Hebert-Croteau, N.; Yaffe, M.; Cote, G.; Berube, S. & Brisson, J. (2005a). Levels of C-peptide and mammographic breast density. *Cancer Epidemiol Biomarkers Prev,* Vol.14, No.11 Pt 1, pp.2661-2664, ISSN 1055-9965

Diorio, C.; Pollak, M.; Byrne, C.; Masse, B.; Hebert-Croteau, N.; Yaffe, M.; Cote, G.; Berube, S.; Morin, C. & Brisson, J. (2005b). Insulin-like growth factor-I, IGF-binding protein-3, and mammographic breast density. *Cancer Epidemiol Biomarkers Prev,* Vol.14, No.5, pp.1065-1073, ISSN 1055-9965

Diorio, C.; Brisson, J.; Berube, S. & Pollak, M. (2008). Genetic polymorphisms involved in insulin-like growth factor (IGF) pathway in relation to mammographic breast density and IGF levels. *Cancer Epidemiol Biomarkers Prev,* Vol.17, No.4, pp.880-888, ISSN 1055-9965

El-Bastawissi, A. Y.; White, E.; Mandelson, M. T. & Taplin, S. H. (2000). Reproductive and hormonal factors associated with mammographic breast density by age (United States). *Cancer Causes Control,* Vol.11, No.10, pp.955-963, ISSN 0957-5243

Finak, G.; Sadekova, S.; Pepin, F.; Hallett, M.; Meterissian, S.; Halwani, F.; Khetani, K.; Souleimanova, M.; Zabolotny, B.; Omeroglu, A. & Park, M. (2006). Gene expression signatures of morphologically normal breast tissue identify basal-like tumors. *Breast Cancer Res,* Vol.8, No.5, pp.R58, ISSN 1465-542

Fleishman, S. J.; Schlessinger, J. & Ben-Tal, N. (2002). A putative molecular-activation switch in the transmembrane domain of erbB2. *Proc Natl Acad Sci U S A,* Vol.99, No.25, pp.15937-15940, ISSN 0027-8424

Garbett, E. A.; Reed, M. W.; Stephenson, T. J. & Brown, N. J. (2000). Proteolysis in human breast cancer. *Mol Pathol,* Vol.53, No.2, pp.99-106, ISSN 1366-8714

Graham, J. D. & Clarke, C. L. (1997). Physiological action of progesterone in target tissues. *Endocr Rev,* Vol.18, No.4, pp.502-519, ISSN 0163-769

Greendale, G. A.; Palla, S. L.; Ursin, G.; Laughlin, G. A.; Crandall, C.; Pike, M. C. & Reboussin, B. A. (2005). The association of endogenous sex steroids and sex steroid binding proteins with mammographic density: results from the Postmenopausal Estrogen/Progestin Interventions Mammographic Density Study. *Am J Epidemiol,* Vol.162, No.9, pp.826-834, ISSN 0002-9262

Guillemette, C.; Belanger, A. & Lepine, J. (2004). Metabolic inactivation of estrogens in breast tissue by UDP-glucuronosyltransferase enzymes: an overview. *Breast Cancer Res,* Vol.6, No.6, pp.246-254, ISSN 1465-542

Guo, Y. P.; Martin, L. J.; Hanna, W.; Banerjee, D.; Miller, N.; Fishell, E.; Khokha, R. & Boyd, N. F. (2001). Growth factors and stromal matrix proteins associated with mammographic densities. *Cancer Epidemiol Biomarkers Prev,* Vol.10, No.3, pp.243-248, ISSN 1055-9965

Haakensen, V. D.; Biong, M.; Lingjaerde, O. C.; Holmen, M. M.; Frantzen, J. O.; Chen, Y.; Navjord, D.; Romundstad, L.; Luders, T.; Bukholm, I. K.; Solvang, H. K.; Kristensen, V. N.; Ursin, G.; Borresen-Dale, A. L. & Helland, A. (2010). Expression levels of uridine 5'-diphospho-glucuronosyltransferase genes in breast tissue from healthy women are associated with mammographic density. *Breast Cancer Res,* Vol.12, No.4, pp.R65, ISSN 1465-542

Haiman, C. A.; Stram, D. O.; Pike, M. C.; Kolonel, L. N.; Burtt, N. P.; Altshuler, D.; Hirschhorn, J. & Henderson, B. E. (2003). A comprehensive haplotype analysis of CYP19 and breast cancer risk: the Multiethnic Cohort. *Hum Mol Genet,* Vol.12, No.20, pp.2679-2692, ISSN 0964-6906

Hankinson, S. E.; Willett, W. C.; Colditz, G. A.; Hunter, D. J.; Michaud, D. S.; Deroo, B.; Rosner, B.; Speizer, F. E. & Pollak, M. (1998). Circulating concentrations of insulin-like growth factor-I and risk of breast cancer. *Lancet,* Vol.351, No.9113, pp.1393-1396, ISSN 0140-6736

Hankinson, S. E. & Eliassen, A. H. (2007). Endogenous estrogen, testosterone and progesterone levels in relation to breast cancer risk. *J Steroid Biochem Mol Biol,* Vol.106, No.1-5, pp.24-30, ISSN 0960-0760

Harvey, J. A.; Santen, R. J.; Petroni, G. R.; Bovbjerg, V. E.; Smolkin, M. E.; Sheriff, F. S. & Russo, J. (2008). Histologic changes in the breast with menopausal hormone therapy use: correlation with breast density, estrogen receptor, progesterone receptor, and proliferation indices. *Menopause,* Vol.15, No.1, pp.67-73, ISSN 1072-3714

Heine, J. J. & Malhotra, P. (2002). Mammographic tissue, breast cancer risk, serial image analysis, and digital mammography. Part 1. Tissue and related risk factors. *Acad Radiol,* Vol.9, No.3, pp.298-316, ISSN 1076-6332

Henson, D. E. & Tarone, R. E. (1994). Involution and the etiology of breast cancer. *Cancer,* Vol.74, No.1 Suppl, pp.424-429, ISSN 0008-543

Howard, B. A. & Gusterson, B. A. (2000). Human breast development. *J Mammary Gland Biol Neoplasia,* Vol.5, No.2, pp.119-137, ISSN 1083-3021

Hunter, D. J. & Willett, W. C. (1993). Diet, body size, and breast cancer. *Epidemiol Rev,* Vol.15, No.1, pp.110-132, ISSN 0193-936

Imagawa, W.; Pedchenko, V. K.; Helber, J. & Zhang, H. (2002). Hormone/growth factor interactions mediating epithelial/stromal communication in mammary gland development and carcinogenesis. *J Steroid Biochem Mol Biol,* Vol.80, No.2, pp.213-230, ISSN 0960-0760

Irahara, N.; Miyoshi, Y.; Taguchi, T.; Tamaki, Y. & Noguchi, S. (2006). Quantitative analysis of aromatase mRNA expression derived from various promoters (I.4, I.3, PII and I.7) and its association with expression of TNF-alpha, IL-6 and COX-2 mRNAs in human breast cancer. *Int J Cancer,* Vol.118, No.8, pp.1915-1921, ISSN 0020-7136

Jemal, A.; Thomas, A.; Murray, T. & Thun, M. (2002). Cancer statistics, 2002. *CA Cancer J Clin,* Vol.52, No.1, pp.23-47, ISSN 0007-9235

Jiang, Y.; Goldberg, I. D. & Shi, Y. E. (2002). Complex roles of tissue inhibitors of metalloproteinases in cancer. *Oncogene,* Vol.21, No.14, pp.2245-2252, ISSN 0950-9232

Kelemen, L. E.; Couch, F. J.; Ahmed, S.; Dunning, A. M.; Pharoah, P. D.; Easton, D. F.; Fredericksen, Z. S.; Vierkant, R. A.; Pankratz, V. S.; Goode, E. L.; Scott, C. G.; Rider,

D. N.; Wang, X.; Cerhan, J. R. & Vachon, C. M. (2008). Genetic variation in stromal proteins decorin and lumican with breast cancer: investigations in two case-control studies. *Breast Cancer Res,* Vol.10, No.6, pp.R98, ISSN 1465-542

Krajcik, R. A.; Borofsky, N. D.; Massardo, S. & Orentreich, N. (2002). Insulin-like growth factor I (IGF-I), IGF-binding proteins, and breast cancer. *Cancer Epidemiol Biomarkers Prev,* Vol.11, No.12, pp.1566-1573, ISSN 1055-9965

Lebovic, G. S.; Hollingsworth, A. & Feig, S. A. (2010). Risk assessment, screening and prevention of breast cancer: A look at cost-effectiveness. *Breast,* Vol.19, No.4, pp.260-267, ISSN 1532-3080

Lei, H.; Hemminki, K.; Altieri, A.; Johansson, R.; Enquist, K.; Hallmans, G.; Lenner, P. & Forsti, A. (2007). Promoter polymorphisms in matrix metalloproteinases and their inhibitors: few associations with breast cancer susceptibility and progression. *Breast Cancer Res Treat,* Vol.103, No.1, pp.61-69, ISSN 0167-6806

Leygue, E.; Dotzlaw, H.; Watson, P. H. & Murphy, L. C. (1998a). Altered estrogen receptor alpha and beta messenger RNA expression during human breast tumorigenesis. *Cancer Res,* Vol.58, No.15, pp.3197-3201, ISSN 0008-5472

Leygue, E.; Snell, L.; Dotzlaw, H.; Hole, K.; Hiller-Hitchcock, T.; Roughley, P. J.; Watson, P. H. & Murphy, L. C. (1998b). Expression of lumican in human breast carcinoma. *Cancer Res,* Vol.58, No.7, pp.1348-1352, ISSN 0008-5472

Leygue, E.; Snell, L.; Dotzlaw, H.; Troup, S.; Hiller-Hitchcock, T.; Murphy, L. C.; Roughley, P. J. & Watson, P. H. (2000). Lumican and decorin are differentially expressed in human breast carcinoma. *J Pathol,* Vol.192, No.3, pp.313-320, ISSN 0022-3417

Li, F.; Ren, G. S.; Li, H. Y.; Wang, X. Y.; Chen, L. & Li, J. (2009). A novel single nucleotide polymorphism of the cyclooxygenase-2 gene associated with breast cancer. *Clin Oncol (R Coll Radiol),* Vol.21, No.4, pp.302-305, ISSN 0936-6555

Li, T.; Sun, L.; Miller, N.; Nicklee, T.; Woo, J.; Hulse-Smith, L.; Tsao, M. S.; Khokha, R.; Martin, L. & Boyd, N. (2005). The association of measured breast tissue characteristics with mammographic density and other risk factors for breast cancer. *Cancer Epidemiol Biomarkers Prev,* Vol.14, No.2, pp.343-349, ISSN 1055-9965

Lin, S. J.; Cawson, J.; Hill, P.; Haviv, I.; Jenkins, M.; Hopper, J. L.; Southey, M. C.; Campbell, I. G. & Thompson, E. W. (2011). Image-guided sampling reveals increased stroma and lower glandular complexity in mammographically dense breast tissue. *Breast Cancer Res Treat,* Vol.128, No.2, pp.505-516, ISSN 1573-7217

Liu, D.; Shriver, Z.; Qi, Y.; Venkataraman, G. & Sasisekharan, R. (2002a). Dynamic regulation of tumor growth and metastasis by heparan sulfate glycosaminoglycans. *Semin Thromb Hemost,* Vol.28, No.1, pp.67-78, ISSN 0094-6176

Liu, M. M.; Albanese, C.; Anderson, C. M.; Hilty, K.; Webb, P.; Uht, R. M.; Price, R. H., Jr.; Pestell, R. G. & Kushner, P. J. (2002b). Opposing action of estrogen receptors alpha and beta on cyclin D1 gene expression. *J Biol Chem,* Vol.277, No.27, pp.24353-24360, ISSN 0021-9258

Lofgren, L.; Sahlin, L.; Jiang, S.; Von Schoultz, B.; Fernstad, R.; Skoog, L. & Von Schoultz, E. (2007). Expression of syndecan-1 in paired samples of normal and malignant breast tissue from postmenopausal women. *Anticancer Res,* Vol.27, No.5A, pp.3045-3050, ISSN 0250-7005

Lundstrom, E.; Sahlin, L.; Skoog, L.; Hagerstrom, T.; Svane, G.; Azavedo, E.; Sandelin, K. & von Schoultz, B. (2006). Expression of Syndecan-1 in histologically normal breast tissue from postmenopausal women with breast cancer according to mammographic density. *Climacteric,* Vol.9, No.4, pp.277-282, ISSN 1369-7137

Macaulay, V. M.; Nicholls, J. E.; Gledhill, J.; Rowlands, M. G.; Dowsett, M. & Ashworth, A. (1994). Biological effects of stable overexpression of aromatase in human hormone-dependent breast cancer cells. *Br J Cancer,* Vol.69, No.1, pp.77-83, ISSN 0007-0920

Maeda, T.; Alexander, C. M. & Friedl, A. (2004). Induction of syndecan-1 expression in stromal fibroblasts promotes proliferation of human breast cancer cells. *Cancer Res,* Vol.64, No.2, pp.612-621, ISSN 0008-5472

Marshman, E. & Streuli, C. H. (2002). Insulin-like growth factors and insulin-like growth factor binding proteins in mammary gland function. *Breast Cancer Res,* Vol.4, No.6, pp.231-239, ISSN 1465-5411

Martin, L. J. & Boyd, N. F. (2008). Mammographic density. Potential mechanisms of breast cancer risk associated with mammographic density: hypotheses based on epidemiological evidence. *Breast Cancer Res,* Vol.10, No.1, pp.201, ISSN 1465-542

Martin, M. B. & Stoica, A. (2002). Insulin-like growth factor-I and estrogen interactions in breast cancer. *J Nutr,* Vol.132, No.12, pp.3799S-3801S, ISSN 0022-3166

McCormack, V. A. & dos Santos Silva, I. (2006). Breast density and parenchymal patterns as markers of breast cancer risk: a meta-analysis. *Cancer Epidemiol Biomarkers Prev,* Vol.15, No.6, pp.1159-1169, ISSN 1055-9965

Menashe, I.; Maeder, D.; Garcia-Closas, M.; Figueroa, J. D.; Bhattacharjee, S.; Rotunno, M.; Kraft, P.; Hunter, D. J.; Chanock, S. J.; Rosenberg, P. S. & Chatterjee, N. (2010). Pathway analysis of breast cancer genome-wide association study highlights three pathways and one canonical signaling cascade. *Cancer Res,* Vol.70, No.11, pp.4453-4459, ISSN 1538-7445

Moscatello, D. K.; Santra, M.; Mann, D. M.; McQuillan, D. J.; Wong, A. J. & Iozzo, R. V. (1998). Decorin suppresses tumor cell growth by activating the epidermal growth factor receptor. *J Clin Invest,* Vol.101, No.2, pp.406-412, ISSN 0021-9738

Mundhenke, C.; Meyer, K.; Drew, S. & Friedl, A. (2002). Heparan sulfate proteoglycans as regulators of fibroblast growth factor-2 receptor binding in breast carcinomas. *Am J Pathol,* Vol.160, No.1, pp.185-194, ISSN 0002-9440

Nilsson, S.; Makela, S.; Treuter, E.; Tujague, M.; Thomsen, J.; Andersson, G.; Enmark, E.; Pettersson, K.; Warner, M. & Gustafsson, J. A. (2001). Mechanisms of estrogen action. *Physiol Rev,* Vol.81, No.4, pp.1535-1565, ISSN 0031-9333

Olson, J. E.; Ma, C. X.; Pelleymounter, L. L.; Schaid, D. J.; Pankratz, V. S.; Vierkant, R. A.; Fredericksen, Z. S.; Ingle, J. N.; Wu, Y.; Couch, F.; Sellers, T. A.; Weinshilboum, R. M. & Vachon, C. M. (2007). A comprehensive examination of CYP19 variation and breast density. *Cancer Epidemiol Biomarkers Prev,* Vol.16, No.3, pp.623-625, ISSN 1055-9965

Page, D. L. & Winfield, A. C. (1986). The dense mammogram. *AJR Am J Roentgenol,* Vol.147, No.3, pp.487-489, ISSN 0361-803

Perrimon, N. & Bernfield, M. (2000). Specificities of heparan sulphate proteoglycans in developmental processes. *Nature,* Vol.404, No.6779, pp.725-728, ISSN 0028-0836

Peterson, N. B.; Beeghly-Fadiel, A.; Gao, Y. T.; Long, J.; Cai, Q.; Shu, X. O. & Zheng, W. (2009). Polymorphisms in tissue inhibitors of metalloproteinases-2 and -3 and breast cancer susceptibility and survival. *Int J Cancer,* Vol.125, No.4, pp.844-850, ISSN 1097-0215

Pike, M. C.; Pearce, C. L. & Wu, A. H. (2004). Prevention of cancers of the breast, endometrium and ovary. *Oncogene,* Vol.23, No.38, pp.6379-6391, ISSN 0950-9232

Pollak, M.; Costantino, J.; Polychronakos, C.; Blauer, S. A.; Guyda, H.; Redmond, C.; Fisher, B. & Margolese, R. (1990). Effect of tamoxifen on serum insulinlike growth factor I levels in stage I breast cancer patients. *J Natl Cancer Inst,* Vol.82, No.21, pp.1693-1697, ISSN 0027-8874

Preston-Martin, S.; Pike, M. C.; Ross, R. K.; Jones, P. A. & Henderson, B. E. (1990). Increased cell division as a cause of human cancer. *Cancer Res,* Vol.50, No.23, pp.7415-7421, ISSN 0008-5472

Roger, P.; Sahla, M. E.; Makela, S.; Gustafsson, J. A.; Baldet, P. & Rochefort, H. (2001). Decreased expression of estrogen receptor beta protein in proliferative preinvasive mammary tumors. *Cancer Res,* Vol.61, No.6, pp.2537-2541, ISSN 0008-5472

Russo, J.; Gusterson, B. A.; Rogers, A. E.; Russo, I. H.; Wellings, S. R. & van Zwieten, M. J. (1990). Comparative study of human and rat mammary tumorigenesis. *Lab Invest,* Vol.62, No.3, pp.244-278, ISSN 0023-6837

Saceda, M.; Lippman, M. E.; Chambon, P.; Lindsey, R. L.; Ponglikitmongkol, M.; Puente, M. & Martin, M. B. (1988). Regulation of the estrogen receptor in MCF-7 cells by estradiol. *Mol Endocrinol,* Vol.2, No.12, pp.1157-1162, ISSN 0888-8809

Santen, R. J.; Martel, J.; Hoagland, M.; Naftolin, F.; Roa, L.; Harada, N.; Hafer, L.; Zaino, R. & Santner, S. J. (1994). Stromal spindle cells contain aromatase in human breast tumors. *J Clin Endocrinol Metab,* Vol.79, No.2, pp.627-632, ISSN 0021-972

Santra, M.; Mann, D. M.; Mercer, E. W.; Skorski, T.; Calabretta, B. & Iozzo, R. V. (1997). Ectopic expression of decorin protein core causes a generalized growth suppression in neoplastic cells of various histogenetic origin and requires endogenous p21, an inhibitor of cyclin-dependent kinases. *J Clin Invest,* Vol.100, No.1, pp.149-157, ISSN 0021-9738

Schernhammer, E. S.; Holly, J. M.; Pollak, M. N. & Hankinson, S. E. (2005). Circulating levels of insulin-like growth factors, their binding proteins, and breast cancer risk. *Cancer Epidemiol Biomarkers Prev,* Vol.14, No.3, pp.699-704, ISSN 1055-9965

Scollen, S.; Luccarini, C.; Baynes, C.; Driver, K.; Humphreys, M. K.; Garcia-Closas, M.; Figueroa, J.; Lissowska, J.; Pharoah, P. D.; Easton, D. F.; Hesketh, R.; Metcalfe, J. C. & Dunning, A. M. (2011). TGF-{beta} Signaling Pathway and Breast Cancer Susceptibility. *Cancer Epidemiol Biomarkers Prev,* Vol.20, No.6, pp.1112-1119, ISSN 1538-7755

Shekhar, M. P.; Pauley, R. & Heppner, G. (2003). Host microenvironment in breast cancer development: extracellular matrix-stromal cell contribution to neoplastic phenotype of epithelial cells in the breast. *Breast Cancer Res,* Vol.5, No.3, pp.130-135, ISSN 1465-542

Shin, A.; Cai, Q.; Shu, X. O.; Gao, Y. T. & Zheng, W. (2005). Genetic polymorphisms in the matrix metalloproteinase 12 gene (MMP12) and breast cancer risk and survival: the Shanghai Breast Cancer Study. *Breast Cancer Res,* Vol.7, No.4, pp.R506-512, ISSN 1465-542

Shyamala, G.; Chou, Y. C.; Louie, S. G.; Guzman, R. C.; Smith, G. H. & Nandi, S. (2002). Cellular expression of estrogen and progesterone receptors in mammary glands: regulation by hormones, development and aging. *J Steroid Biochem Mol Biol,* Vol.80, No.2, pp.137-148, ISSN 0960-0760

Smigal, C.; Jemal, A.; Ward, E.; Cokkinides, V.; Smith, R.; Howe, H. L. & Thun, M. (2006). Trends in breast cancer by race and ethnicity: update 2006. *CA Cancer J Clin,* Vol.56, No.3, pp.168-183, ISSN 0007-9235

Smith, G. H.; Sharp, R.; Kordon, E. C.; Jhappan, C. & Merlino, G. (1995). Transforming growth factor-alpha promotes mammary tumorigenesis through selective survival and growth of secretory epithelial cells. *Am J Pathol,* Vol.147, No.4, pp.1081-1096, ISSN 0002-9440

Soslow, R. A.; Dannenberg, A. J.; Rush, D.; Woerner, B. M.; Khan, K. N.; Masferrer, J. & Koki, A. T. (2000). COX-2 is expressed in human pulmonary, colonic, and mammary tumors. *Cancer,* Vol.89, No.12, pp.2637-2645, ISSN 0008-543

Starlard-Davenport, A.; Lyn-Cook, B. & Radominska-Pandya, A. (2008). Identification of UDP-glucuronosyltransferase 1A10 in non-malignant and malignant human breast tissues. *Steroids,* Vol.73, No.6, pp.611-620, ISSN 0039-128

Steude, J. S.; Maskarinec, G.; Erber, E.; Verheus, M.; Hernandez, B. Y.; Killeen, J. & Cline, J. M. (2009). Mammographic Density and Matrix Metalloproteinases in Breast Tissue. *Cancer Microenviron,* ISSN 1875-2284 Stone, J.; Gurrin, L. C.; Byrnes, G. B.; Schroen, C. J.; Treloar, S. A.; Padilla, E. J.; Dite, G. S.; Southey, M. C.; Hayes, V. M. & Hopper, J. L. (2007). Mammographic density and candidate gene variants: a twins and sisters study. *Cancer Epidemiol Biomarkers Prev,* Vol.16, No.7, pp.1479-1484, ISSN 1055-9965

Strange, K. S.; Wilkinson, D. & Emerman, J. T. (2002). Mitogenic properties of insulin-like growth factors I and II, insulin-like growth factor binding protein-3 and epidermal growth factor on human breast epithelial cells in primary culture. *Breast Cancer Res Treat,* Vol.75, No.3, pp.203-212, ISSN 0167-6806

Strange, K. S.; Wilkinson, D.; Edin, G. & Emerman, J. T. (2004). Mitogenic properties of insulin-like growth factors I and II, insulin-like growth factor binding protein-3 and epidermal growth factor on human breast stromal cells in primary culture. *Breast Cancer Res Treat,* Vol.84, No.2, pp.77-84, ISSN 0167-6806

Studer, R. K. & Chu, C. R. (2005). p38 MAPK and COX2 inhibition modulate human chondrocyte response to TGF-beta. *J Orthop Res,* Vol.23, No.2, pp.454-461, ISSN 0736-0266

Subbaramaiah, K.; Hudis, C.; Chang, S. H.; Hla, T. & Dannenberg, A. J. (2008). EP2 and EP4 receptors regulate aromatase expression in human adipocytes and breast cancer cells. Evidence of a BRCA1 and p300 exchange. *J Biol Chem,* Vol.283, No.6, pp.3433-3444, ISSN 0021-9258

Tanne, J. H. (2010). Fall in breast density is linked with lower risk of breast cancer, studies say. *BMJ,* Vol.340, pp.c2285, ISSN 1468-5833

Tao, W.; Wang, C.; Han, R. & Jiang, H. (2009). HER2 codon 655 polymorphism and breast cancer risk: a meta-analysis. *Breast Cancer Res Treat,* Vol.114, No.2, pp.371-376, ISSN 1573-7217

Toniolo, P.; Bruning, P. F.; Akhmedkhanov, A.; Bonfrer, J. M.; Koenig, K. L.; Lukanova, A.; Shore, R. E. & Zeleniuch-Jacquotte, A. (2000). Serum insulin-like growth factor-I and breast cancer. *Int J Cancer,* Vol.88, No.5, pp.828-832, ISSN 0020-7136

Trentham-Dietz, A.; Newcomb, P. A.; Storer, B. E.; Longnecker, M. P.; Baron, J.; Greenberg, E. R. & Willett, W. C. (1997). Body size and risk of breast cancer. *Am J Epidemiol,* Vol.145, No.11, pp.1011-1019, ISSN 0002-9262

Trichopoulos, D.; Lagiou, P. & Adami, H. O. (2005). Towards an integrated model for breast cancer etiology: the crucial role of the number of mammary tissue-specific stem cells. *Breast Cancer Res,* Vol.7, No.1, pp.13-17, ISSN 1465-542

Uria, J. A.; Ferrando, A. A.; Velasco, G.; Freije, J. M. & Lopez-Otin, C. (1994). Structure and expression in breast tumors of human TIMP-3, a new member of the metalloproteinase inhibitor family. *Cancer Res,* Vol.54, No.8, pp.2091-2094, ISSN 0008-5472

Ursin, G.; Lillie, E. O.; Lee, E.; Cockburn, M.; Schork, N. J.; Cozen, W.; Parisky, Y. R.; Hamilton, A. S.; Astrahan, M. A. & Mack, T. (2009). The relative importance of genetics and environment on mammographic density. *Cancer Epidemiol Biomarkers Prev,* Vol.18, No.1, pp.102-112, ISSN 1055-9965

Vachon, C. M.; Kuni, C. C.; Anderson, K.; Anderson, V. E. & Sellers, T. A. (2000). Association of mammographically defined percent breast density with epidemiologic risk factors for breast cancer (United States). *Cancer Causes Control,* Vol.11, No.7, pp.653-662, ISSN 0957-5243

Vachon, C. M.; Sasano, H.; Ghosh, K.; Brandt, K. R.; Watson, D. A.; Reynolds, C.; Lingle, W. L.; Goss, P. E.; Li, R.; Aiyar, S. E.; Scott, C. G.; Pankratz, V. S.; Santen, R. J. & Ingle, J. N. (2011). Aromatase immunoreactivity is increased in mammographically dense regions of the breast. *Breast Cancer Res Treat,* Vol.125, No.1, pp.243-252, ISSN 1573-7217

Verheus, M.; Maskarinec, G.; Erber, E.; Steude, J. S.; Killeen, J.; Hernandez, B. Y. & Cline, J. M. (2009). Mammographic density and epithelial histopathologic markers. *BMC Cancer,* Vol.9, pp.182, ISSN 1471-2407

Warren, R. & Lakhani, S. R. (2003). Can the stroma provide the clue to the cellular basis for mammographic density? *Breast Cancer Res,* Vol.5, No.5, pp.225-227, ISSN 1465-542

Warren, R. (2004). Hormones and mammographic breast density. *Maturitas,* Vol.49, No.1, pp.67-78, ISSN 0378-5122

Wolfe, J. N. (1976). Breast patterns as an index of risk for developing breast cancer. *AJR Am J Roentgenol,* Vol.126, No.6, pp.1130-1137, ISSN 0361-803

Woodward, T. L.; Xie, J. W. & Haslam, S. Z. (1998). The role of mammary stroma in modulating the proliferative response to ovarian hormones in the normal mammary gland. *J Mammary Gland Biol Neoplasia,* Vol.3, No.2, pp.117-131, ISSN 1083-3021

Woolcott, C. G.; SenGupta, S. K.; Hanna, W. M. & Aronson, K. J. (2008). Estrogen and progesterone receptor levels in nonneoplastic breast epithelium of breast cancer cases versus benign breast biopsy controls. *BMC Cancer,* Vol.8, pp.130, ISSN 1471-2407

Yang, W. T.; Lewis, M. T.; Hess, K.; Wong, H.; Tsimelzon, A.; Karadag, N.; Cairo, M.; Wei, C.; Meric-Bernstam, F.; Brown, P.; Arun, B.; Hortobagyi, G. N.; Sahin, A. & Chang, J. C. (2010). Decreased TGFbeta signaling and increased COX2 expression in high risk women with increased mammographic breast density. *Breast Cancer Res Treat,* Vol.119, No.2, pp.305-314, ISSN 1573-7217

Yarden, Y. (2001). Biology of HER2 and its importance in breast cancer. *Oncology,* Vol.61 Suppl 2, pp.1-13, ISSN 0030-2414

Yu, K. D.; Chen, A. X.; Yang, C.; Qiu, L. X.; Fan, L.; Xu, W. H. & Shao, Z. M. (2010). Current evidence on the relationship between polymorphisms in the COX-2 gene and breast cancer risk: a meta-analysis. *Breast Cancer Res Treat,* Vol.122, No.1, pp.251-257, ISSN 1573-7217

Zhao, Y.; Agarwal, V. R.; Mendelson, C. R. & Simpson, E. R. (1996). Estrogen biosynthesis proximal to a breast tumor is stimulated by PGE2 via cyclic AMP, leading to activation of promoter II of the CYP19 (aromatase) gene. *Endocrinology,* Vol.137, No.12, pp.5739-5742, ISSN 0013-7227

Zhou, P.; Du, L. F.; Lv, G. Q.; Yu, X. M.; Gu, Y. L.; Li, J. P. & Zhang, C. (2011). Current evidence on the relationship between four polymorphisms in the matrix metalloproteinases (MMP) gene and breast cancer risk: a meta-analysis. *Breast Cancer Res Treat,* Vol.127, No.3, pp.813-818, ISSN 1573-7217

Ziv, E.; Shepherd, J.; Smith-Bindman, R. & Kerlikowske, K. (2003). Mammographic breast density and family history of breast cancer. *J Natl Cancer Inst,* Vol.95, No.7, pp.556-558, ISSN 0027-8874

10

Mammographic Density Under Hormonal and Hormone-Like Treatments

Şerban Nastasia
University of Medicine and Pharmacy "Carol Davila" Bucharest
Romania

1. Introduction

Mammographic screening is the only important intervention for the early detection of breast cancer. The ability of mammography to detect incipient breast cancer depends on breast density. Hormonal treatments, affecting the breast radiological density, are an important risk factor interfering mammography. In the same time, mammographic density is currently being explored as a biomarker of response in primary and secondary prevention trials. Important considerations for chemoprevention studies include maximizing intrareader reliability and minimizing variance resulting from technical and physiologic factors (Fabian & Kimler, 2006). While technical factors for maximizing intrareader reliability and minimizing variance depend on classifications and technology, it is also important to evaluate the impact of physiologic and pharmacological factors

2. Classifications of breast mammographic density

Mammographic breast density reflects mammary gland development and structure. From the multiple methods that have been developed to assess mammographic density, Wolfe`s classification identified four categories: N1, P1, P2 and DY (Wolfe), with density increasing from N1 to DY, the greatest relative risk being associated with the DY pattern (Wolfe, 1976). The BIRADS system developed by the American College of Radiology classifies breasts as 1) almost entirely fatty, 2) scattered fibronodular tissue, 3) heterogeneously dense and 4) extremely dense (American College of Radiology [ACR], 1993). The proportion of women having BIRADS category 3 and 4 dramatically decreases with age. BIRADS semiquantitative classification has a suboptimal intrareader reliability (Fabian & Kimler, 2006). For greater intraobserver reliability, continuous, computer assisted measurements have a better performance, being more suitable for prevention studies (Fabian & Kimler, 2006).

Byrne, using the mammograms from the Breast Cancer Detection Demonstration Project, developed a continuous density measurement system, in which the area of the breast occupied by increased density was measured relative to the total area of the breast (Byrne et al., 1995). Byrne`s classification has 5 categories of relative areas of increased mammographic density and give a better assessment of relative risk for breast cancer than the 4-category Wolfe classification. The authors observed that the area of increased density is a risk factor, while the total breast area is not.

Boyd et al divided breast density measurements into 6 categories similar to those of Byrne, using a similar computer-assisted system for detection of mammographic density (Boyd et al., 1995).

Continuous density measurement system studies reported that the 10% of women who had >75% increased breast density had a 4 to 5-fold greater risk of breast cancer than women with no areas of increased breast density, after corrections for weight, reproductive and family history (Byrne et al.,1995; Boyd et al., 1995). Women with 50–75% area of density have a 2.5 to 3.0-fold increase in risk. Boyd et al. have suggested that the increase in relative risk estimates resulting from a breast density measurement lasts at least a decade (Fabian & Kimler, 2006; Boyd et al., 2002).

This long-lasting influence of breast density further justifies the interest in evaluation of the impact of physiologic and pharmacological factors on mammografic breast density.

Mammographic density category							
Wolfe	Increased breast density	N 1			P 1	P 2	DY
Byrne		0 %	1-24 %		25-49 %	50-74 %	≥ 75 %
Byrne (absolute density)		0 cm^2	1-13.9 cm^2	14-22.9 cm^2	23-33.9 cm^2	34-52.9 cm^2	> 53 cm^2
Boyd		None	< 10 %	10- <25 %	25- <50 %	50- <75 %	≥ 75 %
Wolfe	Percent of women exhibiting breast density patterns	12 %			28 %	48 %	12 %
Byrne		11 %	27 %		25 %	28 %	8 %
Byrne (absolute density)		Control group divided in six approximately equal groups					
Boyd		7 %	17 %	21 %	27 %	19 %	9 %
Wolfe	Adjusted odd ratio	1.0			1.68	2.83	2,73
Byrne (adjusted for all confounding factors)		1.0	1.57		2.47	2.77	4.35
Byrne (absolute density)		1.0	1.48	1.99	2.08	3.24	3.35
Boyd (all ages)		1.0	1.2	2.2	2.4	3.4	5.3

Table 1. Risk of breast cancer development associated with mammographic density in Wolfe`s (Wolfe, 1976), Byrne`s (Byrne et al., 1995) and Boyd`s (Boyd et al., 1995) classifications (adapted from Fabian & Kimler, 2006).

3. Endogenous influences on breast mammographic density

Mammographic parenchymal patterns are a function of breast development. The development of breast is the sum of ducts and lobules genetic-induced development, under the control of endogenous factors, mainly endocrine. Estrogens are responsible for growth and developments of the ducts, while the maturation of the breast acinus is progesteron-dependent. Progesteron is responsible for water accumulation at the end of menstrual cycle, increasing the breast density and whiteness on mammography. Declining in levels of estrogens and progesteron in menopause is associated with a decrease in breast density, making it easier to be examined by mammography.

4. Exogenous influences on breast mammographic density

Exogenous hormonal influences on mammografic breast density are best reflected by positive associations of mammografic breast density with postmenopausal hormone replacement therapy (HRT) and inverse associations with tamoxifen (Ghosh & Vachon, 2010).

4.1 Hormone replacement therapy

Hormone replacement therapy (HRT) increase the breast density (glandular tissue), which appears as white areas on a mammography, making microcalcifications and breast masses more difficult to detect, since breast abnormalities also appear as white areas on a mammography.

HRT is used by perimenopausal and early postmenopausal women, in the age group in which the incidence of breast cancer is maximum. As HRT contains a wide range of therapeutic interventions, its effects on mammography will vary according to several variables: HRT users versus non-users, age and window of opportunity, duration and dose of therapy, estrogen versus estrogen+progestin therapy, continuos combined versus sequential HRT, type of progestin, transdermal versus oral HRT.

The impact of HRT on mammographic screening is decreasing its sensibility, current use of HRT being associated with reduced sensitivity and specificity of mammographic breast cancer screening (Banks, 2001). Many studies suggest that current HRT users are more likely than non-users to have interval breast cancer (cancer occurring in the interval between screenings) (Banks, 2001; Cohen, 1997; Rosenberg et al., Litherland et al., 1999). Therefore, the benefit of mammographic screening may be reduced in HRT users, in terms of breast cancer mortality reduction, compared with non-users. Regarding the specificity of mammographic screening, many studies showed a lower specificity for current HRT users (Laya et al., 1996; Thurfjell et al., 1997), who may experience more false positive recall, compared with non-users (recalled for assessment after initial mammography, but found not to have breast cancer) (Clemons & Goss, 2001). Thurfjell et al (Thurfjell et al., 1997) divided current HRT users into three categories: less than 3 years of use, 3-6 years of use and more than 6 years of use. They reported specificities of 95%, 95%, and 92% respectively ($p=0.046$), revealing a trend for false positive recalls with increasing duration of use of HRT. These data are consistent with the study of Sala et al, who found that starting HRT pre- or perimenopausally and > 5 years of use will increase the probability of a high-risk mammographic density pattern, more difficult to evaluate (Sala et al., 2000).

Current HRT users have an increased probability of having a high risk pattern of breast density (Sala et al., 2000; Persson et al., 1997; McTiernan et al., 2005; Greendale et al., 2003; Chlebowski et al., 2003; Boyd et al., 2006). Current estrogen + progestin therapy users and current estrogen-only therapy users had greater odds of having dense breasts (98% [1.87–

2.09]) and 71%, respectively [1.56–1.87]), compared to never users (Aiello et al., 2006). Type of HRT regimen is an important factor, influencing breast mammographic density. Lundstrom E et al (Lundstrom E et al., 1999) found that increase in mammographic density was much more common among women receiving continuous estrogen + progestin HRT (52%) than among those receiving estrogen + progestin HRT (13%) and estrogen-only (18%) treatment. The increase in density was apparent already at first visit after the start of hormone replacement therapy. There was little change in mammographic status during long-term follow-up (Lundstrom E et al., 1999).

Transdermal HRT use is associated with a significantly lower incidence of increased mammographic breast density and breast tenderness compared with oral HRT (Harvey et al., 2005). In Harvey`s study (2005), 202 postmenopausal women were randomized to transdermal (estradiol+norethindrone) or oral (estradion+norethistron acetate) HRT. Significantly fewer women using transdermal HRT had an increase in mammographic breast density or breast tenderness compared to oral HRT. Of the women using transdermal HRT, 39.1% had no change in breast density compared to 15.7% for women using oral HRT. Only 4% of women using transdermal HRT had a marked increase in density (>25%) compared to 15.7% of women using oral HRT.

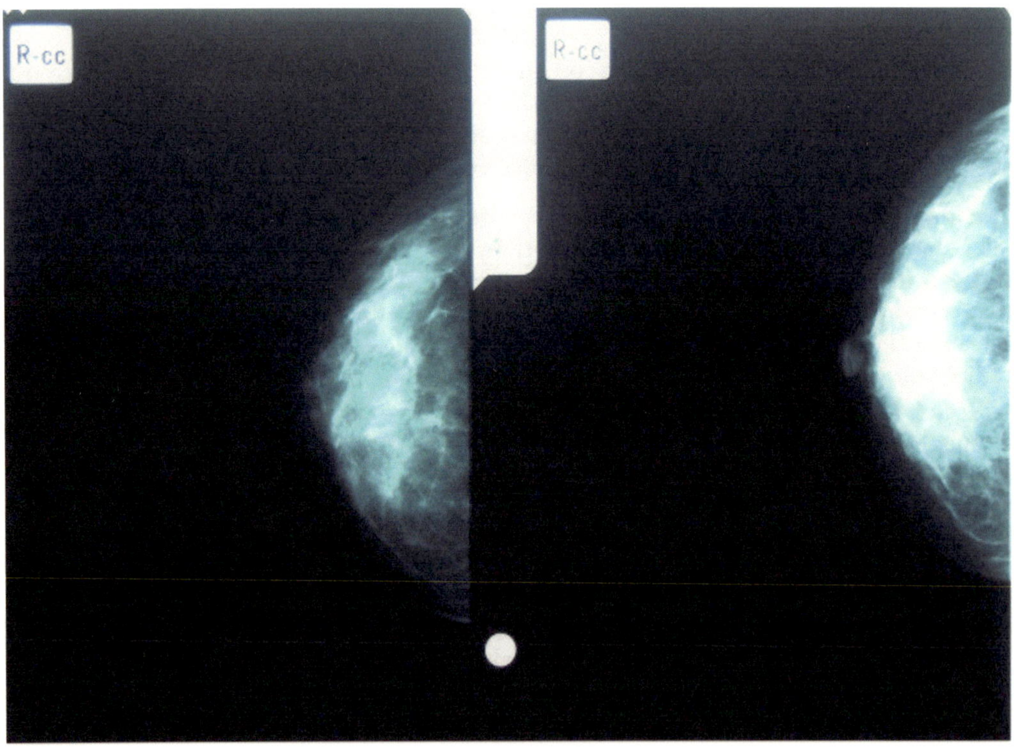

Fig. 1. Increase in mammographic breast density in a 53 years old patient on sequential combined hormonal therapy (1,5 mg estradiol transdermally+20 mg dydrogesterone orally). Left - mammography at baseline; right - mammography after 1 year of treatment. Procentual mammographic density raised from 23% to 55% (Russu et al., 2008).

The randomized, double-blinded PEPI trial (Greendale et al., 1999) compared the mammography before and after twelve months of treatment, for HRT patients versus placebo. Twenty percent of HRT patients had increased mammographic density, as compared to 0 % in placebo group. There was no difference in breast densities between continuous combined and sequential HRT groups. There was also no difference in breast densities with different progestins. Patients with estrogen-only therapy had a very small increase in breast density.

The WHI Study (Chlebowski et al., 2003) found that, after one year of estrogen plus progestin therapy, the percent of abnormal mammography was higher in estrogen plus progestin therapy group, compared with placebo group (9,4% vs 5,4%; P<0.001), and the difference was maintained throughout the duration of the study. In each year thereafter, the percentage of women with abnormal mammograms was significantly higher in the estrogen plus progestin group vs the placebo group. For the whole study, 31.5% of women in the estrogen plus progestin group had at least 1 abnormal mammogram vs 21.2% of women in the placebo group (*P*<.001). Thus, even short-term estrogen plus progestin use resulted in a substantial increase in abnormal mammograms requiring medical evaluation. The risk for breast cancer parallels the percentage of abnormal mammography. The authors concluded that E+P therapy increased the number of breast cancer and the number of not necessary interventions for false positive mammography in this group. However, most of the studies found a lower mortality for HRT users compared with non-users.

The Million Women Study showed that current users of HRT at recruitment were more likely than never users to develop breast cancer (adjusted relative risk 1.66 [95% CI 1.58-1.75], p<0.0001) and die from it (1.22 [1.00-1.48], p=0.05). Stopping HRT reduces breast cancer risk, as demonstrated in WHI study (Chlebowski et al., 2003), where the authors found that past users of HRT were not at an increased risk of incident or fatal disease (1.01 [0.94-1.09] and 1.05 [0.82-1.34], respectively).

Patients with estrogen-only therapy tend to have a small increase in breast density and lower risk for invasive breast cancer. In WHI study follow-up (La Croix et al., 2011), after 6 years of equine estrogens use and a mean 10,7 years after baseline, estrogen-only therapy was associated with a lower risk for invasive breast cancer than the placebo group (hazard ratio, 0.77; 95% confidence interval, 0.62–0.95); moreover, among younger women, estrogen use was associated with lower risk for CHD (HR, 0.59; 95% CI, 0.38–0.90). However, this does not imply that estrogen-only therapy should be recommended at this time for breast cancer chemoprophylaxis (Beral et al., 2003; Kaunitz, 2011; Jungheim & Colditz, 2011).

Progestin-releasing intrauterine devices are a type of hormone therapy addressed to women younger than 50 years of age, especially with associated uterine pathology (e.g., fibroids, menorrhagia).

A retrospective, population-based, case-control study (Dinger et al., 2011), performed on 25565 women (5113 breast cancer cases and 20452 controls) failed to observe any increase of breast cancer risk in levonorgestrel intrauterine device users.

Combination of levonorgestrel intrauterine device and low-dose oral estradiol valerate was associated with a slight increase in mammographic breast density. Lundstrom et al (Lundstrom et al., 2006) assessed 20 healthy patients with levonorgestrel intrauterine device and 2 mg oral estradiol valerate and they found an apparent increase in breast density in only 3 women (15%). However, there was no increase in proliferation, as expressed by the percentage of MIB-1-positive breast cells in fine-needle aspiration biopsies. Given the small number of cases, these results need to be confirmed by larger studies.

Timing of HRT initiation influences the mammographic parenchymal patterns. Analizing a subgroup from EPIC-Norfolk cohort, Sala et al (Sala et al., 2000) found that women who are starting HRT, while still menstruating, were more likely to have a high-risk breast density pattern compared to women not exposed to HRT or to those who started HRT after menopause. A recent Million Women Study analysis update (Beral et al., 2011) focused on the influence of timing on breast cancer risk for the different treatment regimens. Relative risks were found to be higher if therapy was started before or soon after menopause than in the case of a longer interval between menopause and starting HRT ($p < 0.001$). Among current users of estrogen-only therapy, there was little or no increase in risk if use began 5 years or more after menopause (RR 1.05, 95% CI 0.89–1.24), whereas risk was increased if use began before or within 5 years after menopause (RR 1.43, 95% CI 1.35–1.51). A similar pattern was seen for users of E+P (RR 1.53, 95% CI 1.38–1.70 vs. RR 2.04, 95% CI 1.95–2.14). The timing of initiation of HRT relative to that of menopause appears to be an important factor that modulates the risk of breast cancer.

HRT effects on breast and mammography are reversible. After discontinuing hormone therapy, breast density decrease rapidly. Discontinuation of HRT a few weeks prior to mammography may improve mammographic performances. The rapid decrease in breast density after stopping HRT suggest that increased breast density in HRT users is different from increased breast density in non-users. Increased breast density in non-users reflects a genetic increased quantity of glandular and fibrous tissue, whereas increased breast density in HRT users may suggest a water retention at breast level, probably due to stromal changes, under hormonal influence (Alowami et al., 2003). In a retrospective study, Harvey at al analyzed breast density modifications after stopping HRT (Harvey et al., 1997). HRT-induced mammographic changes disappeared two weeks after HRT discontinuation. However, twelve patients in their study did not experienced mammographic reversal after HRT discontinuation, and, on biopsy, one case of atypical hyperplasia and one case of ductal invasive carcinoma were found. More recent studies failed to observe an improvement in mammographic diagnostic accuracy, following HRT suspension. The Buist`s randomised trial revealed that HT suspension was associated with small changes in breast density and did not affect recall rates. There was no evidence to support short-term HT suspension before mammography (Buist et al., 2009).

A few studies addressed the issue of reducing breast cancer risk in HRT population. Adding aromatase inhibitors to HRT may lower mammographic breast density in postmenopausal women. A small retrospective study (Mousa et al., 2008) demonstrated a statistically significant reduction in mammographic breast density occurred in the women who received hormone therapy plus an aromatase inhibitor letrozole, whereas no significant change was observed in the women receiving hormone therapy alone. Aromatase inhibitors could be good candidates for primary chemoprevention of breast cancer in postmenopausal women using hormone therapy (Mousa et al., 2008).

4.2 Oral contraceptive

A special type of exogenous hormonal therapy is oral contraceptive (OC) use. Modern OC consist in a combination of ethinilestradiol (20µg or 30 µg) and different types of progestins. Oral contraceptive use is an issue of young women, mostly before age of 40, a time when mammographic screening begins. Therefore, studies evaluating the impact of COC on mammographic breast density are lacking.

A Norwegian study (Gram et al., 2002) examined the relationship between oral contraceptive ever use and mammographic patterns among 3218 women, aged 40-56 years, who fulfilled a questionnaire about ever OC use, duration, and starting age of OC. Women ever having used OCs had an increased risk for high-risk mammographic patterns [OR 1.27; 95% CI (1.0-1.6)], compared with those reporting never having used OCs. There was no relationship between different types of OC use (different doses) and high-risk patterns. Nulliparous women, who ever used OCs, were four times more likely [OR 4.65; 95% CI (2.1-10.3)] to have high-risk patterns, compared with never users.

Breast cancer lifetime-risk of oral contraceptive use was addressed in a large study (Hunter et al., 2010), performed on 116.608 female nurses, aged 25 to 42 years at enrollment in 1989, among which 1.344 cases of invasive breast cancer were diagnosed until 2001. There was no relationship between past use of any oral contraceptive and breast cancer risk [RR= 1.12; 95% confidence interval (0.95-1.33)]. Current use of any oral contraceptive was only marginally related to a higher risk of breast cancer [RR=1.33; 95% confidence interval (1.03-1.73)]. However, users of triphasic oral contraceptive, with levonorgestrel as the progestin, were exposed to an excess risk of breast cancer, as high as 3.05 [95% confidence interval (2.00-4.66); $P < 0.0001$]. The authors (Hunter et al., 2010) concluded that current use of oral contraceptives is associated with an excess risk of breast cancer, levonorgestrel-based triphasic contraceptives accounting for this risk elevation.

4.3 Gonadotropin-releasing hormone agonists

Gonadotropin-releasing hormone agonist (GnRHA) suppress ovarian function, decreasing circulating levels of estrogens, so it could be assumed that their administration would influence breast density. A special designed contraceptive study (Spicer et al., 1994) randomly assigned 21 patients, 27–40 years of age, with a 5-fold greater than normal risk of breast cancer, in a 2:1 ratio to special contraceptive group (14 women who received GnRHA (leucoprolide acetate) plus very low doses add-back conjugated estrogen and medroxy-progesterone acetate) or to a control group (7 women). The authors found that women on the contraceptive regimen showed significant ($P = 0.039$) reduction in mammographic densities between the baseline and 1-year mammograms, compared with control group. In a follow-up of this study (Spicer et al., 1994), 12 months after completion of treatment, the mean percentage of mammographic density in the treated group was no different from that at baseline ($P = 0.73$). Reductions in mammographic density for this special contraceptive regimen (GnRHA plus low-dose add-back estrogen-progestin) persist only during treatment period. The densities return to baseline when the women resume normal menstrual cycles.

A more recent study (Weitzel et al., 2007) performed on BRCA1 mutation high-risk patients, using GnRHA deslorelin, confirmed these data. Twelve months treatment with deslorelin, plus low-dose add-back steroids, significantly decreased mammographic percent density in BRCA1 mutation carriers. This regimen may reduce breast cancer risk and improve the usefulness of mammographic surveillance by reducing density.

4.4 Selective tissue estrogenic activity regulator

Other forms of sistemic therapy for relief of climacteric symptoms and prevention of osteoporosis in postmenopausal women include selective tissue estrogenic activity regulator (STEAR), the most known being tibolone. Tibolone, a tissue-specific compound, constitutes an alternative for treatment in postmenopausal women (Moore, 1999).

It appears that tibolone exerts minimal effects of the breast tissue and mammographic density. In a prospective, randomized, double-blind, placebo-controlled study (Lundström et al., 2002), breast density was increased in 46-50% of oral continuous combined HRT users, as opposed to only 2-6% in oral tibolone users and 0% in placebo group. The authors concluded that in contrast to estrogen/progestogen treatment, tibolone seems to exert little stimulation of breast tissue.

According to Asia Pacific Tibolone Consensus Group, symptomatic HRT users with increased breast density that result in an unreadable mammogram could be switched on tibolone, in order to decrease mammographic density without losing the beneficial effects of HRT (Huang & Baber, 2010).

However, the relationship between tibolone use and increased risk of breast cancer remains inconclusive (Opatrny et al., 2008). A population-based case-control study, GPRD database (Opatrny et al., 2008), found that tibolone do not increase the risk for breast cancer in postmenopausal women (RR 0.86; 95% CI 0.65-1.13). Even more, LIFT trial (Cummings et al., 2008), which included 4538 osteoporotic postmenopausal women with no history of breast cancer, treated with tibolone, 1,25 mg/day, demonstrated a decreased risk of invasive breast cancer (RR = 0.32; 95% CI, 0.13 to 0.80; P=0.02).

However, in women with a history of breast cancer, data from the LIBERATE (Kenemans et al., 2009) study show that tibolone (2,5 mg/day) does increase the risk of breast cancer recurrence. LIBERATE population of women is mostly using adjuvant systemic therapy, 67% of women being on tamoxifen and 6.5% on aromatase inhibitors. Tibolone may interfere with the protective action of these agents, especially with the aromatase inhibitors, through an estrogen-agonistic action on dormant tumor cells. To date, tibolone should be contraindicated for women with a history of breast cancer.

Although comparison is not possible between LIFT and LIBERATE study, dose seems to be an important issue with respect to breast cancer risk, when using tibolone for vasomotor symptoms relief and osteoporosis treatment.

4.5 Selective estrogen-receptor modulators

Selective estrogen-receptor modulators (SERMs), previously called antiestrogens, are drugs that competitively inhibit estrogen binding to estrogen receptors (ERs), and have mixed agonist and antagonist activity (depending on the target tissue). SERMs affect a variety of biologic processes regulated by activated estrogen receptor. Depending on the target tissue, levels and types of ERs, and their structure, SERMs may exhibit either estrogen antagonist or estrogen agonist effects (Fabian & Kimler, 2005).

Tamoxifen is a SERM with estrogen antagonist effects in the breast, weak estrogen agonist activity in the bone, cardiovascular system and CNS, and important estrogen agonist effects in the uterus, liver, and vagina.

Most of the data regarding tamoxifen effects on mammographic breast density came from prevention studies, performed on populations at high-risk for breast cancer or with a history of breast cancer. In the National Surgical Adjuvant Breast and Bowel Project (NSABP) randomized clinical trial of high-risk women, 5 years of tamoxifen therapy was shown to reduce invasive breast cancer risk by 49% and noninvasive breast cancer risk by 50% compared with placebo (Fisher et al., 1998).

Treatment with tamoxifen is associated with a reduction in breast density in both premenopausal and postmenopausal women (Ursin et al., 1996). However, the reduction in breast density in association with these factors has not yet been correlated with the reduction in the risk of breast cancer.

Slanetz (Slanetz et al., 2004) described mammographic density decrease on tamoxifen and return to the baseline density following termination of the drug, so they postulated that decrease in breast density could reflect the sensitivity to tamoxifen and be a marker of therapeutic benefit associated with tamoxifen. The more radiolucent pattern by tamoxifen allow enhanced mammographic detection and may further add benefit for women. After discontinuation of tamoxifen, breast density is returning to its initial pattern. The clinical significance of resumption of a dense breast pattern following discontinuation of tamoxifen remains to be determined (Ursin et al., 1996).

In high-risk populations (women with known breast cancer on adjuvant tamoxifen or women at high risk for breast cancer on tamoxifen for chemoprevention), tamoxifen produced a statistically significant reduction in mammmographic breast density and this reduction occurred more frequent in premenopausal than in postmenopausal women (54).

In a study (Son & Oh, 1999), performed on breast cancer patients who have undergone surgery, 87% of premenopausal women with breast cancer had a decrease in parenchymal area with tamoxifen use, whereas only 29% of postmenopausal women experienced a decrease.

A similar trend was observed in the Brisson`s study, performed on women with high-risk for breast cancer. Women younger than 50 experienced a decrease in parenchymal pattern classification in 67% of cases compared with 13% of postmenopausal women aged 50 or older (Brisson et al., 2000).

The duration of tamoxifen treatment is important. In a nested case-control study performed for IBIS-1 participants, Cuzick et al. noticed that the reduction in dense area for women treated for 4,5 years with tamoxifen is double compared with women given placebo (Cuzick et al., 2004). The majority of breast density reduction occurred in the first 18 months of treatment. There was a significant interaction with age such that a minimal decrease in area of density was observed for women over 55 treated with tamoxifen, that is, 1% compared to 13% for women younger than 45 (Cuzick et al., 2004). Importantly, reduction in breast density predicted only one-third of the reduction in breast cancer incidence seen in prevention trials.

While tamoxifen is mostly recommended by the oncologists, both for curative or preventive breast cancer treatment, other SERM`s, like raloxifen, are largely recommended by general practitioners for the treatment of postmenopausal osteoporosis. Raloxifene has higher affinity for estrogen receptor and more intense antagonistic effects (by blocking ER-activating function domains, AF-1 and AF-2), than tamoxifen (which blocks only AF-2, but not AF-1) (Howell et al., 2001; Katzenellenbogen et al., 1996).

In the STAR trial (Vogel et al., 2006), tamoxifen and raloxifene had equivalent effects in reducing risk of invasive breast cancer in all examined subgroups, including women with a history of atypical hyperplasia or LCIS, who had the highest annual rates of invasive breast cancer. Most of the STAR cases were diagnosed as a result of mammograms demonstrating increasing calcifications, in conditions of reducted breast density. Because the lesions were early detected and small, most were treated surgically with lumpectomy.

In a retrospective analysis, performed on a subset of women enrolled in a multicenter, double-blind, randomized, placebo- and active-controlled phase 3 trial evaluating bazedoxifene for the treatment of postmenopausal osteoporosis, Harvey et al found that the changes in breast density with the newer SERM bazedoxifene 20 or 40 mg were similar to those with raloxifene 60 mg or placebo (Harvey et al., 2009).

The analysis of extraskeletal outcomes (Gennari et al., 2009) of PEARL study indicated that lasofoxifene 0.25 mg and 0.5 mg reduces the risk of ER positive breast cancer (by 84% and 67%, respectively). This effect was also evident for all breast cancers (a composite endpoint consisting of ER+, ER–, invasive, and ductal cancer in situ) with lasofoxifene 0.5 mg dose (65% and 79% risk reduction compared to placebo through 3 and 5 years, respectively) (Cummings et al., 2008).

4.6 Aromatase inhibitors

The aromatase inhibitors reduce breast and circulating estrogen levels in postmenopausal women. As a consequence, aromatase inhibitors may reduce mammographic breast density.

Vachon et al randomized 106 postmenopausal women to either aromatase inhibitor letrozole or placebo after 5 years of tamoxifen (Vachon et al., 2007). After 9 to 15 months, no difference breast mammographic density was found between the 2 groups.

MAP1 was a multicenter, randomized, double-blind, placebo-controlled, feasibility trial in which postmenopausal women with or without prior invasive breast cancer were randomized in a 2:1 ratio of letrozole (2.5 mg daily) or placebo for 12 months and followed for a total of 24 months. After one year treatment, letrozole does not appear to have a significant effect on mammographic percent breast density, compared with placebo (Cigler et al., 2010). Same author performed MAP 2 trial (Cigler et al., 2011) randomizing healthy postmenopausal women to exemestan (25 mg daily) or placebo for 12 months and followed them for a total of 24 months. The primary endpoint was change in percent breast density between the baseline and 12-month mammograms. For exemestan-treated patients, there was no significant difference in percent breast density from baseline to 6, 12, or 24 months; in the same time, there was no difference between exemestan and placebo group.

It was postulated that aromatase inhibitors could reduce mammographic breast density in women taking HRT. Two studies examined the influence of letrozole on MBD among postmenopausal women taking HRT: one found no change in percent MBD among 42 high-risk women on either estrogen alone or combination HRT (estrogen and progestins) after taking 2.5 mg letrozole per day for 6 months (64), whereas the other study found a reduction among women on low-dose combination therapy who were taking letrozole (2.5 mg) 3 times weekly for a median of 24 (range, 2-63) months (6.8% vs 1.4% reduction) (Mousa et al., 2008).

The effects of aromatase inhibitors on breast density, as well as on breast cancer risk, still require further investigation (Becker & Kaas, 2009).

4.7 Phytoestrogens

Phytoestrogens are plant derived substances that are structurally and functionally similar to estrogens and are found in many foods. They exhibit both weak estrogen and anti-estrogenic activity; therefore, they act as natural SERMs. There are 3 classes of phytoestrogens: isoflavonoids, coumestans and ligans (Malik & Prakash, 2004).

Maskarinec et al randomly assigned 220 premenopausal women, aged 39 - 46 years old, to soy intake intervention group or control group (Maskarinec et al., 2004). After 2 years of intervention, the authors observed no significant differences in mammographic densities by intervention status.

Association between regular green tea intake and high soy intake may have beneficial effects on the breast density. Wu, Ursin et al assessed the effects of the effects of regular green tea and soy intake on mammographic density, in a cross-sectional study performed on 3315 Chinese women in Singapore (Wu et al., 2008). For daily green tea drinkers, percent mammographic density was statistically significantly lower than for non-tea drinkers (19.5 % versus 21.7%; P = 0.002), even after adjustment for soy (P = 0.002). There was no association between black tea intake and percent mammographic density. Very high soy intake was associated with lower percent density only among postmenopausal women (compared normal or low soy intake; 18.9% versus 20.5%, P = 0.035); however, after adjustment for green tea intake, this association was no longer statistically significant (P = 0.52).

5. Conclusion

Mammographic density is a well-known risk factor for breast cancer, although the biologic basis of the relationship between breast cancer risk and increased mammographic density is not yet completely understood. Nor is the mechanism by which hormonal therapy influences mammographic breast density. Despite the beneficial effects on menopausal symptoms and osteoporosis, it is the fear of breast cancer that make menopausal women reluctant to take hormone therapy. Characterizing the association between breast density and hormonal influences may enhance the understanding of how mammographic density influences breast cancer risk for both pre- and postmenopausal women. Mammographic density reflecting directly the changes at the breast level, the influences generated by the associated therapies should be taken into account in screening and diagnostic programs.

6. References

Aiello, EJ; Buist, DSM; White, E. Do breast cancer risk factors modify the association between hormone therapy and mammographic breast density? *Cancer Causes and Control* Vol.17, No.10, (Dec 2006), pp.1227-35, Print ISSN 0957-5243, Online ISSN 1573-7225

Alowami, S; Troup, S; Al-Haddad, S; Kirkpatrick, I; Watson, PH. Mammographic density is related to stroma and stromal proteoglycan expression. *Breast Cancer Research* Vol.5No.5, (Jul 2003), pp.129–35. Available from http://breast-cancer-research.com/content/5/6/R129

American College of Radiology. Breast imaging reporting and data system (BIRADS). Reston, VA: American College of Radiology, 1993

Arthur, JE; Ellis, IO; Flowers, C; Roebuck, E; Elston, CW; Blamey, RW. The relationship of "high risk" mammographic patterns to histological risk factors for development of cancer in the human breast. *The British Journal of Radiology* Vol.63No.755, (Nov 1990), pp. 845–9.

Banks, E. Hormone replacement therapy and the sensitivity and specificity of breast cancer screening: a review. (Statistical Data Included). *Journal of Medical Screening* Vol.8, No.1, (Oct 2001), pp.29-34. Available from http://jms.rsmjournals.com/content/8/1/29.long

Becker, S; Kaaks, R. Exogenous and endogenous hormones, mammographic density and breast cancer risk: Can mammographic density be considered an intermediate marker of risk? *Recent Results in Cancer Research* Vol.181, No.5, (2009), pp.135-57, Print ISSN 0080-0015

Beral, V; Million Women Study Collaborators. Breast cancer and hormone-replacement therapy in the Million Women Study. *The Lancet* Vol.362, No.9382, (Aug 2003) pp.419-27, Print ISSN 0140-6736, Online ISSN 1474-547X

Beral, V; Reeves, G; Bull, D; Green, J; Million Women Study Collaborators. Breast cancer risk in relation to the interval between menopause and starting hormone therapy. *Journal of the National Cancer Institute* Vol.103, No.4, (Feb 2011), pp.296-305, Print ISSN 1052-6773, Online ISSN 1745-6614

Boyd, NF; Jensen, HM; Cooke, G; Han, HL. Relationship between mammographic and histological risk factors for breast cancer. *Journal of the National Cancer Institute* Vol.84, No.15, (1992), pp.1170-1179.

Boyd, NF; Byng, JW; Jong, RA; Fishell, EK; Little, LE; Miller, AB; Lockwood, GA; Tritchler, DL; Yaffe, MJ. Quantitative classification of mammographic densities and breast cancer risk: results from the Canadian National Breast Screening Study. *Journal of the National Cancer Institute* Vol.87, No.9, (May 1995), pp.670-5, Print ISSN 1052-6773, Online ISSN 1745-6614

Boyd, NF; Stone, J; Martin, LJ; Jong, R; Fishell, E; Yaffe, M; Hammond, G; Minkin, S. The association of breast mitogens with mammographic densities. *British Journal of Cancer* Vol.87, No.8, (Oct 2002), pp.876-82

Boyd, NF; Martin, LJ; Li, Q; Sun, L; Chiarelli, AM; Hislop, G; Yaffe, MJ; Minkin, S. Mammographic density as a surrogate marker for the effects of hormone therapy on risk of breast cancer. *Cancer Epidemiology, Biomarkers and Prevention* Vol.15, No.5, (May 2006), pp.961-6, Print ISSN 1055-9965, Online ISSN 1538-7755

Brisson, J; Brisson, B; Cote, G; Maunsell, E; Bérubé, S; Robert, J. Tamoxifen and mammographic breast densities. *Cancer Epidemiology, Biomarkers & Prevention* Vol.9, No.9, (Sep 2000), pp.911-5, Print ISSN 1055-9965, Online ISSN 1538-7755

Buist, DS; Anderson, ML; Reed, SD; et al. Short-term hormone therapy suspension and mammography recall: a randomized trial. *Annals of Internal Medicine* Vol.150, No.11, (Jun 2009), pp.752-65, Print ISSN 0003-4819, Online ISSN 1539-3704

Byrne, C; Schairer, C; Wolfe, J; Parekh, N; Salane, M; Brinton, LA; Hoover, R; Haile, R. Mammographic features and breast cancer risk: effects with time, age, and menopause status. *Journal of the National Cancer Institute* Vol.87, No.21, (Nov 1995), pp.1622-9, Print ISSN 1052-6773, Online ISSN 1745-6614

Byrne, C; Schairer, C; Brinton, LA; Wolfe, J; Parekh, N; Salane, M; Carter, C; Hoover, R. Effects of mammographic density and benign breast disease on breast cancer risk (United States). *Cancer Causes Control* Vol.12No.2, (Feb 2001), pp.103–10.

Chlebowski, RT; Hendrix, SL; Langer, RD; Stefanick, ML; Gass, M; Lane, D; Rodabough, RJ; Gilligan, MA; Cyr, MG; Thomson, CA; et al. Influence of estrogen plus progestin on breast cancer and mammography in healthy postmenopausal women: the Women's Health Initiative Randomized Trial. *JAMA* Vol.289, No.24, (Jan 2003), pp.3243-53, Print ISSN 0098-7484, Online ISSN 1538-3598

Chlebowski, RT; Hendrix, SL; Langer, RD; Stefanick, ML; Gass, M; Lane, D; Rodabough, RJ; Gilligan, MA; Cyr, MG; Thomson, CA; et al. Influence of estrogen plus progestin on breast cancer and mammography in healthy postmenopausal women: the Women's Health Initiative Randomized Trial. *JAMA* Vol.289, No.24, (Jan 2003), pp.3243-53, Print ISSN 0098-7484, Online ISSN 1538-3598

Cigler, T; Tu, D; Yaffe, MJ; Findlay, B; Verma, S; Johnston, D; Richardson, H; Hu, H; Qi, S; Goss, PE. A randomized, placebo-controlled trial (NCIC CTG MAP1) examining the effects of letrozole on mammographic breast density and other end organs in postmenopausal women. *Breast Cancer Research and Treatment* Vol.120, No.2, (Apr 2010), pp.427-35, Print ISSN 0167-6806, Online ISSN 1573-7217

Cigler, T; Richardson, H; Yaffe, MJ; Fabian, CJ; Johnston, D; Ingle, JN; Nassif, E; Brunner, RL; Wood, ME; Pater, JL; Hu, H; Qi, S; Tu, D; Goss, PE. A randomized, placebo-controlled trial (NCIC CTG MAP.2) examining the effects of exemestane on mammographic breast density, bone density, markers of bone metabolism and serum lipid levels in postmenopausal women. *Breast Cancer Research and Treatment* Vol.126, No.2, (Apr 2011), pp.453-61, Print ISSN 0167-6806, Online ISSN 1573-7217

Clemons, M; Goss, P. Estrogen and the risk of breast cancer. *New England Journal of Medicine* Vol.344, No.4, (Jan 2001), pp.276-285, Print ISSN 0028-4793, Online ISSN 1533-4406

Cohen, MEL. Effect of hormone replacement therapy on cancer detection by mammography. *The Lancet* Vol.349, No.9065, (May 1997) p1624

Cummings, SR; Eastell, R; Ensrud, K; Reid, DM; Vukicevic, S; LaCroix, A; Sriram, U; Thompson, S; Thompson, JR; Delmas, PD. The effects of lasofoxifene on fractures and breast cancer: 3-year results from the PEARL Trial. *Journal of Bone and Mineral Research* Vol.23, No Suppl S1, pp.81, (Aug 2008), Abstract 1288, Print ISSN 0884-0431, Online ISSN 1523-4681

Cummings, SR; Ettinger, B; Delmas, PD; Kenemans, P; Stathopoulos, V; et al. LIFT Trial Investigators. The effects of tibolone in older postmenopausal women. *The New*

England Journal of Medicine Vol.359, No.7, (Aug 2008), pp.697-708, Print ISSN 0028-4793, Online ISSN 1533-4406

Cuzick, J; Warwick, J; Pinney, E; Warren, RM; Duffy, SW. Tamoxifen and breast density in women at increased risk of breast cancer. *Journal of the National Cancer Institute* Vol.96, No.8, (Apr 2004), pp.621-8, Print ISSN 1052-6773, Online ISSN 1745-6614

Dinger, J; Bardenheuer, K; Minh, TD. Levonorgestrel-releasing and copper intrauterine devices and the risk of breast cancer. *Contraception* Vol.83, No.3, (Mar 2011), pp.211-7, Print ISSN 0010-7824, Online ISSN 1879-0518, Epub 2011 Jan 7

Fabian, CJ; Kimler, BF. Selective estrogen-receptor modulators for primary prevention of breast cancer. *Journal of Clinical Oncology* Vol.23, No.8, (Mar 2005), pp.1644-55, Print ISSN 0732-183X, Online ISSN 1527-7755

Fabian, CJ; Kimler, BF. Biomarkers as indicators of cancer risk reduction following dietary manipulation. Mammographic density: use in risk assessment and as a biomarker in prevention trials. *The Journal of Nutrition* 2006;136:S2705–2708. Available from http://jn.nutrition.org/content/136/10/2705S.full.pdf

Fabian, CJ; Kimler, BF; Zalles, CM; Khan, QJ; Mayo, MS; Phillips, TA; Simonsen, M; Metheny, T; Petroff, BK. Reduction in proliferation with six months of letrozole in women on hormone replacement therapy. *Breast Cancer Research and Treatment* Vol.106, No.1, (Nov 2007), pp.75-84, Print ISSN 0167-6806, Online ISSN 1573-7217

Fisher, B; Costantino, JP; Wickerham, DL; Redmond, CK; Kavanah, M; Cronin, WM; Vogel, V; Robidoux, A; Dimitrov, N; Atkins, J; Daly, M; Wieand, S; Tan-Chiu, E; Ford, L; Wolmark, N. Tamoxifen for prevention of breast cancer: report of the National Surgical Adjuvant Breast and Bowel Project P-1 Study. *Journal of the National Cancer Institute* Vol.90, No.18, (Sep 1998), pp.1371-88, Print ISSN 1052-6773, Online ISSN 1745-6614

Gennari, L; Merlotti, D; De Paola, V; Nuti, R. Lasofoxifene: the evidence of its therapeutic value in osteoporosis. *Core Evidence* Vol.4, (Jun 2010), pp.113-29, Print ISSN 1555-1741, Online ISSN 1555-175X

Ghosh, K; Vachon, CM. Mammographic breast density, endocrine therapies, and breast cancer risk. Menopausal Medicine Vol.18, No.1, (Feb 2010), pp.34-9

Gram, IT; Funkhouser, E; Nordgård, L; Tabár, L; Ursin, G. Oral contraceptive use and mammographic patterns. *European Journal of Cancer Prevention* Vol.11, No.3, (Jun 2002), pp.265-270, Print ISSN 0959-8278, Online ISSN 1473-5709

Greendale, GA; Reboussin, BA; Sie, A; et al. Effects of estrogen and estrogen-progestin on mammographic parenchymal density. Postmenopausal Estrogen/Progestin Interventions (PEPI) Investigators. *Annals of Internal Medicine* Vol.130, No.4, (Feb 1999), pp.262-9, Print ISSN 0003-4819, Online ISSN 1539-3704

Greendale, GA; Reboussin, BA; Slone, S; Wasilauskas, C; Pike, MC; Ursin, G. Postmenopausal hormone therapy and change in mammographic density. *Journal of the National Cancer Institute* Vol.95, No.1, (Jan 2003), pp.30-37, Print ISSN 1052-6773, Online ISSN 1745-6614

Harvey, JA; Pinkerton, JV; Herman, CR. Short-term cessation of hormone replacement therapy and improvement of mammographic specificity. *Journal of the National Cancer Institute* Vol.89, No.21, (Nov 1997), pp.1623-5, Print ISSN 1052-6773, Online ISSN 1745-6614

Harvey, J; Scheurer, C; Kawakami, FT; Quebe-Fehling, E; de Palacios, PI; Ragavan, VV. Hormone replacement therapy and breast density changes. *Climacteric* Vol.8, No.2, (Jun 2005), pp. 185-92, Print ISSN 1369-7137, Online ISSN 1473-0804

Harvey, J; Holm, M; Ranganath, R; Guse, PA; Trott, EA; Helzner, E. The effects of bazedoxifene on mammographic breast density in postmenopausal women with osteoporosis. *Menopause* Vol.16, No.6, (Nov-Dec 2009), pp.1193-6, Print ISSN 1072-3714, Online ISSN 1530-0374

Howell, A; Howell, SJ; Clarke, R; et al. Where do selective estrogen receptor modulators (SERMs) and aromatase inhibitors (AIs) now fit into breast cancer treatment algorithms? *The Journal of Steroid Biochemistry and Molecular Biology* Vol.79, No.1-5, (Dec 2001), pp.227-37, Print ISSN 0960-0760, Online ISSN 1879-1220

Huang, KE; Baber, R; Asia Pacific Tibolone Consensus Group. Updated clinical recommendations for the use of tibolone in Asian women. *Climacteric* Vol.13, No.4, (Aug 2010), pp.317-27, Print ISSN 1369-7137, Online ISSN 1473-0804

Hunter, DJ; Colditz, GA; Hankinson, SE; Malspeis, S; Spiegelman, D; Chen, W; Stampfer, MJ; Willett, WC. Oral contraceptive use and breast cancer: a prospective study of young women. *Cancer Epidemiology, Biomarkers & Prevention* Vol.19, No.10, (Oct 2010), pp. 2496-502, Print ISSN 1055-9965, Online ISSN 1538-7755

Jungheim, ES; Colditz, GA. Short-term use of unopposed estrogen: A balance of inferred risks and benefits. *JAMA* Vol.305, No.13, (Apr 2011), pp.1354-5, Print ISSN 0098-7484, Online ISSN 1538-3598

Katzenellenbogen, JA; O'Malley, BW; Katzenellenbogen, BS. Tripartite steroid hormone receptor pharmacology: Interaction with multiple effector sites as a basis for the cell- and promoter-specific action of these hormones. *Molecular Endocrinology* Vol.10, No.2, (Feb 1996), pp.119-31, Print ISSN 0888-8809, Online ISSN 1944-9917

Kaunitz, AM. Lengthened WHI Follow-up: Postmenopausal Estrogen Therapy. *Journal Watch Women's Health,* (Apr 2011). Print ISSN 1521-4710

Kenemans, P; Bundred, NJ; Foidart, JM; et al. LIBERATE Study Group. Safety and efficacy of tibolone in breast-cancer patients with vasomotor symptoms: a double-blind, randomized, non-inferiority trial. *The Lancet Oncology* Vol.10, No.2, (Feb 2009), pp.135-46, Print ISSN 1470-2045, Online ISSN 1474-5488

LaCroix, AZ; Chlebowski, RT; Manson, JE; Aragaki, AK; Johnson, KC; Martin, L; Margolis, KL; Stefanick, ML; Brzyski, R; Curb, JD; Howard, BV; Lewis, CE; Wactawski-Wende, J; WHI Investigators. Health outcomes after stopping conjugated equine estrogens among postmenopausal women with prior hysterectomy: A randomized controlled trial. *JAMA* Vol.305, No.13, (Apr 2011), pp.1305-14, Print ISSN 0098-7484, Online ISSN 1538-3598

Laya, MB; Larson, EB; Taplin, SH; et al. Effect of estrogen replacement therapy on the specificity and sensitivity of screening mammography. *Journal of the National Cancer Institute* Vol.88, No.10, (1996), pp.643-9, Print ISSN 1052-6773, Online ISSN 1745-6614

Litherland, JC; Stallard, S; Hole, D; et al. The effect of hormone replacement therapy on the sensitivity of screening mammograms. *Clinical Radiology* Vol.54, No.5, (May 1999), pp. 285-288

Lundström, E; Wilczek, B; von Palffy, Z; Söderqvist, G; von Schoultz, B. Mammographic breast density during hormone replacement therapy: Differences according to treatment. *American Journal of Obstetrics & Gynecology* Vol.181, No.2, (Aug 1999), pp. 348-52, Print ISSN 0002-9378, Online ISSN 1097-6868

Lundström, E; Christow, A; Kersemaekers, W; Svane, G; Azavedo, E; Söderqvist, G; Mol-Arts, M; Barkfeldt, J; von Schoultz, B. Effects of tibolone and continuous combined hormone replacement therapy on mammographic breast density. *American Journal of Obstetrics & Gynecology* Vol.186, No.4, (Apr 2002), pp.717-22, Print ISSN 0002-9378, Online ISSN 1097-6868

Lundström, E; Söderqvist, G; Svane, G; Azavedo, E; Olovsson, M; Skoog, L; von Schoultz, E; von Schoultz, B. Digitized assessment of mammographic breast density in patients who received low-dose intrauterine levonorgestrel in continuous combination with oral estradiol valerate: a pilot study. *Fertility and Sterility* Vol.85, No.4, (Apr 2006), pp.989-95, Print ISSN 0010-7824, Online ISSN 1556-5653

Malik, S; Prakash, V. Phytoestrogen and herbs. *Obstetrics Gynaecology Today* Vol.9, No.11, (2004), pp.733-40

Maskarinec, G; Takata, Y; Franke, AA; Williams, AE; Murphy, SP. A 2-Year Soy Intervention in Premenopausal Women Does Not Change Mammographic Densities. *The Journal of Nutrition* Vol.134, No.11, (Nov 2004), pp.3089-94, Print ISSN 0022-3166, Online ISSN 1541-6100

McTiernan, A; Martin, CF; Peck, JD; Aragaki, AK; Chlebowski, RT; Pisano, ED; Wang, CY; Brunner, RL; Johnson, KC; Manson, JE; et al. Estrogen-plus-progestin use and mammographic density in postmenopausal women: women's health initiative randomized trial. *Journal of the National Cancer Institute* Vol.97, No.18, (Sept 2005), pp.1366-1376, Print ISSN 1052-6773, Online ISSN 1745-6614

Moore, RA. Livial: a review of clinical studies. *British Journal of Obstetrics and Gynaecology* Vol.106, Suppl No.19, (Mar 1997), pp.1-21, Print ISSN 0306-5456

Mousa, NA; Crystal, P; Wolfman, WL; Bedaiwy, MA; Casper, RF. Aromatase inhibitors and mammographic breast density in postmenopausal women receiving hormone therapy. *Menopause* Vol.15, No.5, (Jun 2009), pp.875-84, Print ISSN 1072-3714, Online ISSN 1530-0374

Opatrny, L; Dell'Aniello, S; Assouline, S; Suissa, S. Hormone replacement therapy use and variations in the risk of breast cancer. *British Journal of Obstetrics and Gynaecology* Vol.115, No.2, (Jan 2008), pp.169-75, Print ISSN 0306-5456

Persson, I; Thurfjell, E; Holberg, L. Effect of estrogen and estrogen-progestin replacement regimens on mammographic breast parenchymal density. *Journal of Clinical Oncology* Vol.15, No.10, (Oct 1997), pp.3201-7, Print ISSN 0732-183X, Online ISSN 1527-7755

Rosenberg, RD; Hunt, WC; Williamson, MR; et al. Effects of age, breast density, ethnicity, and estrogen replacement therapy on screening mammographic sensitivity and cancer stage at diagnosis: review of 183 134 screening mammograms in Albuquerque, New Mexico. *Radiology* Vol.209, No.2, (1998), pp.511-18, Print ISSN 0033-8419, Online ISSN 1527-1315

Russu, M; Nastasia, S; Mubarak, N; Marin, JA; Hudita, D. Two years of lipid profile monitoring on transdermal estrogens and vaginal micronised progesterone compared to oral route of hormone therapy in healthy postmenopausal women. *Climacteric* Vol.11 No.2, (2008), Abstract Book, pp.232, Print ISSN 1369-7137, Online ISSN 1473-0804

Sala, E; Warren, R; McCann, J; Duffy, S; Luben, R; Day, N. High risk mammographic parenchymal patterns, hormone replacement therapy and other risk factors: a case-control study. *International Journal of Epidemiology* Vol.29, No.4, (Aug 2000), pp.629-636, Print ISSN 0300-5771, Online ISSN 1464-3685

Slanetz, PJ; Grandpre, LE; Yeh, ED; Kopans, DB; Mendel, JB. Effect of tamoxifen on breast tissue density in premenopausal breast cancer. *The Breast Journal* Vol.10, No.1, (Jan-Feb 2004), pp.27-32, Print ISSN 1075-122X, Online ISSN 1524-4741

Son, HJ; Oh, KK. Significance of follow-up mammography in estimating the effect of tamoxifen in breast cancer patients who have undergone surgery. American Journal of Roentgenology Vol.173, No.4, (Oct 1999), pp.905-9, Print ISSN 0361-803X, Online ISSN 1546-3141

Spicer, DV; Ursin, G; Parisky, YR; Pearce, JG; Shoupe, D; Pike, A; Pike, MC. Changes in mammographic densities induced by a hormonal contraceptive designed to reduce breast cancer risk. *Journal of the National Cancer Institute* Vol.86, No.6, (Mar 1994), pp.431-436, Print ISSN 1052-6773, Online ISSN 1745-6614

Thurfjell, E; Holmberg, L; Persson, I. Screening mammography: sensitivity and specificity in relation to hormone replacement therapy. *Radiology* Vol.203, No.2, (May 1997), pp.339-41, Print ISSN 0033-8419, Online ISSN 1527-1315

Ursin, G; Pike, MC; Spicer, DV; Porrath, SA; Reitherman, RW. Can mammographic densities predict effects of tamoxifen on the breast? *Journal of the National Cancer Institute* Vol.88, No.2, (Jan 1996), pp.128-9, Print ISSN 1052-6773, Online ISSN 1745-6614

Vachon, CM; Ingle, JN; Suman, VJ; Scott, CG; Gottardt, H; Olson, JE; Goss, PE. Pilot study of the impact of letrozole vs. placebo on breast density in women completing 5 years of tamoxifen. *Breast* Vol.16, No.2, (Apr 2007), pp.204-10, Print ISSN 0960-9776, Online ISSN 1532-3080

Vogel, VG; Costantino, JP; Wickerham, DL; Cronin, WM; Cecchini, RS; Atkins, JN; Bevers, TB; Fehrenbacher, L; Pajon, ER Jr; Wade, JL 3rd; Robidoux, A; Margolese, RG; James, J; Lippman, SM; Runowicz, CD; Ganz, PA; Reis, SE; McCaskill-Stevens, W; Ford, LG; Jordan, VC; Wolmark, N. National Surgical Adjuvant Breast and Bowel Project (NSABP). Effects of Tamoxifen vs Raloxifene on the Risk of Developing Invasive Breast Cancer and Other Disease Outcomes: The NSABP Study of Tamoxifen and Raloxifene (STAR) P-2 Trial. *JAMA* Vol.295, No.23, (Jun 2006), pp.2727-41, Print ISSN 0098-7484, Online ISSN 1538-3598

Warren, R; Lakhani, SR. Can the stroma provide the clue to the cellular basis for mammographic density? *Breast Cancer Research* Vol.5No.5, (Jul 2003), pp.225-7.

Weitzel, JN; Buys, S; Sherman, WH; Daniels, AM; Ursin, G; Daniels, JR; MacDonald, DJ; Blazer, KR; Pike, MC; Spicer, DV. Reduced mammographic density with use of a gonadotropin-releasing hormone agonist-based chemoprevention regimen in BRCA 1 carriers. *Clinical Cancer Research* Vol.13, No.1-2, (Jan 2007), pp.654-8, Print ISSN 1078-0432

White, E; Velentgas, P; Mandelson, MT; Lehman, CD; Elmore, JG; Porter, P; Yasui, Y; Taplin, SH. Variation in Mammographic Breast Density by Time in Menstrual Cycle Among Women Aged 40–49 Years. *Journal of the National Cancer Institute* Vol.90, No.12, (Jun 1998), pp.906-10, Print ISSN 1052-6773, Online ISSN 1745-6614

Wolfe, JN. Risk for breast cancer development determined by mammographic parenchymal pattern. *Cancer* Vol.37, No.5, (May 1976), pp.2486-92

Wu, AH; Ursin, G; Koh, WP; Wang, R; Yuan, JM; Khoo, KS; Yu, MC. Green tea, soy, and mammographic density in Singapore Chinese women. *Cancer Epidemiology, Biomarkers & Prevention* Vol.134, No.11, (Nov 2008), pp.3358-65, Print ISSN 1055-9965, Online ISSN 1538-7755

11

Evaluation of Mammographic Segmentation and Risk Classification Based on Tabár Tissue Modelling

Wenda He[1], Erika Denton[2] and Reyer Zwiggelaar[1]
[1] *Department of Computer Science, Aberystwyth University, SY23 3DB*
[2] *Department of Radiology, Norfolk & Norwich University Hospital, NR4 7UY*
United Kingdom

1. Introduction

This chapter evaluates recently proposed computer vision methodologies for mammographic segmentation and risk classification based on Tabár tissue modelling (Tabár et al., 2004). The overall objective is to bridge the gap between the theoretical work and their clinical usefulness, with respect to mammographic risk assessment for early breast cancer detection.

In the computer vision literature, there are two lines of scientific investigation into automated mammographic risk assessment. The first focuses on the correlation between mammographic risk and the parenchymal; and the second focuses on the correlation with the overall breast density. In addition, the sensitivity of mammography is significantly reduced by increased breast density which can mask some tumours due to dense fibroglandular tissue (Sickles, 2007). Whilst computer aided mammographic density estimation has been widely investigated as a two-class (i.e. dense and non-dense breast tissue) problem, Tabár breast components composition estimation as a four-class (i.e. nodular, linear, homogeneous densities and radiolucent) problem seems to be overlooked in computer aided mammography. Despite the current standard which is favouring breast density based risk estimation, clinical evidence has shown that the mammographic parenchymal appearances (*e.g.* distribution of various breast tissues) may provide more information than percent density alone (Astley, 2004).

2. Background

Breast density varies from one woman to another. These variations are related to the risk of developing breast cancer; the denser the breast appearance the higher the risk. Mammographic breast density also has a strong association with mammographic screening sensitivity (Couto et al., 2001). Women with high risk density patterns are advised to undergo screening mammography more frequently, and may require additional views (Ciatto et al., 2004).

2.1 Mammographic risk assessment

To assess breast cancer risk, different methods have been developed to measure mammographic density patterns. Two most frequently used classification methods for measuring breast density include Wolfe's mammographic parenchymal patterns (Wolfe, 1976a), and the percentage of the breast densities (Brisson et al., 2003). In Wolfe's scheme, breast cancer risk (i.e. N1, P1, P2 and DY) is assessed based on four mammographic features, including the extent of dense breast tissue in the mammogram, and characteristics of densities (*e.g.* shape and texture). Several other classification methods use parenchymal patterns, including BIRADS classification (i.e. BIRADS I-IV) proposed by the American College of Radiology (American College of Radiology, 2004), and Tabár's scheme (i.e. Tabár I-V) (see Section 2.2). Breast percentage density based scheme, such as Boyd's six-class categories (Boyd et al., 1995) assesses the extent of fibroglandular breast densities in the mammogram, without taking into account the various types of fibroglandular densities, and is expressed by the percentage of the breast showing dense tissue (Boyd et al., 2006).

Experts' subjective appraisal of mammograms can lead to inter and intra observer variability. Automated mammographic risk assessment may be beneficial in a clinical environment, because computerised processes can produce unbiased and consistent results as a means of aiding diagnosis.

2.2 Tabár tissue modelling

In mammographic risk assessment, Tabár *et al.* have proposed a mixture model of four mammographic building blocks, representing nodular, linear, homogeneous and radiolucent tissues (Tabár et al., 2004). These four building blocks compose the normal breast anatomy. Nodular densities mainly correspond to Terminal Ductal Lobular Units (TDLUs). Linear structures correspond to either ducts, fibrous tissue or blood vessels. Homogeneous structureless densities correspond to fibrous tissues which appearance could hide the underlying normal TDLUs and ducts, as well as their alterations due to hyperplastic breast changes. Radiolucent areas are related to adipose fatty tissues, which appear as dark areas in mammographic images (Tabár et al., 2004).

Tabár's tissue modelling is strongly influenced by Wolfe's original work, which divided mammograms, using parenchymal patterns, into four classes (Wolfe, 1976b). For Tabár's risk assessment model, the relative proportions of the tissues belonging to the four building blocks are used to subdivide mammograms into five risk classes. Patterns I to V indicate low to high mammographic risk. The relative composition of the four building blocks, nodular, linear, homogeneous and radiolucent (in that order) are as follows:

- Pattern I has composition [25%, 15%, 35%, 25%]. This pattern is the most common mammographic pattern in premenopausal woman (Tabár et al., 2004). All four building blocks are fairly equally distributed in this pattern. *However, with involution, pattern I will change to either pattern II or pattern III; on the other hand, hormone-replacement therapy often reverses the process of involution. Mammograms of pattern I show normal fibroglandular tissue with partial fatty replacement, and pathological changes can be easily perceived in pattern I, although these breasts can be radiologically "dense"* (Tabár et al., 2004). This pattern is considered the lowest mammographic risk.

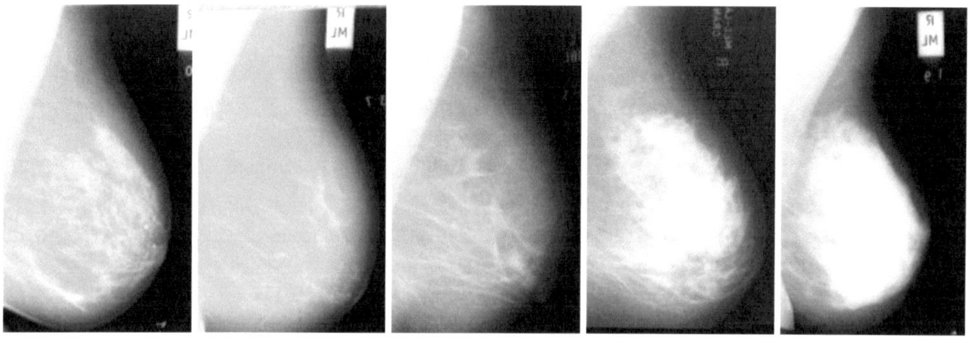

Fig. 1. Mammographic risk patterns with respect to Tabár's risk classification. From left to right showing patterns I-V, corresponding from low to high mammographic risk.

- Pattern II has composition [2%, 14%, 2%, 82%]. This pattern represents the end results of the process of involution, and is characterised by the over representation of radiolucent fatty tissue, which provides excellent background for radiologists to visualise any process of disease (Tabár et al., 2004). Therefore, the detection of abnormalities in mammograms of pattern II is relatively easier.
- Pattern III is similar in composition to pattern II. In this pattern the retroareolar prominent ducts are often associated with periductal fibrosis (Tabár et al., 2004). *Neither of these patterns (i.e. patterns II and III) has nodular densities or diffuse fibrosis; the over representation of radiolucent fatty tissue makes pathological lesions being detected relatively easier on the mammogram* (Tabár et al., 2004).
- Pattern IV has composition [49%, 19%, 15%, 17%]. This pattern is dominated by prominent nodular and linear densities. *Their presence often makes perception of pathological lesions difficult. Also this pattern appears to be resistant to the process of involution* (Tabár et al., 2004). This pattern is considered higher mammographic risk.
- Pattern V has composition [2%, 2%, 89%, 7%]. *This patten is dominated by extensive fibrosis. The overwhelming dominance of this homogeneous, structureless fibrous tissue limits the capabilities of mammography to demonstrate the details of normal anatomy and to reveal small pathological lesions. The radiology reports often state such a mammogram as "extensive fibrosis", which is the only demonstrable feature* (Tabár et al., 2004). This pattern is considered the highest mammographic risk.

Fig. 1 shows example mammographic images with respect to Tabár's five mammographic risk patterns.

3. Literature review

Automatic mammographic risk assessment is expected to play a significant role in the development of breast screening programs and computer-aided detection/diagnosis systems. As mentioned, strong evidence has indicated a correlation between mammographic parenchymal patterns and mammographic risk. This section reviews the existing representative methodologies used for mammographic risk assessment, and related techniques used in computer-aided mammography, with discussions of their merits and shortcomings.

3.1 Textons representation

Recent research has demonstrated the use of textons (Varma & Zisserman, 2004) based mammographic segmentation. Petroudi *et al.* (Petroudi et al., 2003) applied such a technique directly to mammographic images for risk classification. A total of 40 textons were generated via clustering over the filter response space; that is 10 textons for each of the four BIRADS categories. Mammograms were modelled as texton frequency histograms; and by comparing the texton distribution of a mammogram to the learned models using the χ^2 (chi-square) method, the mammographic risk was determined as the BIRADS risk category corresponding to the nearest neighbour model. The evaluation was conducted on a small Oxford database (not publicly available) (Evertsz et al., 2000), the exact agreement with the ground truth was 76% accuracy.

Gong *et al.* (Gong et al., 2006) used a similar statistical approach for mammographic segmentation and risk classification. Instead of using image filtering to obtain the feature vectors, the raw pixel intensities of a $N \times N$ square neighbourhood image patch around a pixel were taken and row reordered, to form a N^2 dimensional feature vector. Four mammographic risk classes were learned based on Wolfe's scheme (Wolfe, 1976b). The same processes used in (Petroudi et al., 2003) were employed for the texton generation, mapping, and risk classification. The Oxford database was again used in the evaluation, and an average classification accuracy of 87% was achieved for 43 randomly selected mammograms.

The statistical texture based classification method (Petroudi et al., 2003) was combined with the multi-vector Markov random fields based approach (Gong et al., 2006) in (Petroudi & Brady, 2006), to perform mammographic density segmentation using textural and structural information based on Wolfe's scheme. At the evaluation stage, 32 mammograms were selected from the Oxford database. The segmentation results show a strong correspondence between the texture variations and the radiologists perception of the different breast density patterns. Despite the use of a small dataset, the breast density segmentation is considered anatomically plausible from an expert radiologist's point of view. It is concluded that texton based statistical modelling is able to generalise the data, and overcome noise issues related to image acquisition and involution of the breast.

Muhimmah *et al.* (Muhimmah et al., 2007) applied a texton related technique for mammographic segmentation based on Tabár's tissue modelling; a texton selection strategy is incorporated using a combination of visual assessment (probability maps) and minimum spanning tree topological information. The initial number of textons (cluster centres) for each tissue type (i.e. nodular, linear, homogeneous and radiolucent) was empirically chosen to be 25. In the texton selection process, the (Euclidean) minimum spanning tree was used to indicate a topologically probable correct connectivity, in high dimensional spaces. Distinct textons (higher discriminative power) tend to be situated towards the outer edges of the tree; common texture, noise and intensity aspects tend to be modelled by textons in the central part of the tree. A visual assessment was employed to determine the appropriate textons, based on the distinctiveness of the textons spatial displacements. Subsequently, a model driven based mammographic segmentation was performed based on the selected textons. A similar approach was applied in (He et al., 2008) with an alternative texton selection process. Both studies have shown realistic segmentation results, but no risk classification experiments were conducted.

3.2 Co-occurrence matrix representation

Arnau *et al.* (Oliver et al., 2007) applied co-occurrence matrices as a means of extracting texture features directly from mammographic images for automatic classification of breast density. A total of 216 features were computed from the co-occurrence matrices and used at the classification stage. The classification accuracy achieved was 78% using a K-Nearest-Neighbour ($K = 3$) classifier over the complete set of the MIAS database (Suckling et al., 1994). Further improvement was made in (Oliver et al., 2008) based on the same methodology, where 10 additional morphological features for the fatty and dense tissue regions were calculated. At the classification stage a combined Bayesian classifier was developed based on the K-Nearest-Neighbour and ID3 Decision Tree; the combined classifier achieved 86% and 77% correct classification for the MIAS and DDSM (Heath et al., 1998) database, respectively. The investigation indicated that classification accuracies can be improved by increasing the combination of the orientations and step intervals of the co-occurrence matrices (as well as additional features). However, the dimensionality of the feature space was increased.

Zwiggelaar *et al.* (Zwiggelaar et al., 2003) introduced set-permutation-occurrence matrices (a set of co-occurrence matrices) as texture feature vectors for texture segmentation of mammographic density. The novel texture modelling approach incorporated spatial information implicitly. The segmentation results were used for automatic mammographic risk assessment. Further improvement was made in (Zwiggelaar & Denton, 2004), where a transportation algorithm (Hitchcock, 1941) was used to select the appropriate set of co-occurrence matrices for the segmentation of mammographic density. It should be noted that using the transportation algorithm can lead to a very computational intensive task (Andoni et al., 2008); therefore it may not be practical for use in a clinical environment.

3.3 Moments representation

As breast cancer develops/progresses, statistical information can be gathered with respect to shape related texture (*e.g.* various types of tumours), which may have significant implication for the staging of breast cancer. Inspired by medical diagnosis of malignant breast cancer, where mammogram masses are classified based on the presence of spicular lesions or diffuse stellate appearance (Tavassoly, 1992); Soares *et al.* (Soares et al., 1998) have shown that moment techniques can be used for shape related texture analysis in digitised mammograms. Specifically, moments were used as features for automated classification of masses in mammography (Soares et al., 1998). It is a logical approach to use moments as shape features for mass classification, because stellate tumours can be characterised as an irregular shape with radiating spicules. A similar technique was used in (Mencattini et al., 2007), and additional texture features (i.e. Haralick features (Haralick et al., 1973)) are incorporated for mass classification. Other types of moments, such as discrete orthogonal Chebyshev moments were employed in (Vyas & Priti, 2007) for malignancy texture classification in digitised mammograms. Eisa *et al.* (Eisa et al., 2009) combined moments with texture features to improve content-based image retrieval in mammography. For an image a set of geometric moments (spatial moments) of different orders are computed, as a global shape descriptor to describe different spatial characteristics of the image intensity distribution. The results indicated that the mixture of features is more discriminative than the texture or moments based features alone. Tucceryan (Tucceryan, 1994) demonstrated the efficiency of obtaining texture features by computing moments over local image regions. A set of features with respect to specific texture properties of the image, can be used to derive a set of spatial moments from the second and third-order moments. The spatial moments based texture features are able to capture orientation sensitive texture properties, as well as more complicated textural properties. Substantial evidence has shown that moments based techniques are feasible for texture modelling in mammography. It is especially true when modelling Tabár's mammographic building blocks (i.e. nodular, linear, homogeneous and radiolucent) as different breast tissue types have texture patterns related to not only their periodicity but also shape features.

3.4 Signatures representation

In the computer vision literature, signature (2D histogram) techniques have been applied to texture analysis in mammography as a means of detection and recognition. Guliato *et al.* (Guliato et al., 2008) used signature of a turning angle function to encode features (*e.g.* roughness, complexity) that characterise the contours of masses for breast tumour classification, because malignant breast tumours and benign masses can be distinguished by their shape characteristics. Zwiggelaar *et al.* (Zwiggelaar, 2002; Zwiggelaar et al., 1999) investigated abnormality (*e.g.* the central mass of spiculated lesions) detection in mammography using scale-orientation signatures. Such signatures have been described as rich descriptors of the neighbourhood around each image pixel, and were used to label structures in images, to classify the pixels into linear structures, blob-like structures or background texture. Therefore, signature techniques are also capable of modelling shape related texture.

4. Materials

The Mammographic Image Analysis Society (MIAS) database consists of 322 mammographic images in mediolateral views. The mammographic films were digitised to 50 micron × 50 micron resolution with a Joyce-Loebl scanning microdensitometer, a device linear in the optical density range 0-3.2 and representing each pixel with an 8-bit word (Suckling et al., 1994). The database provides $\{x, y\}$ image-coordinates for the centre of a circle, its approximate radius (in pixels) that encloses the abnormalities, the information about their severities (i.e. benign and malignant), and the abnormality types (*e.g.* calcification, masses, architectural distortion and asymmetry). Ground truth for breast density is classed into three categories (i.e. fatty, glandular, and dense). The ground truth for mammographic risk classification with respect to Tabár and BIRADS was provided by an expert radiologist.

4.1 Mammographic image patches

In order to facilitate the texture modelling and training process, a set of randomly selected mammograms from the MIAS database were subsampled by an expert mammographic screening radiologist to obtain samples representing Tabár's mammographic building blocks, resulting in patches containing (199) nodular, (253) linear, (70) homogeneous and (121) radiolucent tissue examples (Muhimmah et al., 2007). The collection of patches (See Fig. 2 for examples) covers the various mammographic risk classifications. In addition, for 98 subsampled mammographic patches detailed manual annotations were provided by the same radiologist covering (21) nodular, (27) linear structure, (28) homogeneous and (22) radiolucent regions.

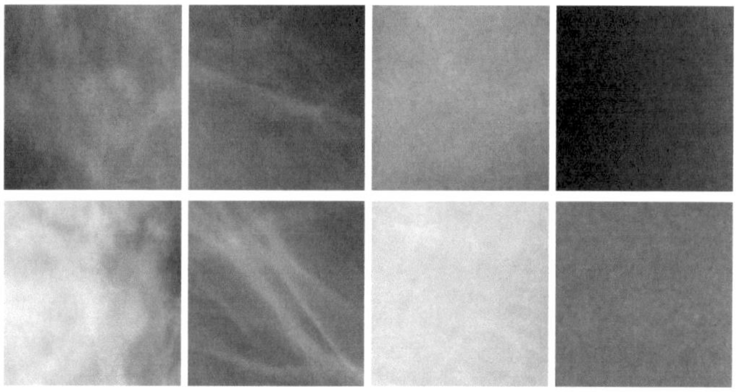

Fig. 2. Subsampled mammographic patches in the top and bottom row belong to the same tissue type. From left to right: nodular, linear, homogeneous, and radiolucent. It should be noted that intra class variation can be seen as large variation in intensity and texture patterns within the same tissue types (Tabár's mammographic building blocks).

5. Methodologies

With respect to mammographic risk assessment using computer vision techniques, there are a few approaches to mammographic segmentation and risk classification using Tabár's scheme, probably because BIRADS is currently more wildly used. However, in computer aided mammography, it is plausible to perform risk assessment based on Tabár's tissue modelling. This section describes two recently developed approaches (He et al., 2009; 2010) for mammographic segmentation and risk estimation based on modelling of various breast components (i.e. nodular, linear, homogeneous and radiolucent tissue) as seen in mammograms. To develop an automated, accurate and repeatable mammographic risk estimation approach based on Tabár's tissue modelling, the major challenge is to segment a given mammographic image according to Tabár's mammographic building blocks, so that the characteristic mixture of these building blocks can be determined, the mammographic risk can be estimated, and the relative proportions of different breast tissue patterns can be quantified. This process is illustrated in Fig. 3.

5.1 Moments based approach

Mammographic segmentation based on spatial moments and prior information (*e.g.* shape related texture features) of mammographic building blocks was investigated. The developed methodology is capable of modelling complex mammographic images and can deal with intra class variation and noise aspects.

5.1.1 Local moments calculation

Moments up to order four are computed within a small local window centred at each pixel (i, j) in an image. This number of moments is capable of capturing sufficient texture geometry information on a low dimensional feature. The coordinates of a local window, with size equal to $W \times W$ (with W being odd so that the pixel (i, j) is at the centre of the window) are normalised to be in the [-1, 1] range. The size of the local window was determined by estimating the position of the first side-band in Fourier space, using Fourier analysis on local patches (Gonzales & Woods, 1992). A series of investigations was conducted on parameter settings based on the full range of anatomical objects; the chosen sampling regions consisted

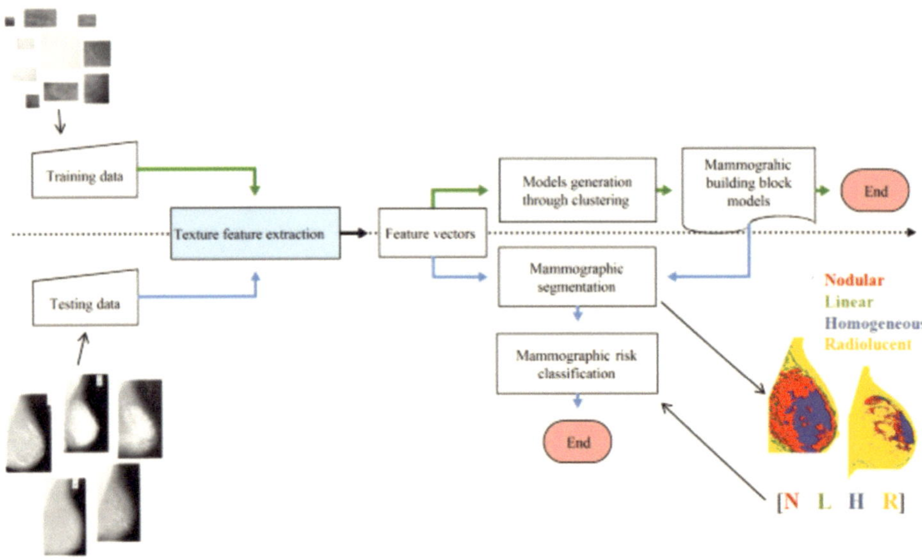

Fig. 3. A flowchart of mammographic segmentation and risk classification methodology. Note that mammographic patches are used at the training (modelling) stage, but full mammographic images are used at the testing (segmentation) stage.

of four square windows with $W = \{7, 13, 33, 63\}$, where the lower limit indicates the feature extraction of small structures (*e.g.* small diameter nodular tissue, thin linear structures), and the upper limit indicates the feature extraction of larger structures. For a pixel (m, n) which falls within the local window $f(m, n)$, the normalised coordinates (x_m, y_n) are defined as $x_m = (m - i)/(W/2)$ and $y_n = (n - j)/(W/2)$. The $(p + q)^{th}$ order moments within the window centred at pixel (i, j) are computed by a discrete sum approximation, which uses the normalised coordinates (x_m, y_n) and is defined as

$$m_{pq} = \sum_{-W/2}^{W/2} \sum_{-W/2}^{W/2} x_m^p y_n^q f(m, n). \tag{1}$$

The lower-order moments $(p + q \leq 1)$ have well defined geometric interpretations. The higher-order moments $(p + q \geq 2)$ give more detailed shape characteristics of the polygons (Tucceryan, 1994). The m_{00} moment is used to identify concentrated density (compact high-intensity) at a point, which can be interpreted as a centre of mass detector. The two first order moments, m_{10} and m_{01} are used to identify image pixels at which the brightness changes sharply or has a discontinuity, which can be interpreted as edge or contrast detectors, respectively. The second order moment m_{11} is used to identify image pixels brightness discontinuities at cross like junctions, which can be interpreted as a cross detector. Local moments are inherently integral-based features, which can reduce the effect of uncorrelated noise. The computation of local moments can be interpreted as a convolution of an image with a set of masks (Tucceryan, 1994), this has been illustrated in Fig. 4. The x and y coordinates of the centre of mass can be computed as $\bar{x} = m_{10}/m_{00}$ and $\bar{y} = m_{01}/m_{00}$ with respect to the normalised coordinates. The central moments are computed for each pixel in the local

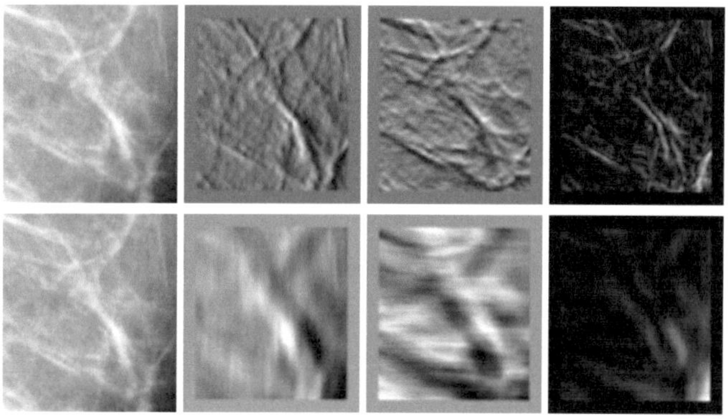

Fig. 4. In both rows, from left to right: original input image, m_{10} moment image, m_{01} moment image, and m_{11} moment image. The local window sizes used were 13 (top) and 63 (bottom).

window, and defined as

$$\mu_{pq} = \sum_{-W/2}^{W/2} \sum_{-W/2}^{W/2} (x_m - \bar{x})^p (y_n - \bar{y})^q f(m,n). \qquad (2)$$

5.1.2 Deriving local image properties

Local image properties are derived from higher order moments (Awcock & Thomas, 1996; Eisa et al., 2009), and determined as

- Variance V_{xy} (spreading) around the centre of mass with respect to the x-axis and y-axis can be computed from normalised 2nd order moments and defined as

$$V_{xy} = \frac{\mu_{11}}{\mu_{00}}, \quad V_x = \frac{\mu_{20}}{\mu_{00}} \quad \text{and} \quad V_y = \frac{\mu_{02}}{\mu_{00}}, \qquad (3)$$

  where V_x and V_y are the variances with respect to the x-axis and y-axis, respectively.
- Skewness (symmetry) around the centre of mass can be characterised by the normalised 3rd order moments and defined as

$$S_x = \frac{\mu_{30}}{(\mu_{00} V_x)^{3/2}} \quad \text{and} \quad S_y = \frac{\mu_{03}}{(\mu_{00} V_y)^{3/2}}. \qquad (4)$$

  Skewness values of $S = 0$, $S < 0$ and $S > 0$ can be interpreted as a Gaussian (normal) distribution, flatter than a normal distribution, and more peaked than a normal distribution, respectively.
- Kurtosis (peakedness) around the centre of mass can be computed from the normalised 4th order moments and defined as

$$K_x = \frac{\mu_{40}}{(\mu_{00} V_x)^2} - 3 \quad \text{and} \quad K_y = \frac{\mu_{04}}{(\mu_{00} V_y)^2} - 3. \qquad (5)$$

  Kurtosis values of $K = 0$, $K < 0$, $K > 0$ and $K < -1.2$ can be interpreted as a Gaussian (normal) distribution, flatter than normal distribution, more peaked than normal distribution, and bimodal (multi-modal) distribution, respectively.

- The ratio of the longest to the shortest distance vectors from the centroid of the local window to its boundaries is considered as a measure of elongation of the region and is defined as

$$elongation = \frac{(\mu_{20} - \mu_{02})^2 + 4{\mu_{11}}^2}{\mu_{00}}. \quad (6)$$

- For elongated objects, the orientation θ (in degrees) of the major ('long') direction with respect to the x-axis is defined as

$$\theta = \frac{1}{2} \arctan \frac{2\mu_{11}}{\mu_{20} - \mu_{02}} \frac{180}{\pi}. \quad (7)$$

For each pixel, 12 attributes were obtained to form a feature vector (i.e. μ_{00}, m_{10}, m_{01}, $\bar{x}$, $\bar{y}$, m_{11}, elongation, θ, S_x, S_y, K_x, K_y) at four scales; this gives a total of 48 features to represent each pixel.

5.1.3 Feature transformation

A nonlinear transformation, namely a hyperbolic tangent function (Caelli & Oguztoreli, 1987), is used to map moment feature M_k with mean $\overline{M}$ to texture feature F_k defined as

$$F_k(i,j) = \frac{1}{L^2} \sum_{(a,b)\in\omega_{ij}} |\tanh(\sigma(M_k(a,b) - \overline{M}_k))|, \quad (8)$$

where ω_{ij} is an $L \times L$ ($L = 55$) averaging window centred at location (i,j), finer textures require a smaller window to detect smaller features, whereas coarser textures require a larger window; the value $\sigma = 0.01$ controls the shape of the logistic function; and $k = \{1, 2, ..., 12\}$. The parameter values were empirically determined to achieve optimal results, and no significant effect on the results were caused by small variations. Fig. 5 shows example moment images before and after transformation; before the nonlinear transformation, the extracted feature images can be interpreted visually as line detection with different orientations and scales. The enhanced feature images show increased differentiation on tissue specific areas. This is expected to lead to more discriminative feature vectors.

5.1.4 Mammographic model generation

Once the transformed feature vectors were obtained, Tabár mammographic building blocks can be modelled using K-means clustering ($K = 10$). A total of 40 cluster centres were generated to represent nodular, linear, homogeneous and radiolucent tissue (10 for each of the four tissue types). The number of cluster centres (K value) was determined empirically based on the assumption that each mammographic building block contains at least 4 to 6 texture primitives according to their visual appearance covering different orientations and scales. A smaller number of cluster centres can lead to less discriminative models; conversely, too many cluster centres can lead to many similar models and redundancy. Visual assessment of the segmentation of mammographic patches using the manual annotations (*e.g.* outlined tissue specific areas) provided by the expert radiologist, was used to heuristically decide the number of cluster centres. It should be noted that there is no rigorous way to determine exactly how many texture primitives should be used for complex texture patterns as seen in mammographic images. However, it is expected that the set of features describes all mammographic anatomical aspects covering lines and regions at various scales.

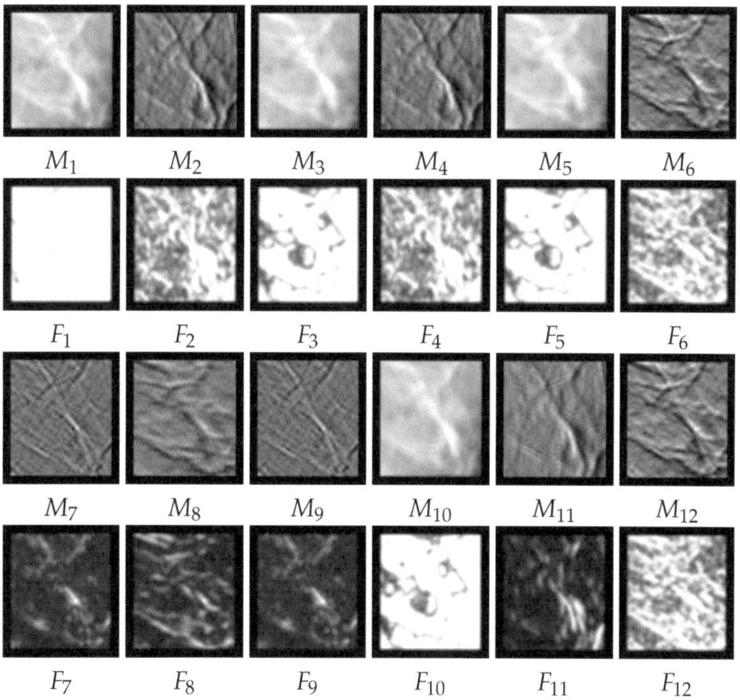

Fig. 5. Example moment images M_k and the corresponding transformed feature images F_k, where $k = 1, 2, ..., 12$. The original linear structure patch is the same as in Fig. 4. The local window $W = 13$.

5.1.5 Model driven segmentation

At the segmentation stage, for each pixel of a mammographic image, the same procedure was applied to obtain transformed feature vectors. For each pixel, the resultant feature vector was compared to the distribution of all the mammographic building block models. A distance weighted K-Nearest-Neighbour (KNN) classifier ($K = 9$) was used, to assign a Tabár mammographic building block class to each pixel, which weighted the contribution of each of the K nearest neighbours with the Mahalanobis distance (Mahalanobis, 1936) to the query point, giving greater weight to closer neighbours to reduce misclassification. The K value was determined empirically, but variation in these parameter indicated robustness.

It is indicated in the computer vision literature that a low intensity background (*e.g.* low or zero grey level values) can lead to meaningless moments (Tucceryan, 1994). When performing texture analysis in mammographic images, this can happen when extracting features of homogeneous regions have high intensity background, and can cause misclassification between high density homogeneous tissue and low density radiolucent tissue. The intensity of homogeneous and radiolucent areas may vary between different mammographic risk patterns; and image normalisation can alter the intensity distribution. To tackle the problem of misclassification due to meaningless moments between high intensity tissues (*e.g.* homogeneous and nodular) and low intensity tissues (*e.g.* radiolucent), a threshold post-processing is incorporated into the classifier to reduce classification errors. This involves reclassifying tissue that is initially classified as radiolucent, but has a very high intensity, to homogeneous or nodular tissue. The threshold values were determined based on prior knowledge of the intensity distribution and variation of mammographic images across the whole MIAS database, and were defined as the mean values of homogenous and nodular tissues from the collection of annotated mammographic patches. It should be noted that in practice, mammographic images may be obtained through different image acquisition processes. Therefore, for an alternative database, the threshold values may need to be re-evaluated using training images obtained from a specific image acquisition process.

5.2 Texture signatures based approach

Mammographic segmentation using texture signatures based methodology was developed in an attempt to incorporate spatial (*e.g.* textons based techniques) and geometric (*e.g.* moments based techniques) texture features.

For each pixel, a texture signature is generated, consisting of three distinct signatures. Each signature of size $L \times L$ was computed within a local window C, to encode different texture features. To ensure computational correctness, it is necessary to use a circular window instead of a more conventional square window to compute local image features. This is because the proposed methodology uses the distance between a pixel and the centre pixel within the sampling window C as a parameter. The upper limit of the parameter is defined as the value of the max distance between these two points, and the radial distance for any point on a circle to the centre has the same max value. A series of investigations was conducted on parameter settings; covering the full range of anatomical objects. Fourier analysis was used to estimate the first side-band (Gonzales & Woods, 1992) which indicated a circular window of 63 pixels in diameter for feature extraction. Whilst, texture signature size was empirically defined in a dimension of 25×25 pixels, which is expected to be able to encode sufficient mammographic features. A significant amount of randomly sampled points ($\geq$ 60,000) from 78 patches (*e.g.* 16 nodular, 22 linear structure, 23 homogeneous and 17 radiolucent) were used at the training stage, regardless of the associated risk class for the original mammogram.

A texture signature is effectively a stack of three 2D histograms, encoding directional texture features (*e.g.* intensity, orientation and elongation variation).

5.2.1 Texture signature - Part I

The first part of a texture signature consists of a cumulative histogram based on the radial distance between the centre pixel and grey-level intensity within the circular window C. The signature's y-axis represents the grey-level intensity, and the x-axis represents the radial distance to the centre pixel. The occurrence values at any $\{x, y\}$ position within the signature are multiplied with the relevant grey-level value. In the grey-level spatial distribution space, the first part of the texture signature represents the roughness of a given circular texture region. The signature configuration varies rapidly with distance in coarse textures (*e.g.* nodular tissues in Fig. 6 A(a)), and steady with distance in fine textures (*e.g.* homogeneous tissues in Fig. 6 C(a)); the accumulated grey-level close to the top of the signature indicates dominance of low intensity pixel presence (*e.g.* radiolucent fatty tissues in Fig. 6 D(a)), whilst the accumulated grey-level close to the bottom of the signature indicates dominance of high intensity pixel presence (*e.g.* homogeneous tissues in Fig. 6 C(a)).

5.2.2 Texture signature - Part II

The second part of a texture signature is a cumulative histogram based on the angle between the tangent at each segment and grey-level intensity within the circular window C. The angle $\theta = 0^\circ$ is defined when a pixel lies on the positive side of the y-axis of the circular window C, and increases counterclockwise. The signature's y-axis represents the grey-level intensity, and the x-axis represents the tangent at segment within the circular window C. The occurrence values at any $\{x, y\}$ position within the signature are multiplied with the relevant grey-level value. The accumulated grey-level values change with the orientation of the linear structures. Visually speaking, texture signature containing many rough peaks indicate the presence of lines (*e.g.* linear structure in Fig. 6 B(b)). A thick band with spreading tendency appearing in the texture signature indicates the presence of nodular tissues (*e.g.* Fig. 6 A(b)). Note that the linear structure patches may contain noise, and have very low contrast between the foreground and background. These issues make it difficult to extract the related linear structure features. However, the spikes as seen in the corresponding signatures indicate the presence of linear structures and their approximate orientations.

5.2.3 Texture signature - Part III

A texture image may contain repeated occurrence of some grey-level configurations, which vary rapidly in fine textures, and slowly in coarse textures (Haralick et al., 1973). These changes can be encoded in co-occurrence matrices. A co-occurrence matrix is constructed by describing how frequently two pixels, separated by a distance d, with grey-level x_1 and x_2 appear. The occurrence of a grey-level configuration may be described by matrices of relative frequencies. The third part of a texture signature is a modified co-occurrence matrix with $d = 1$ and $\theta = 90^\circ$. In this case, the x and y-axes of the signature represent grey-level information. Note that other configurations are possible, but the experimental results indicated variations in these are not significant. Given a pair of values for the x and y-axis, the absolute value of the intensity difference between two pixels is accumulated, and used as the corresponding histogram value. The statistical variations such as the frequency of some grey-level configurations, and the magnitude of the variance of the configurations, can be used to discriminate breast components with different texture properties (*e.g.* Fig. 6 A(c)-D(c)).

5.2.4 Texture signature - combined (I + II + III)

Finally, all the values in the signature were normalised to zero mean and unit variance. The x and y-axes were normalised to L, to ensure the constructed texture signature has a consistent size of $L \times L$ for the three parts. Fig. 6 shows normalised individual signatures, and the resulting combined texture signatures.

5.2.5 Model generation, selection and reduction

Texture signatures generated from the mammographic patches vary due to mammographic images taken under various exposure conditions, linear structures at different orientations, and stochastic parenchymal patterns in nodular tissue. K-means clustering was used to establish initial models based on the assumption that similar models are closely clustered in the feature space, and can be combined through a clustering process. Initially, 30 cluster centres were empirically defined for each mammographic building block. Note

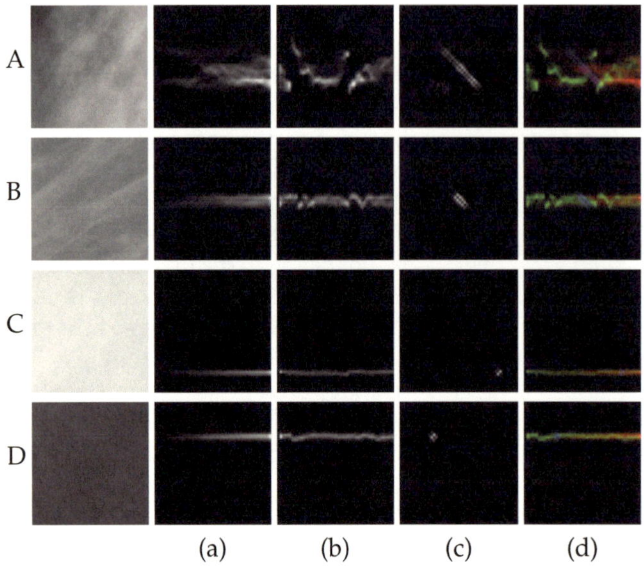

Fig. 6. From top to bottom showing mammographic patches containing nodular, linear structure, homogeneous and radiolucent tissue, respectively. For each row, from left to right showing an mammographic patch, three individual signatures, and the texture signature.

that to predetermine the appropriate number of cluster centres may prove challenging for complicated breast anatomic components. Therefore, the initial number of cluster centres was over-estimated deliberately to facilitate further model selection and reduction. This model generation by clustering resulted in a total of 120 (30×4) cluster centres to represent four types of mammographic building blocks. For each mammographic building block model M_i ($i \in 1, 2, ...120$), a cross voting process was employed to achieve the optimal model subsets, by determining whether it is the nearest neighbour (in a Euclidean sense) of the other models of the same type of mammographic building block. For instance, if model M_i receives votes from a subset of models M_s, it can be interpreted as to be representative of the mammographic building block. Models receiving no or few votes may be outliers, and are removed. The outlier bounds (threshold values) were determined empirically through a series of tests on mammographic patch segmentation. The threshold values for nodular and homogeneous tissue models, were defined as half of the largest standard deviation values of the corresponding models; whereas for linear and radiolucent tissue models, the threshold values were defined as half of the smallest standard deviation values of the corresponding models. As a result, a total of 42 models (i.e. 12 for nodular tissue, 15 for linear tissue, 8 for homogeneous tissue, and 7 for radiolucent tissue) were selected from the initial 120 models.

5.2.6 Model driven segmentation

At the segmentation stage, the same procedure was used to generate a texture signature at each pixel. The resultant texture signatures were compared to the 42 selected mammographic building block models. A distance weighted K-Nearest-Neighbour (KNN) classification ($K = 3$) was used in the Euclidean space, to assign a mammographic building block to each pixel, which weighted the contribution of each of the K nearest neighbours with the distance to the query point, giving greater weight to closer neighbours to reduce misclassification. The

K value was determined empirically, but variation in this parameter indicated robustness, in terms of the number of correctly classified pixels and visual correctness of the segmented tissue specific areas.

6. Evaluation

A comparative evaluation of two mammographic segmentation methods was conducted; evaluation aspects include: 1) mammographic segmentation using the MIAS database, 2) quantitative and qualitatively measurement on the derived tissue compositions from the segmented images, 3) mammographic risk classification based on the tissue compositions, and 4) clinical evaluation of the segmentation to assess the realistic and practical use of the proposed methodologies in a clinical environment.

Customised software was developed for evaluation, to determine the effectiveness of the segmentation methodologies and the potential clinical utilisation for screening mammography or computer aided diagnosis systems. An expert consultant radiologist performed the evaluation by grading a given mammographic segmentation from five available options (i.e. *unacceptable*, *poor*, *acceptable*, *good* and *very good*). In addition, the grades can be combined and referred to as principal grades; the first two grades were considered as *clinically unacceptable* (CUA), the remaining three were considered as *clinically acceptable* (CA)). The statistical results are presented as percentages with respect to the five grades and principal grades, and associated with all Tabár and BIRADS risk classification, as well as the corresponding low and high risk categories. Expert feedback was collected and incorporated in the investigation, including the segmentation accuracy on the tissue specific areas, and the misclassified breast tissues associated with the segmentation methodology issues. All the clinical evaluation aspects were taken into account to conclude the relationship between the risk classification and clinical practice satisfaction.

7. Results and discussion

This section compares the experimental results, and is arranged in line with the evaluation stages described in Section 6. With respect to the mammographic risk classification, both Tabár and BIRADS risk categories are included, in order to facilitate the classification accuracy comparison achieved using existing work in the literature.

7.1 Mammographic segmentation

Mammographic segmentation was performed on the MIAS database using both the moments and texture signatures based methods. Visually speaking, comparing the results achieved using a filter bank based texton approach in (He et al., 2008), the segmentation results produced by both the methods show significant improvements with respect to segmentation on tissue specific areas (see Fig. 7 for examples). In terms of mammographic segmentation accuracy, pectoral muscle and upper abdominal fat are often misclassified as nodular or homogeneous fat within nodular tissues. With respect to segmentation produced using the moments based method, dense areas are often misclassified as radiolucent tissue. Misclassified tissues between nodular and homogeneous classes may be caused by under exposed films. This indicated the lack of discriminative modelling between nodular and homogeneous tissues, as well as between nodular and radiolucent tissues. The segmentation results indicated that both the moments and texture signatures based methods are capable of

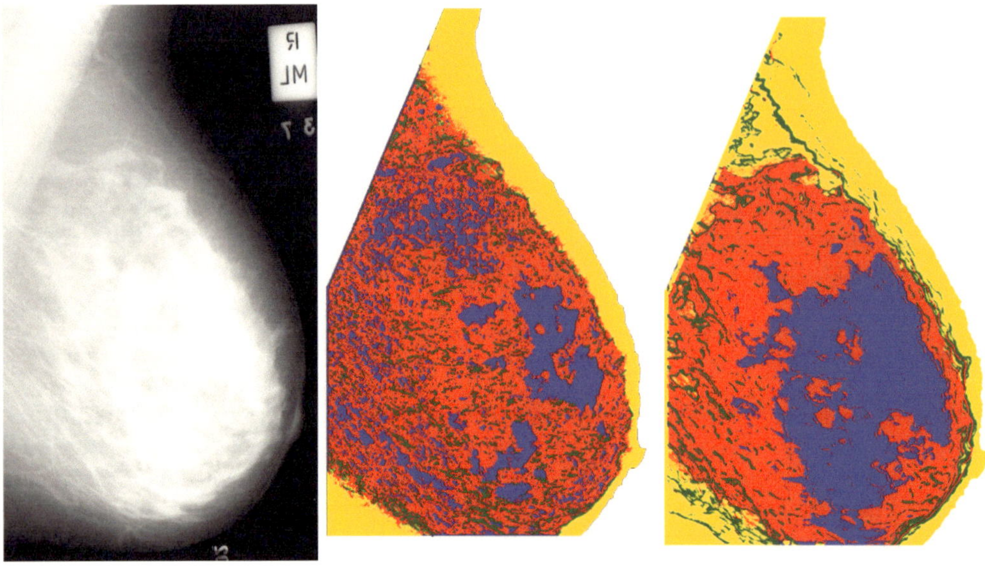

Fig. 7. Example mammographic segmentation. Tabár risk pattern IV; BIRADS risk pattern III. This shows the original mammographic image (left) and the segmentation produced using the moments (middle) and texture signatures (right) based methodologies. The tissue specific areas are: nodular (red), linear (green), homogeneous (blue) and radiolucent (yellow). Note that nodular tissue was over-segmented when using the moments based method.

incorporating shape related texture features during the Tabár tissue modelling. Although the segmentation seems to be less accurate on extremely larger tissue structures. This is due to the use of sampling windows at the feature extraction stage, as the encompassed region for a local window may not be sufficiently large to capture these structures. However, using a larger window can compromise computational efficiency.

With respect to the moments based approach, some of the misclassified pixels within low contrast regions (*e.g.* radiolucent tissue) may be caused by meaningless moments. High intensity homogeneous density regions (*e.g.* homogeneous tissue) can lead to a similar problem. This indicates that the currently used texture features may miss out some discriminative intensity information. It seems necessary to have an approach designed specifically for dealing with intensity variation as seen on digitised mammograms; the zero mean normalisation method used may be too generalised, and can have a direct effect on the model generation. A threshold based post-processing step was used to reduce the false positives using prior knowledge. This process is effective but may require tuning for an alternative database (*e.g.* DDSM (Heath et al., 1998)), because the mammographic image intensity distribution can be affected, due to a different image acquisition process.

7.2 Tissue composition

Table 1 shows the average tissue compositions (the relative proportions of the four mammographic building blocks) achieved, based on the developed segmentation approaches. The differences between the achieved and proposed tissue compositions (see Section 2.2) were measured by the Euclidean distance (ED). The smaller the distance, the more similar

	Nodular	Linear	Homogeneous	Radiolucent	ED
	Tabár pattern I				
Tabár *et al.* (Tabár et al., 2004)	25	15	35	25	
Moment	27±18	15±5	26±17	32±21	11.6
Texture Signature	19±5.8	14±5.3	26±15.6	41±16.3	19.3
	Tabár pattern II/III				
Tabár *et al.* (Tabár et al., 2004)	2	14	2	82	
Moment	14±10	9±4	21±20	56±23	34.7
Texture Signature	10±9.4	12±4.2	10±18.8	68±21.6	18.1
	Tabár pattern IV				
Tabár *et al.* (Tabár et al., 2004)	49	19	15	17	
Moment	38±19	12±5	26±15	24±14	18.4
Texture Signature	44±11.7	11±4.3	13±11.5	32±12.4	17.8
	Tabár pattern V				
Tabár *et al.* (Tabár et al., 2004)	2	2	89	7	
Moment	12±18	4±4	67±27	17±13	26.2
Texture Signature	11±3.3	7 ±4.4	64±11.0	18±10.9	29.2

Table 1. The relative proportions of the four mammographic building blocks and their standard deviations, obtained using the developed mammographic segmentation approaches. The Euclidean distances between the achieved and the tissue compositions proposed by Tabár are shown in the column 'ED'.

the achieved and proposed tissue composition, which also reflects the effectiveness of the developed mammographic segmentation approaches. The ED results indicated that the agreement between the proposed tissue compositions are closer to those achieved using the texture signatures based approach, compared to the moments based approach. The average values of the summations of the variances for the risk patterns for the moments and texture signatures based approach are 90.9 and 84.4, respectively. The smaller average total variance can be linked to the satisfactory classification accuracies achieved using texture signatures based mammographic segmentation (see Sections 7.3 and 7.4).

The resultant tissue composition from each segmented mammographic image was used as a feature vector for the risk classification. With respect to Tabár based risk classification, the feature vectors were compared with Tabár models (risk patterns) and using a Euclidean distance. Whilst BIRADS based risk classification was performed using leave-one (mammographic image)-out methodology. The ground truth was provided by an expert radiologist.

7.3 Risk classification - Tabár's risk categories

In the computer vision literature, very few investigations were conducted with respect to mammographic risk classification based on Tabár's risk categories. These classification results are summarised and compared in Table 3. Details of risk classification confusion matrices are shown in Table 2. A direct comparison with existing mammographic risk assessment methods is not always possible due to differences in databases choice. Jamal *et al.* (Jamal et al., 2006) used 122 mammograms, 30, 21, 20, 27 and 24 for patterns I to IV, respectively. It should be noted that the used dataset is much smaller than the MIAS database and not publicly

	Tabár	Automatic I	II/III	IV	V	Accuracy
Truth	I	33	36	41	9	28%
	II/III	14	66	5	8	71%
	IV	22	6	50	2	63%
	V	1	1	5	21	75%

	Tabár	Automatic I	II/III	IV	V	Accuracy
Truths	I	102	16	1	0	86%
	II/III	7	61	11	14	66%
	IV	9	5	65	1	81%
	V	1	4	0	23	82%

Table 2. Classification confusion matrices based on Tabár risk categories. With respect to the moments based method (left), total accuracy was 53%, $\kappa = 0.36$ (fair agreement). Total accuracy for low and high categories was 71%, $\kappa = 0.40$ (fair agreement). With respect to the texture signatures (right) based method, total accuracy was 78%, $\kappa = 0.7$ (substantial agreement). Total accuracy for low and high categories was 86%, $\kappa = 0.69$ (substantial agreement).

Database		I	II/III	IV	V	$Total_1$	Low	High	$Total_2$
	Jamal (Jamal et al., 2006)	73	90	74	88	83			
MIAS	He_M (He et al., 2009)	28	71	63	75	53	70	72	71
	He_TS (He et al., 2010)	86	66	81	82	78	88	82	86

Table 3. Mammographic risk classification based on Tabár's risk categories. He_M (He et al., 2009) used the developed moments based approach. He_TS (He et al., 2010) used the developed texture signatures based approach.

available. Therefore, the distribution over the inter and intra class variations are expected to be different, which can effect the classification results. With respect to the classification achieved using the developed methods, strong correlation was found between the precision of mammographic segmentation and subsequent risk classification. The segmentation accuracy is particular critical when performing risk classification based on Tabár tissue modelling, because tissue compositions for the segmented images were used as feature vectors at the risk classification stage. The results show overall good classification accuracies, except for Tabár pattern I results achieved using the moments based approach. It should be noted that the latter aspect can be linked to previous published results (Muhimmah et al., 2006), which indicated that Tabár Patten I shows weak correlation between BIRADS and Tabár risk models.

7.4 Risk classification - BIRADS risk categories

The majority of the investigations with respect to mammographic risk classification are based on BIRADS risk categories. The classification results are summarised and compared in Table 5. Details of risk classification confusion matrices are shown in Table 4. Note that Bovis *et al.* (Bovis & Singh, 2002) used mammographic images for 377 patients from DDSM. Petroudi *et al.* (Petroudi et al., 2003) used 132 images selected from the Oxford database (not publicly available). A direct comparison with Oliver *et al.* (Oliver et al., 2008) is probably the closest option. Oliver *et al.* (Oliver et al., 2008) shows divergence in the opinion of three expert radiologists, and the inter observer variation is dealt with using the majority vote from the three radiologists. In the experiment, the consensus classification was used and superior classification was achieved. It should be noted that the inter observer variation seems to be minimised by using the consensus classification. In (Oliver et al., 2008) the MIAS database was used, and 82% correct classification was obtained based on 'expert C' (Oliver et al., 2008).

		Automatic				
	BIRADS	I	II	III	IV	Accuracy
Truth	I	65	10	1	11	75%
	II	0	71	21	11	69%
	III	0	18	63	12	68%
	IV	0	5	7	25	68%

		Automatic				
	BIRADS	I	II	III	IV	Accuracy
Truths	I	41	5	10	3	70%
	II	1	68	12	5	79%
	III	0	11	101	29	71%
	IV	0	0	5	29	85%

Table 4. Classification confusion matrices based on BIRADS risk categories. With respect to the moments based method (left), total accuracy was 70%, $\kappa = 0.59$ (moderate agreement). Total accuracy for low and high categories was 79%, $\kappa = 0.58$ (moderate agreement). With respect to the texture signatures (right) based method, total accuracy was 75%, $\kappa = 0.75$ (substantial agreement). Total accuracy for low and high categories was 87%, $\kappa = 0.74$ (substantial agreement).

Database		I	II	III	IV	$Total_1$	Low	High	$Total_2$
MIAS	Oliver(A) (Oliver et al., 2008)	80	60	67	46	66	79	77	79
	Oliver(B) (Oliver et al., 2008)	89	75	69	59	75	92	77	85
	Oliver(C) (Oliver et al., 2008)	91	84	89	73	86	89	94	91
	He_M (He et al., 2009)	47	73	87	65	73	73	91	83
	He_TS (He et al., 2010)	70	79	72	85	75	79	94	87
DDSM	Oliver (Oliver et al., 2008)	55	88	77	69	77	89	79	84
	Bovis (Bovis & Singh, 2002)					71			97
Oxford	Petroudi (Petroudi et al., 2003)	91	64	70	78	76	91	94	

Table 5. Mammographic risk classification based on BIRADS risk categories and comparison with existing work using: Oliver(A), the segmentation and feature extraction are described in (Karssemeijer, 1998); Oliver(B), the segmentation approach is described in (Karssemeijer, 1998) and the feature extraction is used in (Oliver et al., 2008); Oliver(C), both the segmentation and feature extraction are described in (Oliver et al., 2008). He_M (He et al., 2009) used the developed moments based approach. He_TS (He et al., 2010) used the developed texture signatures based approach.

It should be noted that the proposed mammographic segmentation is specifically designed with respect to Tabár mammographic parenchymal patterns, and has fundamental differences to density based segmentation described in (Oliver et al., 2008). In this study, BIRADS risk classification was obtained to facilitate the classification performance evaluation when using different risk models (i.e. Tabár and BIRADS), as using mammographic parenchymal patterns rather than density information alone.

7.5 Clinical evaluation

The risk classification results (see Tables 2 and 4) show both Tabár and BIRADS related aspects, and indicate that the results for the high risk mammograms are significantly better than those for the low risk mammograms; also show a clear correlation between the Tabár and BIRADS results, and is in line with previous published work (Muhimmah et al., 2006). Table 6 shows the segmentation assessment results with respect to the moments based approach, in which for Tabár II/III and BIRADS I, at about 41%, are especially low. The other individual classes are encouraging, with the Tabár V and BIRADS IV classes reaching 100% clinical acceptable results (note that the number of samples for Tabár V or BIRADS IV are small). The segmentation assessment results based on all the images in both Tabár and BIRADS risk categories indicate the robustness of the segmentation methodology, as both achieved 70% clinical acceptable results. Further details of the segmentation assessment results can be found in Table 7, where the classification results were correlated from the risk classification confusion matrices (see Tables 2 (left) and 4 (left)) and Table 6. Table 7 shows the number of cases which were correctly classified (*e.g.* all the cases on the diagonal of a confusion matrix) in the original mammographic risk assessment experiment against the clinical evaluation of the segmentation results. The results for mammographic risk assessment that were misclassified by a single, two and three classes (*e.g.* +/- 1 to II would be I and III) are also included (it should be noted that the misclassification by three classes only happens with a few cases).

The same clinical satisfaction study was conducted with respect to the results obtained using the texture signatures based approach. Table 8 shows the segmentation assessment results, which for Tabár I, at 42% is especially low; however, the clinical acceptable rate increases as the risk level gets higher which is particularly encouraging, with the Tabár V class reaching over 96% clinical acceptable results. For BIRADS risk classes I-III, the clinical acceptable rate for segmentation is about 55%; and 92% clinical acceptable rate is achieved for BIRADS risk class IV. It should be noted that the number of samples for Tabár V or BIRADS IV are small. These aspects are also clear for the low/high risk results, which show a relative better clinical acceptable result for high risk categories, where the high risk results based on Tabár risk modelling are promising as over 76% are considered clinically acceptable results. Further details of the segmentation assessment results can be found in Table 9, where the classification results from the risk classification confusion matrices (see Tables 2 (right) and 4 (right)) and Table 8 are correlated. Table 9 shows the number of cases which were correctly classified (*e.g.* all the cases on the diagonal of a confusion matrix) in the mammographic risk assessment experiments against the clinical evaluation of the segmentation results.

The results in Tables 7 and 9 show strong correlations between the level of correctness of the mammographic risk classification and clinical evaluation of the segmentation results: i.e. correct mammographic risk classification is associated with the *good* and *very good* segmentation results, whilst misclassification by two and three classes is mainly associated with the *poor* and *unacceptable* segmentation results. This is especially true for the BIRADS based results, where the (almost) correctly classified images each have a clinical acceptable segmentation, as opposed to only a few cases that are in the clinical acceptable segmentation category for the images associated with significant misclassification for mammographic risk assessment.

The decreasing accuracies in all the individual low risk classes indicates the precision of the segmentation are not all up to the clinical standard. From a clinical point of view, a mathematically correct risk classification (possibly due to a robust classifier), does not necessarily reflect the correctness of the associated segmentation. Even though, the clinical evaluation still show strong positive correlations with the automatic risk classification. It is interesting to see the accuracies increased in the individual high risk classes. This seems to indicate an apparent difference between the way in which radiologists perceive mammographic risk and how the segmentation performs, with especially the segmentation of radiolucent tissues maybe less robust. However, in associating the correct classification

Tabár	♯images	U	P	A	G	VG	CA
I	119	8%	11%	14%	29%	37%	81 %
II/III	93	32%	24%	8%	9%	28%	44 %
IV	80	5%	20%	14%	20%	41%	75 %
V	28	0%	0%	4%	43%	54%	100 %
Low	212	19%	17%	11%	20%	33%	65 %
High	108	4%	15%	11%	26%	44%	81 %

BIRADS	♯images	U	P	A	G	VG	CA
I	59	35%	24%	11%	8%	22%	41 %
II	86	20%	20%	9%	19%	32%	60 %
III	141	4%	14%	15%	26%	41%	82 %
IV	34	0%	0%	3%	38%	59%	100 %
Low	145	26%	22%	10%	14%	28%	52 %
High	175	3%	12%	13%	29%	43%	85 %

Table 6. Clinical grading of satisfaction regarding the mammographic segmentation using the moments approach. 'U', 'P', 'A', 'G' and 'VG' denote *unacceptable*, *poor*, *acceptable*, *good* and *very good*, respectively.

Tabár	♯images	U	P	A	G	VG	CA
correct	251	8%	17%	13%	25%	37%	75%
+/- 1	40	28%	20%	3%	5%	45%	53%
+/- 2	28	46%	4%	7%	18%	25%	50%
+/- 3	1	0%	0%	0%	100%	0%	100%
(LH) correct	275	9%	16%	12%	24%	39%	75%
(LH) incorrect	45	42%	13%	4%	13%	27%	44%

BIRADS	♯images	U	P	A	G	VG	CA
correct	239	9%	18%	10%	23%	40%	73%
+/- 1	63	14%	8%	16%	25%	37%	78%
+/- 2	15	80%	13%	7%	0%	0%	7%
+/- 3	3	33%	67%	0%	0%	0%	0%
(LH) correct	279	9%	16%	12%	24%	38%	75%
(LH) incorrect	41	46%	12%	5%	10%	27%	41%

Table 7. Clinical grading of satisfaction regarding the mammographic segmentation using the moments approach, associated with the level of the automatic mammographic risk classification. 'LH' denotes low and high risk.

Tabár	♯imgs	U	P	A	G	VG	CA
I	119	31%	27%	16%	18%	8%	42 %
II/III	93	23%	19%	22%	22%	14%	58 %
IV	80	14%	17%	24%	25%	20%	69 %
V	28	4%	0%	14%	21%	61%	96 %
Low	212	27%	24%	19%	19%	11%	49 %
High	108	11%	13%	21%	24%	31%	76 %

BIRADS	♯imgs	U	P	A	G	VG	CA
I	87	19%	24%	29%	25%	3%	57 %
II	103	28%	16%	20%	17%	19%	56 %
III	93	24%	24%	16%	21%	15%	52 %
IV	37	2%	6%	21%	21%	50%	92 %
Low	190	24%	19%	23%	22%	12%	57 %
High	130	20%	20%	17%	21%	22%	60 %

Table 8. Clinical grading of satisfaction regarding the mammographic segmentation using the texture signatures approach. 'U', 'P', 'A', 'G' and 'VG' denote *unacceptable*, *poor*, *acceptable*, *good* and *very good*, respectively.

Tabár	♯imgs	U	P	A	G	VG	CA
correct	170	11%	21%	22%	24%	22%	68%
+/- 1	68	16%	13%	22%	29%	20%	71%
+/- 2	72	50%	21%	14%	8%	7%	29%
+/- 3	10	40%	40%	20%	0%	0%	20%
(LH) correct	227	11%	20%	22%	26%	21%	69%
(LH) incorrect	93	48%	20%	13%	10%	9%	32%

BIRADS	♯imgs	U	P	A	G	VG	CA
correct	224	16%	16%	23%	25%	20%	68%
+/- 1	68	24%	32%	13%	15%	16%	44%
+/- 2	17	58%	24%	12%	0%	6%	18%
+/- 3	11	82%	9%	9%	0%	0%	9%
(LH) correct	253	15%	19%	22%	25%	19%	66%
(LH) incorrect	67	48%	25%	10%	7%	10%	27%

Table 9. Clinical grading of satisfaction regarding the mammographic segmentation using the texture signatures approach, associated with the level of automatic mammographic risk classification. 'LH' denotes low and high risk.

of mammograms with the assessment of the segmentation results, Tables 7 and 9 indicated a strong correlation between these. This might also indicate that the tissue modelling associated with the segmentation process, does not cover the various tissue classes appropriately, and there might be a strong non-linear component in the expert assessment (*e.g.* when the areas of dense tissues are significant, the areas of linear and radiolucent tissues play a less important role), which is not present in the tissue modelling approach. It is encouraging to see in Table 8 that the accuracies increased in high risk classes (i.e. Tabár V and BIRADS IV). It is also interesting to notice small classification variation between BIRADS risk classes I, II and III. This may indicate that the presented methodology is able to discriminate mammographic parenchymal patterns well based on Tabár risk modelling, but less robust in extracting density information (possible due to meaningless moments) based on BIRADS risk models.

The major concerns from the radiologist who participated in the clinical evaluation include: 1) pectoral muscle and upper abdominal fat are often misclassified as nodular or homogeneous fat within nodular tissues; 2) radiolucent areas are often misclassified as dense tissue; and 3) misclassification of tissue between nodular and homogeneous classes may be caused by (apparently) under exposed films. Clinical feedback indicates some segmentation methodology issues, such as the lack of discriminative modelling between nodular and homogeneous tissues, as well as between nodular and radiolucent tissues. Intra and inter observer variation is noticeable; however, it should be noted that the issue of experts' subjective assignment of risk classification can be dealt with using multiple readers, and the majority risk classifications can be considered as 'final', but full evaluation of these aspects is seen as future work. For automatic mammographic risk assessment based on parenchymal pattern segmentation, it is encouraging that applying advanced machine learning techniques achieves an improved risk classification. At the same time, a follow up clinical evaluation linking the risk classification and segmentation should be emphasised, to ensure a realistic practical usage in a clinical environment.

8. Conclusions

It is possible to use computer vision techniques to estimate the mammographic risk based on the composition of the four mammographic building blocks (i.e. nodular, linear, homogeneous and radiolucent) described by Tabár. The presented results using the moments and texture signatures based methodologies show realistic segmentation on tissue specific areas, improved estimation of the relative proportions of the four building blocks when compared to the results achieved using the textons based approach (He et al., 2008), and leading to promising mammographic risk classification results. The presented clinical evaluation, both quantitative and qualitative, confirms that the technical evaluation of an automatic risk classification based on Tabár's tissue modelling, may not reflect the effectiveness of the methodology in a clinical setting. Even though, the clinical evaluation still shows strong positive correlations with the automatic risk classification. In addition, the segmentation assessment is linked to the correct/incorrect automatic mammographic risk classification, which indicated that anatomically correct segmentation results tend to lead to correct mammographic risk estimation. However, work towards a robust automatic mammographic segmentation using Tabár's tissue modelling is still on going; such an application is expected to be useful as a means of aiding radiologists' diagnosis and treatment planning prior to biopsies.

9. References

American College of Radiology (2004). *Breast Imaging Reporting and Data System BI-RADS*, 4th edn, Reston, VA: American College of Radiology.

Andoni, A., Indyk, P. & Krauthgamer, R. (2008). Earth mover distance over high-dimensional spaces, pp. 343 – 352.

Astley, S. M. (2004). Computer-based detection and prompting of mammographic abnormalities, *The British Journal of Radiology* 77: S194–S200.

Awcock, G. J. & Thomas, R. (1996). *Applied image processing*, McGraw-Hill, Inc., Hightstown, NJ, USA.

Bovis, K. & Singh, S. (2002). Classification of mammographic breast density using a combined classifier paradigm, *In 4th International Workshop on Digital Mammography*, pp. 177–180.

Boyd, N. F., Byng, J. W., Jong, R. A., Fishell, E. K., Little, L. E., Miller, A. B., Lockwood, G. A., Tritchler, D. L. & Yaffe, M. J. (1995). Quantitative classification of mammographic densities and breast cancer risk: results from the canadian national breast screening study, *Journal of the National Cancer Institute* 87: 670–675.

Boyd, N. F., Martin, L. J., Sun, L., Guo, H., Chiarelli, A., Hislop, G., Yaffe, M. & Minkin, S. (2006). Body size, mammographic density, and breast cancer risk, *Cancer Epidemiology Biomarkers & Prevention* 15(11): 2086–2092.

Brisson, J., Diorio, C. & Mâsse, B. (2003). Wolfe's parenchymal pattern and percentage of the breast with mammographic densities: Redundant or complementary classifications?, *Cancer Epidemiology Biomarkers & Prevention* 12(8): 728–732.

Caelli, T. & Oguztoreli, M. N. (1987). Some tasks and signal dependent rules for spatial vsion, *Spatial Vision* 2: 295 – 315.

Ciatto, S., Visioli, C., Paci, E. & Zappa, M. (2004). Breast density as a determinant of interval cancer at mammographic screening, *Journal of Medical Screening* 90: 393–396.

Couto, E., Harrison, D., Duffy, S., Myles, J., Sala, E., Warren, R., Day, N., Luben, R. & Chen, H. (2001). Estimation of disease progression parameters from case-control data: application to mammographic patterns and breast cancer natural history, *Journal of Epidemiology and Biostatistics* 6: 235–242.

Eisa, M., Refaat, M. & El-Gamal, A. F. (2009). Preliminary diagnostics of mammograms using moments and texture features, *International Journal on Graphics, Vision and Image Processing* 9: 21–27.

Evertsz, C. J. G., Bodicker, A., Hendricks, J. H. C. L., Karssemeijer, N., Weber, U., Bohnenkamp, S., Dechow, D., Berger, L., Woudend, S. van., Brady, M., Holland, R. & Peitgen, H. -O. (2000). High throughput soft-copy reading system for digital mammography in nationwide european screening mammography programs: Requirements and first solutions, *Proceedings of the Radiographic Society of North America*.

Gong, Y. C., Brady, M. & Petroudi, S. (2006). Texture based mammogram classification and segmentation, *8th International Workshop on Digital Mammography*, pp. 616–625.

Gonzales, R. & Woods, R. (1992). *Digital Image Processing*, Addison-Wesley Publishing Company.

Guliato, D., de Carvalho, J. D., Rangayyan, R. M. & Sergio, S. A. (2008). Feature extraction from a signature based on the turning angle function for the classification of breast tumors, *Journal of Digital Imaging* 21: 129–144.

Haralick, R. M., Shanmugam, K. & Dinstein, I. (1973). Textural features for image classification., *IEEE Transactions on Systems, Man and Cybernetics*, Vol. 3, pp. 610–621.

He, W., Denton, E. R. E. & Zwiggelaar, R. (2009). Mammographic segmentation based on mammographic parenchymal patterns and spatial moments, *9th International Conference on Information Technology and Applications in Biomedicine*, pp. 1–4.

He, W., Denton, E. R. E. & Zwiggelaar, R. (2010). Mammographic image segmentation and risk classification using a novel texture signature based methodology, *Lecture Notes in Computer Science*, Vol. 6136, Springer, pp. 526–533.

He, W., Muhimmah, I., Denton, E. R. E. & Zwiggelaar, R. (2008). Mammographic segmentation based on texture modelling of Tabár mammographic building blocks, *Lecture Notes in Computer Science*, Vol. 5116, pp. 17–24.

Heath, M., Bowyer, K., Kopans, D., Kegelmeyer, W. P., Moore, R., Chang, K. & MunishKumaran, S. (1998). Current status of the digital database for screening mammography, *International Workshop on Digital Mammography*, pp. 457–460.

Hitchcock, F. L. (1941). The distribution of a product from several sources to numerous localities, *Journal of Mathematical Physics* 20: 224 – 230.

Jamal, N., Ng, K. H., Looi, L. M., McLean, D., Zulfiqar, A., Tan, S. P., Liew, W. F., Shantini, A. & Ranganathan, S. (2006). Quantitative assessment of breast density from digitized mammograms into Tabár's patterns, *Physics in Medicine and Biology* 51(22): 5843–5857.

Karssemeijer, N. (1998). Automated classification of parenchymal patterns in mammograms, *Physics in Medicine and Biology* 43(2): 365–378.

Mahalanobis, P. C. (1936). On the generalised distance in statistics, *In Proceedings National Institute of Science* 2: 49 – 55.

Mencattini, A., Salmeri, M., Lojacono, R., Rabottino, G. & Romano, S. (2007). Mammographic image analysis for tumoral mass automatic classification, *European Conference on Medical Physics*, Castelvecchio Pascoli, Italy.

Muhimmah, I., He, W., Denton, E. R. E. & Zwiggelaar, R. (2007). Segmentation based on textons and mammographic building blocks, *Medical Image Understanding and Analysis*, pp. 228–232.

Muhimmah, I., Oliver, A., Denton, E., Pont, J., Perez, E. & Zwiggelaar, R. (2006). Comparison between Wolfe, Boyd, BI-RADS and Tabár based mammographic risk assessment, *8th International Workshop on Digital Mammography*, pp. 407–415.

Oliver, A., Freixenet, J., Marti, R., Pont, J., Perez, E., Denton, E. R. E. & Zwiggelaar, R. (2008). A novel breast tissue density classification framework, *IEEE Transactions on Information Technology in BioMedicine* 12: 55–65.

Oliver, A., Lladó, X., Martí, R., Freixenet, J. & Zwiggelaar, R. (2007). Classifying mammograms using texture information, *Medical Image Understanding and Analysis*, pp. 223–227.

Petroudi, S. & Brady, M. (2006). Breast density segmentation using texture, *8th International Workshop on Digital Mammography*, pp. 609–615.

Petroudi, S., Kadir, T. & Brady, M. (2003). Automatic classification of mammographic parenchymal patterns: A statistical approach, *Engineering in Medicine and Biology Society*, Vol. 1, pp. 798–801.

Sickles, E. A. (2007). Wolfe mammographic parenchymal patterns and breast cancer risk, *American Journal of Roentgenology* 188(2): 301–303.

Soares, L. M., Conci, A. & Vianna, A. D. (1998). Automated classification of masses on mammography, *International Symposium on Computer Graphics, Image Processing and Vision*, pp. 1–4..

Suckling, J., Parker, J., Dance, D., Astley, S., Hutt, I., Boggis, C., Ricketts, I., Stamatakis, E., Cerneaz, N., Kok, S., Taylor, P., Betal, D. & Savage, J. (1994). The mammographic images analysis society digital mammogram database, *in* Dance, Gale, Astley & Gairns (eds), *Excerpta medica. International Congress Series*, Vol. 1069, Elsevier, pp. 375–378.

Tabár, L., Tot, T. & Dean, P. B. (2004). *Breast Cancer: The Art And Science Of Early Detection With Mamography: Perception, Interpretation, Histopatholigic Correlation*, 1 edn, Georg Thieme Verlag.

Tavassoly, F. A. (1992). *Pathology of the Breast*.

Tucceryan, M. (1994). Moment-based texture segmentation, *Pattern Recognition Letters* 15(7): 659–668.

Varma, M. & Zisserman, A. (2004). Unifying statistical texture classification frameworks, *Image and Vision Computing* 22: 1175 – 1183.

Vyas, V. S. & Priti, P. R. (2007). Malignancy texture classification in digital mammograms based on Chebyshev moments and logpolar transformation, *ICGST International Journal on Bioinformatics and Medical Engineering* 7: 29 – 35.

Wolfe, J. N. (1976a). Breast patterns as an index of risk for developing breast cancer, *American Journal of Roentgenology* 126(6): 1130–1137.

Wolfe, J. N. (1976b). Risk for breast cancer development determined by mammographic parenchymal pattern, *Cancer* 37: 2486–2492.

Zwiggelaar, R. (2002). Image processing in scale-orientation space, *British Machine Vision Conference*, pp. 203–212.

Zwiggelaar, R., Blot, L., Raba, D. & Denton, E. R. E. (2003). Set-permutation-occurrence matrix based texture segmentation, *Iberian Conference on Pattern Recognition and Image Analysis*, pp. 1099–1107.

Zwiggelaar, R. & Denton, E. R. E. (2004). Optimal segmentation of mammographic images, *International Workshop on Digital Mammography*, pp. 751–757.

Zwiggelaar, R., Taylor, C. J. & Rubin, C. M. E. (1999). Detection of the central mass of spiculated lesions - signature normalisation and model data aspects, *Information Processing in Medical Imaging*, Springer-Verlag, London, UK, pp. 406–411.

12

MIDAS – Mammographic Image Database for Automated Analysis

Fabiano Fernandes[1], Rodrigo Bonifácio[2], Lourdes Brasil[3], Renato Guadagnin[4] and Janice Lamas[5]
[1]*Instituto Federal de Brasília,*
[2]*Computer Science Department, University of Brasília,*
[3]*Post-Graduate Program in Biomedical Engineering, University of Brasília at Gama*
[4]*Post-Graduate Program in Knowledge Management and Information Technology, Catholic University of Brasília,*
[5]*Janice Lamas Radiology Clinic*
Brazil

1. Introduction

The CAD (Computer-aided Diagnosis) systems have been experiencing an exponential growth in the last decades. Since the mid-1980s of time consuming film digitization on a limited number of cases to its present status on large FFDM (Full-Field Digital Mammography) databases Giger et al. (2008). The current usage of CAD systems has brought about the need for breast cancer detection and classification efficient mechanisms. The CAD algorithm sensitivity and specificity are influenced directly by database characteristics such as image size, lesion distribution, and location of the lesion, biopsy results, BI-RADS™ classification and consensus opinion Giger et al. (2008). The use of existing mammographic databases such as DDSM (Digital Database for Screening Mammography) Heath et al. (2001b) with female patients mainly from the Massachusetts General Hospital mammography program with the statistics of 56.18% (whites), 30.34% (unknown races), 2.06% (asians), 4.12% (blacks), 6.55% (spanish surnames), 0.75% (other races), to tune the CAD algorithms can avoid time consuming and expensive achievement but on the other hand can bias the CAD algorithm to a women population not reflected in the image database, therefore causing a ripple effect in the results Heath et al. (2001a). In the current study, we developed an unprecedented database, the MIDAS (Mammographic Image Database for Automated Analysis) covering a sample of Brazilian women population - such sample is primarily based on FFDM images and whereas the population are not divides by races but on the other hand are formed by a Brazilian unique mixing of indian south american, africans and european populations along with genetic informations. The initial database contains about 600 digital mammograms including two images of each breast, associated patient information, masses, architectural distortion, special cases, calcification, associated findings, breast composition, BI-RADS™ categories and overall impression. The MIDAS mammogram images are obtained from the Janice Lamas Radiology Clinic.

1.1 The Janice Lamas Radiology Clinic

The Janice Lamas Radiology Clinic is a image diagnosis clinic founded in 1993 that performs mammography exams for diagnosis and screening, general ultrasound exams, biopsies and bone densitometry exams. The medical director is Janice Magalhães Lamas, M.D., PhD. and her clinical interests include all aspects of breast imaging and intervention including digital mammography with the use of CAD systems, breast ultrasound and dedicated breast MRI (Magnetic Resonance Imaging). Dr. Janice's expertise is requested regularly to speak at brazilian meetings dedicated to radiology. In addition to her speaking engagements, she has developing scientific research in breast cancer area and bone mineral density evaluation, and she has published numerous articles on breast imaging. The clinic is also certified by the Brazilian College of Radiology and Image Diagnosis.

1.2 The MIDAS approach

Unlike the others well established mammographic databases, the MIDAS database approach includes all mammogram images covering a sample of Brazilian women population, patient genome sequences data, open source image processing algorithms available, open access and open collaborative environment. The unique characteristic of containing mammographic imagens covering the Brazilian women population associated with the genomic sequences is a brand new inovation that enhances the scientific research and discovery. The MIDAS database also welcomes existing and new open source image processing algorithms that allow the tests and validation on the mammographic images. All scientists worldwide can participate in the MIDAS database with new algorithms and tools in a open and collaborative environment.

1.3 Motivation

The lack of a genuine brazilian mammographic database and the collaborative and open use and test of new CAD tools are the main motivation for MIDAS project. The MIDAS database is an innovative database that integrates phenotypes - the mammograms and increasingly their respective genotypes, according to patient biopsy and subsequent genome sequencing. Complex studies for mapping the effect of distinct genes and their results in the mammogram image pattern will enable the discovery of unknown cancer genes and help to understand their pathways of behavior. The BI-RADS™ assessment for all mammograms is an additive factor that enables better algorithm tunning.

2. Mammography screening

Screening to control chronic-degenerative diseases and diseases of neoplastic nature can be defined as an examination on asymptomatic women, carried out with the intent of classifying them as likely or unlikely to develop the disease Morrison (1992). The goal of screening is to define women with preclinical disease as positive and women without preclinical disease as negative. The result from the screening - positive or negative definition - reflects the efficacy of the test in showing the signs of preclinical disease as well as correct interpretation of the findings. An error, i.e. a positive definition for someone without preclinical disease, or a negative definition for someone with the condition, can result from either low test efficacy or incorrect interpretation Morrison (1992) Barratt et al. (2005). In a screening test, the matter that is under investigation is the capability to correctly distinguish between diseased and healthy individuals. Thus, to be certain that the disease is really present or absent, it is frequently the case that elaborate, expensive or risky tests, such as biopsies, surgical exploration or autopsy, must be carried out Fletcher et al. (1996). Estimation of diagnostic test validity in relation to a standard is certified by knowing the proportions of right diagnoses (true positives and true negatives) and wrong ones (false positives and false negatives) Pereira (2000b). In relation to mammography, the level of logic validity is based on consensus and expert opinions Basset et al. (1994) Fletcher & Elmore (2005), and evaluations of accuracy are based on histopathological examination of the suspected lesion. The ability of mammography to define women with preclinical diseases as positive is referred to as its sensitivity. If measured, it is around 78 to 85%. The specificity of the test is its ability to define as negative women who do not have the disease. If measured, it should be greater than 90% Morrison (1992). The sensitivity of the screening test is a determining factor for disease control programs and the specificity directly influences the costs and feasibility of the screening program Morrison (1992) Fletcher et al. (1996) Basset et al. (1994). All mammograms must be categorized as one of the alternatives below Basset et al. (1994):

- True Positive: when cancer is diagnosed within a one-year period after a biopsy is recommended.
- True Negative: when no cancer is diagnosed up to one year after a normal mammogram is reported.
- False Positive: when no cancer is diagnosed within a one-year period after an abnormal mammogram from which a biopsy is recommended; and when there is a benign finding in a biopsy within a one-year period after an abnormal mammogram Fletcher & Elmore (2005).
- False Negative: when cancer is diagnosed within a one-year period after a normal mammogram is reported.
- Positive Predictive Value: refers to diferent rates, depending on the definition of false positive. Based on an abnormal screening examination: 5-10%. Based on a recommendation for biopsy or surgery: 25-40%. Based on the result from biopsies carried out at the clinic, from an abnormal mammogram or from another diagnostic procedure carried out on the breast, after a negative mammogram Basset et al. (1994); Sickles et al. (2002).

2.1 Prevalence and incidence

A program for early detection and treatment is applicable in the case of diseases that present a preclinical phase that cannot be diagnosed but is detectable, and for which the treatment must offer some advantage over late treatment. The proportion of the population that has a detectable preclinical phase is the prevalence. Prevalence depends, primarily, on the incidence rate of the condition, which, in turn, reflects the action of causal factors. Prevalence varies with the length of the preclinical phase. The greater the duration is, greater the proportion of affected women will be Pereira (1996) Fletcher & Wagner (1996). Finally, prevalence depends on whether or not previous screenings have been carried out Morrison (1992). A screening test with greater sensitivity can detect tumors at the beginning of this phase. Prevalence represents the stock of cases, new and old, and usually expresses damage of a chronic nature Fletcher & Wagner (1996), such as breast cancer. Incidence is recognized as the most important measurement in epidemiology because it relates to the dynamics of occurrence of a certain event, over a specific observation time Pereira (1996). For example, among asymptomatic women with previous mammography examinations that showed no suspicious signs of malignancy, it informs how many of them present subclinical breast cancer. Incidence is one of the determining factors of prevalence Fletcher & Wagner (1996). In reality, estimation of both incidence and prevalence enables better knowledge of the situation and consequently enables adequate orientation of actions, with regard to implementation of new programs. Implementation of an early detection program for breast cancer by means of mammography must be preceded by studies that can evaluate the existing situation. Thus, before the possible beneficial impact on mortality of early detection of malignant but asymptomatic lesions can be measured, it is important to ascertain the breast cancer rate among women who are apparently healthy Warren-Burhenne (1996). In Brazil, there are few reports measuring the distribution of malignant lesions detected by mammography screening among asymptomatic women Koch (1998) Lamas & Pereira (1998).

2.2 Factors related to detection of breast cancer

Several factors influence early detection through mammography or delayed diagnosis of malignant lesions among apparently normal women. Among these are the biological behavior of the tumor, the type of equipment used, the technical ability of those who produce and interpret the mammograms, the time interval between subsequent screenings and the existence of a quality control program at the clinic Koch (1998) Sickles (1995). Technological advances and greater knowledge of breast radiology have made it possible to identify breast lesions with suspected malignancy earlier on Haus et al. (1990) Taplin et al. (2004). The biological behavior of the tumor, which is inherent to each type of neoplasia and the relationships established with the human organism, is one of the factors that determine the length of the subclinical phase and hence favors or hinders early detection Taplin et al. (2004). Length bias The growth speed of the tumor is a crucial matter, since the likelihood of cancer detection during the preclinical phase depends on the length of this phase. There is little chance of detecting tumors with a short preclinical phase before they are manifested clinically. On the other hand, tumors with preclinical phases that last for years are more likely to be discovered through screening Morrison (1992). Studies have shown that the mean duration of the preclinical phase of cases diagnosed through mammography screening tends to be longer than the mean duration of the cases that are routinely identified through the appearance of symptoms Warren-Burhenne (1996) and that tumors that grow slowly during the preclinical phase have the same behavior when symptomatic. Thus, screening would tend to detect tumors with good prognoses, as a result of the bias from the length of the preclinical phase, regardless of how much time is gained through early detection or how much benefit comes from early treatment Black & Ling (1990) Zelen (1976). Prevalence bias Breast cancer has faster growth among young women and slower growth among older women. It can remain in the subclinical phase for an indeterminate length of time Moskowitz (1986). Research has indicated that older women, aged over 50 years, have a longer preclinical phase of the disease, compared with women aged less than 50 years, in whom the biological behavior of the tumor is more aggressive Baker (1982) Kopans (1995).

However, mammography examinations contribute towards elevation of the prevalence rate, through indiscriminately detecting tumors with progressive growth and those that may remain without clinical manifestation for indeterminate periods Morrison (1992). This constitutes a distortion, known as prevalence bias, caused by excessive representation of long-duration cases and can occur in cross-sectional studies Fletcher & Wagner (1996). Although these distortions can contribute towards high prevalence of subclinical lesions, these rates have not been shown to be statistically different at ages of under and over 50 years in Brazil, which seems to indicate that prevalence bias is not the only explanation for the measurement found, especially among younger women Lamas & Pereira (1998). These results are consistent with some other studies that observed that there was no drastic change in cancer rates from under to over the age of 50 years Kopans (1995). Since the duration of subclinical disease is greater among older women, it is expected that there will be a proportionally greater number of affected women over the age of 50 years, represented by the prevalence rates. The data from Brazil do not show statistically significant differences in the proportion of women with cancer at the subclinical phase, at an initial stage of development, comparing women under and over 50 years of age (P = 0.52). These studies in Brazil indicate that detection of a greater number of tumors with slow growth and good prognostics is not, in this particular case, related to age Lamas (2000). By contributing towards a higher detection rate for malignant tumors, mammography includes lesions of different biological behavior with distinguishing between them: lesions with rapid growth and those with slow development Liff et al. (1991). The latter may remain asymptomatic for an indeterminate period of time Feuer & Wun (1992). Regarding the frequency of malignant lesions, there is a consensus that the tumor prevalence rate among asymptomatic women is between six and ten cases per thousand women screened using mammography Warren-Burhenne & Burhenne (1992) . Rates lower than this standard range indicate that mammography is adding little to clinical examination of breasts, in which case there could be many false negatives. In Brazil, the data indicate high rates, in relation to population-based studies Vizcaíno et al. (1998) Thurfjell & Lindgren (1994). The measurements are similar to the rates observed by some institutional studies in developed countries at the beginning of their early detection programs Warren-Burhenne & Burhenne (1992) Maya et al. (2006). Proposals that are feasible for the public healthcare system need to be drawn up from quantitative data on disease frequency. Such knowledge provides information on the magnitude and importance of the damage to health Pereira (1996). The decision on whether it is appropriate or not to begin mammography screening as a secondary prevention strategy must be based on relevant measurements of breast cancer frequency among asymptomatic women.

2.3 Limitation of epidemiological studies

The variation in morbidity due to breast cancer, for which there are multiple causal factors and some are still little known, limits epidemiological studies, even in populations with similar characteristics, which may invalidate comparisons between studies Pereira (1996) Sickles (1992). It has to be borne in mind, regarding the distribution of morbidity, that the disease affects women who are less favored in socioeconomic terms. As also seen with infectious diseases, chronic-degenerative diseases and especially the advanced stages of breast cancer are a greater scourge among less favored individuals. In Brazil, breast cancer is diagnosed at advanced stages: more than 70 % of the cases are found in stages II to VI, a situation in which the chances of cure are much smaller Maya et al. (2006) . According to data from the National Cancer Institute, the estimated risk is 50 cases of this disease for every 100,000 women, including asymptomatic and symptomatic patients. It is therefore important to have public policies that establish nationwide strategies for diagnosing breast cancer, such as the breast cancer information system (SISMAMA) that has been implemented since 2008, and the Mammography Quality Program. There are still flaws in screening for breast cancer in Brazil. SISMAMA has not yet been implemented in all public clinics, and the quality control program is not available in all clinics. However, some important tools for implementing public policy regarding breast cancer prevention have been developed within the Brazilian National Health System (SUS) . Higher social classes are better informed about primary and secondary prevention mechanisms, as well as having greater access to health services, which influences morbidity Pereira (1996). This unequal access is in addition to unequal quality at diagnostic centers, which is another condition responsible for the distorted picture of morbidity. Screening attracts people who are more conscious about healthcare, among whom the disease tends to take a more favorable clinical course, regardless of the time gained through early detection or the benefit of timely treatment. This might not have such an influence on the results if all members of the population were screened. One important point that also influences the measurement of prevalence is sample selection. Samples composed by women who seek medical care or are referred to a clinic dedicated to mammography do not constitute a random sample, but rather, attendance of the demand. One important point to be discussed in investigations from which the aim is to extrapolate the results is the use of randomization for selection of elements for a sample. Age, social levels and ethnic characteristics are factors associated with diseases, and thus, comparisons between groups with different characteristics will be biased. Differences relating to sample selection The institutional nature of some studies may introduce distortions and be responsible for differences in rates, because they constitute attendance of the demand. To minimize this sample selection bias, one option is to use women who undergo mammography examinations as periodic routine examinations required by the companies in which they work. The higher breast cancer prevalence rate at clinics that attend to the demand Sickles (1995) is explained by the greater incidence of the disease in such groups, which expresses the presence of causal factors Kopans (1995) Lopes et al. (1996). There is evidence that women exposed to a greater number of risk factors more frequently seek specialized clinics, which explains some of the differences in the frequencies of breast cancer between populations Smith (1993) Colditz et al. (1993). Women from privileged economic classes are exposed to a greater number of risk situations, such as stress, lack of breastfeeding, use of hormones, nulliparity and use of oral contraceptives, as well as other factors that are associated with greater risk of developing other diseases, including diets rich in animal fat and alcohol, among other factors Koch (1998) MacPherson et al. (1983). These conditions are associated with greater risk of having breast cancer, and personal antecedents of this neoplasia are the factor most strongly related to the disease Roubidoux et al. (1997). Atypical hyperplasia, also known as a high-risk type of lesion, is similarly strongly associated, and it has been estimated that the risk of developing in situ carcinoma or subsequent invasive carcinoma is five to ten times greater Dupont et al. (1993) Boecker et al. (2002). To affirm the causal relationship between the two events, it is necessary to rule out alternative explanations, in order to avoid erroneous conclusions. Confounding factors are one of these explanations, and therefore should be a matter of constant concern during the development of a study: in its planning, in the statistical analysis and in the interpretation of the results Pereira (1996). Differences relating to the existence of previous screenings Another factor that influences the results is the absence of previous screenings. In Brazil, unlike what is found in developed countries, there is no early detection program on a national scale, and only recently has there been any encouragement for asymptomatic women to undergo periodic mammography examinations, as a form of secondary prevention. This explains the small percentage of women who had already undergone screening in the samples of studies published on this issue. The yield from a screening test decreases proportionally as it is repeated among a given group of people Chamberlain (1984). Prevalence studies may differ in relation to the proportion of the women in the sample who had already undergone mammography examinations, since the prevalence measurement includes both new and old cases. The length bias that was described by some English authors Smith (1995) Fletcher & Wagner (1996) may contribute to the high cancer rate found in samples composed predominantly by older women, a situation in which the tumor presents slow growth. Length bias is greater among the cases detected through the initial screening, a situation in which the prevalence of the tumors in this phase is predominantly represented by lesions that have long preclinical phases. As the control examinations are repeated, especially at short intervals, the distribution of the preclinical phase duration among the detected subclinical cases becomes more similar to the distribution routinely diagnosed in a population that did not undergo screening. In these circumstances, it could be that the length bias is less important in the selection of the prognostic factors. However, if the preclinical phase of the disease is short, continuous screenings would be necessary to reach the objective of detecting lesions at these stages Morrison (1992). Differences relating to the measurement procedures Methodological errors can give false interpretations to the results. Although the possibility is smaller, the prevalence rate may be altered by distortions introduced into the measurement of the procedures. Thus, in frequency investigations, these measurement biases appear when the findings obtained from the sample data differ from those of the population, simply through measurement problems. These deviations can occur when the event lacks definition, when poorly elaborated questionnaires are used, when uncalibrated low-resolution equipment is used, and when several data-gatherers, interviewers or observers are used, among other situations Pereira (2000a) Sickles et al. (2002). Randomized clinical trials are considered to be the standard of excellence, because they produce direct and unequivocal evidence to explain a cause-effect relationship between two events Pereira (1996).

2.4 Comparative efficacy of self-examination, clinical breast examination and mammography in screening for breast cancer

There is no way to separate the effects of mammography and clinical breast examination in relation to reduction of mortality. Even with technological advances, there are no reasons to suppose that a mammography screening program, in isolation from a clinical examination, would have the same effect as when they are combined. Since the time of the first randomized study, which began in 1960, a time at which the equipment used had low resolution, mammography has been shown to be 1.6 times more sensitive than the examination carried out separately, for mammography screening Baker (1982). It is important to emphasize that clinical examination has been recommended as an early detection method for breast cancer . Clinical breast examination is important for ruling out clinically evident tumors that do not have a corresponding mammographic configuration. Although mammography is more sensitive than clinical breast examination, 9% of tumors are only detected through palpation Baker (1982). Nevertheless, with the technological evolution of mammography equipment, some studies have observed a decrease in the rate of negative mammograms among patients with palpable nodules . In these cases, non-visualization of the tumor through mammography may result from a variety of factors, but in most cases is a consequence of increased breast density Tabár (1993) Kopans et al. (1996) Fitzgerald (2001). There is evidence that clinical breast examination contributes towards the screening of suspected lesions Baker (1982) Miller et al. (1992) Chu & Connor (1991). However, on a larger scale, it does not have an impact relating to decreased risk of mortality due to cancer Humphrey et al. (2002).

3. Database image and data aquisition

All images are generated in DICOM format by digital mammography equipments at Janice Lamas Radiology Clinic. At first moment the MIDAS database is available to general public containing about 100 mammograms and 600 images and an image sample is shown in Figure 1. The high definition images are available under personal request, after MIDAS team approval. The low definition images are freely available to the general public. All

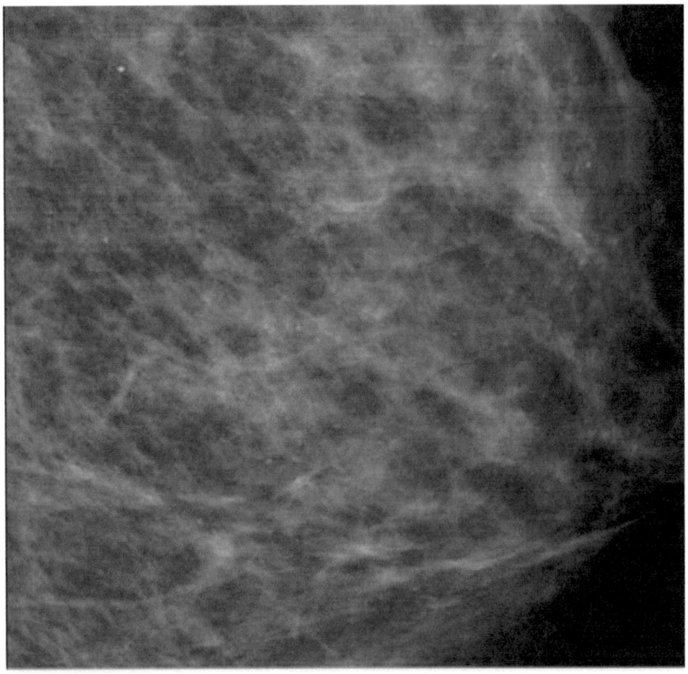

Fig. 1. A Reduced Example of MIDAS Dicom Image

the genomic information will be extracted after breasts biopsies and genomic sequencing at Genome Analyser Illumina GAIIx. All the images are obtained from the following equipment:

- Equipment: Mammomat Inspiration
- Voltage: 23 Kv to 35 Kv
- Large focus: 0.3 mm and small focus: 0.15 mm
- Pixel size: 85 μm and 70 μm
- Samples per pixel: 1
- Image size 2082 x 2800
- Bits allocated: 16
- Photometric interpretation: monochrome-1

The DBMS open source object-relational database system PostgreSQL is used to receive the MIDAS database. The database conceptual modeling is presented in Figure 2.

4. Software tools

We provide a Web application (Midas-Web) for getting access to the database content and for manipulating the database' images through several digital image processing algorithms. Therefore, at a high-level point of view, Midas-Web is both an information system (with CRUD[1] operations for the mammography database) as well as an extensible environment for

[1] In the software community, CRUD operations correspond to basic functions that allow users to create, update, delete, and query data base content

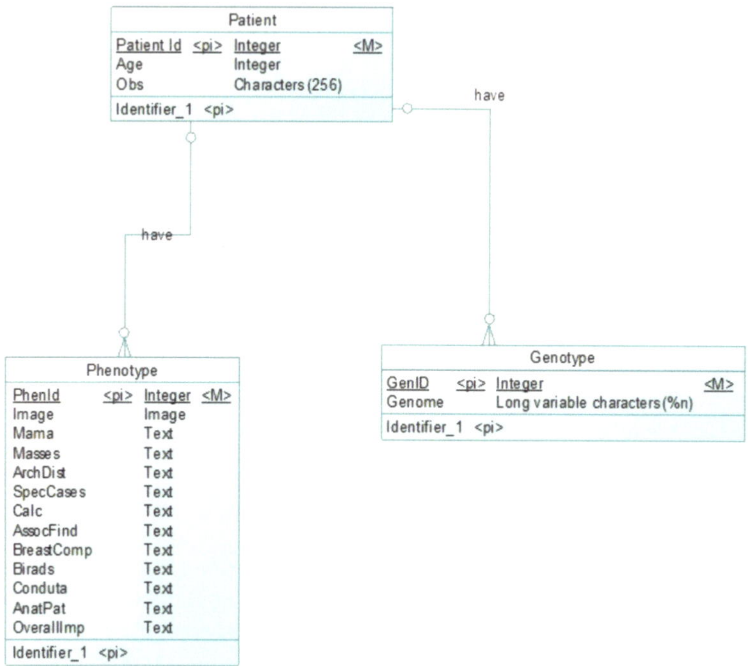

Fig. 2. MIDAS Database Conceptual Model

playing with and experimenting digital image processing algorithms. Some goals have been used to guide the design and development of Midas-Web:

- Basic mechanisms for authentication and authorization.
- Rapid application development cycle
- Extensible set of algorithms for digital image processing and interpretation

We realize three main usage profiles within the Midas-Web context. First, medical practitioners might access Midas-Web to compare, through analogy, their diagnosis with existing BI-RADS™ diagnosis present in the Midas database. Such a comparison is useful for the purpose of increasing diagnosis' confidence and teaching. Another usage profile also corresponds to medical practitioners who want to share their findings, introducing new cases in the Midas database. This usage profile is restricted by security policies, and Midas administrators analyze all requests related to the introduction of new cases before making them publicly available. Another usage profile correspond to researchers that want to apply their algorithms for digital image processing and interpretation using the Midas database images.

In the remaining of this section we detail some design decisions related to the Midas-Web architecture, database schema and extensibility support for introducing new algorithms for digital image processing.

4.1 Architecture

Midas-Web follows a standard web based architecture, in which the system is decomposed in three principal layers Fowler (2002): the *web layer*, the *business logic layer* and the *data source layer*. The web layer provides the presentation logic, processing the user requests, calling business operations, and forwarding to a proper *graphical user interface* (GUI) component that should render the results of a user request.

The business logic layer is responsible for implementing the application transactional logic, which usually involves algorithms for data validation and calculation. Actually, in the case of Midas-Web, this layer is really thin, once Midas-Web basically provides CRUD operations to the Midas database. Nevertheless, it is still important to consider this layer in the architecture, since it increases the opportunities for code reuse.

Finally, the data source layer provides an abstraction over the underlying Midas database system. Therefore, components in this layer implement services for accessing the database, in such a way that we are able to evolve the database (for instance from a SQL based to a non SQL database) without breaking the upper layers of the Midas-Web application.

Figure 3 presents the logical view of the Midas-Web architecture. In order to reduce the development cycle, and also motivated by the low complexity of the business logic, we developed Midas-Web using Grails Smith & Ledbrook (2009). Grails (or Groovy on Rails) is a web development framework focused on productivity gains through the confluence of the Groovy dynamic language Koenig et al. (2007) and the prevalence of *source code structure convention* over *configuration through XML files*. The main components of a Grails application are: (a) the Controller Classes, which handle user inputs and forward business' responses to suitable views; (b) The Grails Server Pages, which renders the graphical user interface; (c) the Service Classes, which implements the business logic; and (d) the Domain Classes, which describe the domain concepts and implement the data access layer to perform queries and updates into the database.

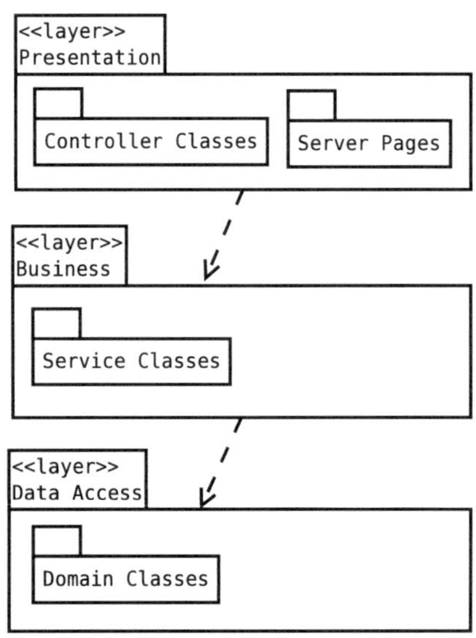

Fig. 3. Logical view of the Midas-Web architecture

Grails offers a powerful integration with the Java language, so that it is possible to call existing Java code from Grails, as well as Grails applications are package as a standard Java Web Archive (WAR) and, as such, they could be deployed into Java Application Servers (like Tom

Cat or JBOSS). The Java integration is useful because it supports the extensible architecture for digital image processing, one of the contributions of Midas-Web (Section 4.3).

4.2 Database structure

The Midas database schema was influenced, at a great extent, by the BI-RADS™ classification D'Osri et al. (2003). For this reason, each patient, whose identity must be preserved, might be associated with different studies (representing clinical cases or investigations); and each study has properties such as:

- breast composition
- histology
- date in which the exam was conducted
- the main findings of the exam

In addition, and also according to the BI-RADS™ classification, each study must provide a *lesion description* and at least four images (mammograms). Table 1 shows the attributes used to describe a lesion, whereas Figure 4 presents part of the Midas database schema.

Attribute	Domain
Assessment	Negative Benign Finding Probably Benign Finding Suspicious Abnormality Highly Suggestive of Malignancy
Mass Shape	Round Oval Lobulated Irregular Architectural distortion
Mass Margins	Circumscribed Microlobulated Obscured Ill Defined Spiculated
Calcification Type	Punctate Amorphous Pleomorphic Round and Regular Luscent Center Fine Linear Branching
Calcification Distribution	Clustered Linear Segmental Regional Diffuse

Table 1. Attributes of a lesion description according to BI-RADS™

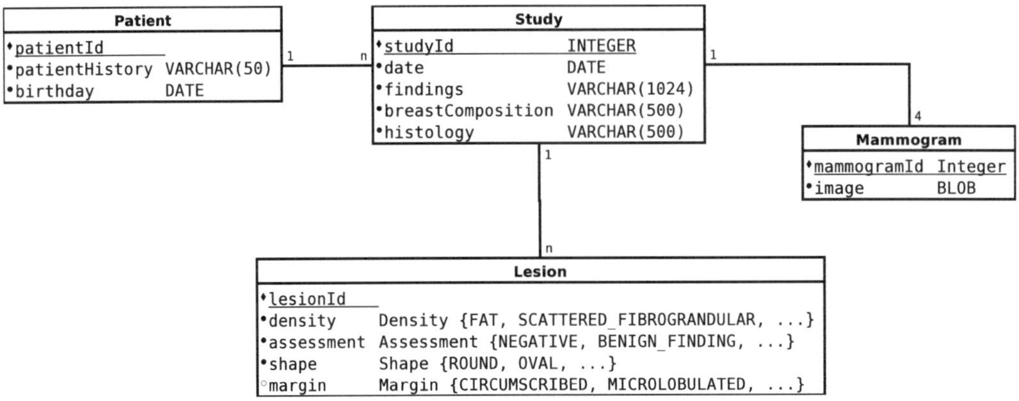

Fig. 4. Core relations of the Midas database schema

4.3 Extensibility support and collaborative environment

The MIDAS project group is a collaborative effort between Instituto Federal de Brasília, University of Brasília Computer Science Department, University of Brasília Post-Graduate Program in Biomedical Engineering, Catholic University of Brasília Post-Graduate Program in Knowledge Management and Information Technology and Janice Lamas Radiology Clinic. The MIDAS open and collaborative environment allows the users and developers to participate in the research process. After MIDAS team validating all new image processing algorithms, artifical intelligence tools, pattern recognition tools, and new findings can be added to MIDAS database.

5. Assessment and automated analysis

5.1 MIDAS assessment

The MIDAS database and application has been tested during the startup process and along its business life. The Information Technology infrastructure provided to MIDAS includes a Cyber Data Center host service and hardware usage monitoring. All the image processing algorithms and pattern recognition tools has been tested by Janice Lamas Radiology Clinic experts and reports will be generated in order to improve the software tools.

5.2 Automated analysis: Breast cancer image assessment using an adaptive network-based fuzzy inference system

The MIDAS database provides an ANFIS model algorithm Fernandes et al. (2010) for automated analysis through every 600 mammogram images. This algorithm presents an ANFIS model for a CAD (Computer Aided Diagnosis) prototype system to classify calcifications in mammograms, in order to aid the medical expert in breast cancer diagnosis. The proposed model embodies pre processing, detection, features extraction and classification phases, which proved adequate for the study domain, obtaining similar results to the indicated in the literature. This approach might be complemented with micro calcification shape analysis and image segmentation techniques. The neuro fuzzy ANFIS model, utilized in the mammogram ROI's classification phase, reached a maximum accuracy rate of 99.75% with Mini MIAS database and now can be tested with MIDAS database. This can be observed in the results presented by Fernandes et al. (2010), when the sigmoidal membership function

PSIGMF was chosen, with the training algorithm in back propagation, employing small values for epochs. The other membership functions analyzed also showed satisfactory accuracy rates, however they were not the best ones. The cross validation method allowed a higher formalism in the division of entry data (estimation, validation and test sets), which is necessary due to the small quantity of images with calcifications available in the database Mini MIAS, to prevent excessive training of the network and, consequently, a better generalization of the system. The proposed system is available as a knowledge management tool. This allows the dissemination of tacit and explicit knowledge of medical experts and their past experience in the field, allowing still a better performance in the evaluation of routine exams by means of a graphical tool.

6. Related work

The Mammographic Image Analysis Society (MIAS) is a database of digital mammograms where the films are from the U.K. National Breast Screening Programme and they have been digitised to 50 micron pixel edge with a Joyce-Loebl scanning microdensitometer, a device linear in the optical density range 0-3.2 and representing each pixel with an 8-bit word Suckling et al. (1994). The database contains 322 digitised films and it also includes radiologist's "truth"-markings on the locations of any abnormalities that can be present. The database has been reduced to a 200 micron pixel edge and padded/clipped so that all the images are 1024x1024 Suckling et al. (1994). The Digital Database for Screening Mammography (DDSM) is a collaborative effort between Massachusetts General Hospital, Sandia National Laboratories and the University of South Florida Computer Science and Engineering Department. The database contains approximately 2,500 mammograms each includes two images of each breast, along with some associated patient information (age at time of study, ACR breast density rating, subtlety rating for abnormalities, ACR keyword description of abnormalities) and image information. Images containing suspicious areas have associated pixel-level "ground truth" information about the locations and types of suspicious regions. The DDSM also provides software for accessing the mammogram and truth images and for calculating performance figures for automated image analysis algorithms Heath et al. (2001b).

7. Future work

7.1 Genotypes and phenotypes

The search of new genes of cancer and its epigenomics implications are the main areas of future investigation. Discovering the human genomic variability and its complexes phenotypes are the major obstacles and where the efforts will be concentrated. New image processing algorithms and also new artificial intelligence methods will be used in order to offer the physicians more technical support in the breast cancer treatment.

7.2 Breast cancer visual modeling

7.2.1 Motivation

Visual characteristics of human body components are highly relevant as an input for a variety of decisions on health concerning activities. One can promptly access and eventually perform adjustments on information upon some injury or physiological change through user-friendly devices, as a valuable resource for therapeutic procedures and specialized training too.

One should remark that visualization is supposed to convey information compatible with viewer's perception and cognition skills Agrawala et al. (2011). Visual modeling of cells growth is an instance of data visualization that allows a fast information analysis for problem solving. This kind of data processing more and more becomes an efficient way to support decision-making. Visualization can be understood as a low-cost human cognitive process to create an image about a domain space. It enables insights about some context, say, qualitative and quantitative answers to existing problems and facts recognition that were previously not possible Fayyad & Grinstein (2002) Konofagou (2004). Although visual models are able to express just part of the features of the real object, they are enough informative and useful for an effective subsequent decision process. Typical instances of lesion that require visual information for treatment are cells abnormal growth that may constitute cancerous tissues as a result of an evolutionary process with genetic mutations Beckmann et al. (1997) Evan & Vousden (2001) Lux et al. (2006). Images provide relevant information about size and tonalities irregularities that may express different kinds of existing lesions. The availability of a non-invasive and inexpensive computational technique to model evolutionary process of breast cancer thus becomes highly relevant. Hence one expects to develop models of breast cancer, to recognize their properties, for supporting therapeutic processes and decisions, with experimental validation in mammography clinics. Its results should be suitable for actual use in units of health care.

7.2.2 Visual modeling

A visualization system is developed according to the following steps Agrawala et al. (2011). Initially, the principles of design-oriented field of interest are identified. Then the algorithms are developed to implement these principles. Afterwards the results are validated based on users' perception of visually modeled information. Segmentation is based on certain characteristic features that are common to the pixels that should make up each segment. If the image contains multiple objects with similar characteristics, as in the case of breast duct anatomy, the approximate tones of pixels belonging to the object are a segmentation criterion. After properly separated and identified the object or region, it becomes possible to capture information that can be used for subsequent classification according known categories. Thus it is essential to know all the properties that are necessary and sufficient to characterize an object. The image of an object is a projection of a three-dimensional object on a plane. Through the image we might infer the size of the projection of the object and thus estimate the size of the object. The position of the object is useful for the activation of devices able to perform any procedure directly on the scene, for example, microsurgery or application of medication. Each property should be able to unambiguously characterize the objects belonging to different classes and at the same time be able to accommodate all the variations that can occur for objects belonging to the same class. The decision about membership of an object to some class can be deterministic or probabilistic. In fact the value of a property in a set of standards can be a random variable with estimated mean and standard deviation. So such decision is based on the membership of the measured property in a pattern to a range of the known model. More accurate procedures for statistical classification also consider the cost of misclassification, which can be quite relevant, for example, at diseases diagnosis based on recognition of images of tissue samples. Concerning therapeutic procedures it is often necessary to recognize tissues with different textures, in order to assess the extent of changes in these tissues. This is the case of analysis of the development of breast cancer. Project activities are shown in Figure 5.

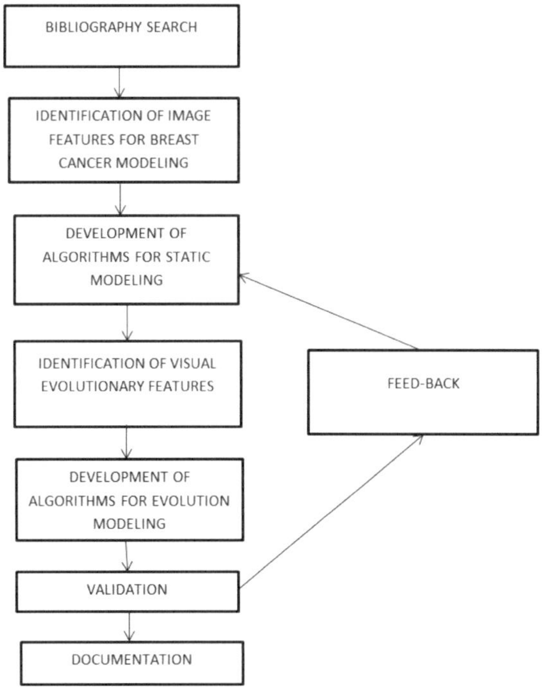

Fig. 5. Visual Modeling Project flow adapted from Guadagnin et al. (2011)

7.2.3 Expected results

One expects to have a system for visual modeling of evolutionary process of breast tumorous tissues. It will also identify the main requirements for training professionals in monitoring and management of patients supposed an appropriate use of computing resources.

7.2.4 Perspectives

Simulations could be used to advise patients and professionals about cancerous lesions evolution as well as to examine evolving response to specific treatments. The model could be also adjusted to simulate different cells mutation types Bankhead & Heckendorn (2007). The amount of image processing and analysis applications in medical diagnosis is very extent. Otherwise there are several other areas where these techniques are useful or even indispensable too, for instance, in computer-assisted surgery, post-surgery follow-up or therapy and monitoring of potentially dangerous evolution. Simulated images are helpful for healing supported by computational processes and medical diagnosis, and applications of telemedicine.

8. Conclusions

The MIDAS (Mammographic Image Database for Automated Analysis) is an innovative database containing mammogram images covering a sample of Brazilian women population, patient genome sequences data, open source image processing algorithms, open access and open collaborative environment. After its initial tunning and legal procedures it will be available to the Internet to worldwide access and collaboration. The MIDAS database project aims to enhance the scientific activity regarding breast cancer research among brazilian women population and therefore raising the health prognosis.

9. References

Agrawala, M., Li, W. & Berthouzoz, F. (2011). Design principles for visual communication, *1.Communications of the ACM* 54(4): 60–69.

Baker, L. (1982). Breast cancer detection demonstration project: five - years summary report, *Cancer Clin.* Vol. 4(No. 32): 194–225.

Bankhead, A. & Heckendorn, R. (2007). Using evolvable genetic cellular automata to model breast cancer, *1.Proceedings of Genetic Programming and Evolvable Machines* pp. 381–393.

Barratt, A., Howard, K., Irwig, L., Salked, G. & Houssami, N. (2005). Model of outcomes of screening mammography: information to support informed choices, *Br Med J* 1(330): 936–941.

Basset, L., Hendrick, R. E. & Bassford, T. L. (1994). Quality determinants of mammography, *Technical report*, U.S. Department of Health and Human Services.

Beckmann, M. W., Niederacher, D., Schnurch, H. G., Gusterson, B. A. & Bender, H. G. (1997). Multistep carcinogenesis of breast cancer and tumour heterogeneity, *1.Journal of Molecular Medicine* 1(75): 429–439.

Black, W. C. & Ling, A. (1990). ls earlier diagnosis really better? the misleading effects of lead time and length biases, *AJR Am J Roentgenol* 1(No. 155): 625–630.

Boecker, W. et al. (2002). Usual ductal hyperplasia of breast is a committed stem (progenitor) cell lesion distinct from atypical ductal hyperplasia and ductal carcinoma in situ, *J. Pathol.* 1(No. 198): 458–467.

Chamberlain, J. (1984). Repeated screening for breast cancer, *J. Epidemiol Com Health* 1(No. 38): 54–57.

Chu, K. & Connor, R. (1991). Analysis of the temporal patterns of benefits in the health insurance plan of new york crial by stage and age, *Am. J. Epidemiol.* 1(No. 133): 1039–1049.

Colditz, G. A. et al. (1993). Family history, age, and risk of breast cancer, *JAMA* 1(No. 270): 338–343.

D'Osri, C., Bassett, L., Berg, W. et al. (2003). Breast imaging reporting and data system: Acr bi-rads, *Technical report*, American College of Radiology.

Dupont, W. D. et al. (1993). Breast cancer risk associated with proliferative breast disease and atypical hyperplasia, *Cancer* 1(No. 71): 1258–1265.

Evan, G. I. & Vousden, K. H. (2001). Proliferation, cell cycle and apoptosis in cancer, *Nature* 1(411): 342–348.

Fayyad, U. & Grinstein, G. (2002). *Information Visualization in Data Mining and Knowledge Discovery*, Academic Press.

Fernandes, F., Brasil, L., Lamas, J. & Guadagnin, R. (2010). Breast cancer image assessment using an adaptive network-based fuzzy inference system, *Pattern recognition and Image Analysis* .

Feuer, E. & Wun, L. (1992). How much of the recent rise in breast cancer incidence can be explained by increases in mammography utilization?, *Am J Epidemiol* 1(No. 136): 1423–1436.

Fitzgerald, R. (2001). Error in radiology, *Clin Radiol.* 1(No. 56): 938–946.

Fletcher, R. F. S. & Wagner, E. (1996). Prevenção, *Epidemiologia clinica: elementos essenciais.*, Artes Médicas, Porto Alegre, pp. 174–194.

Fletcher, R. H., Fletcher, S. W. & Wagner, E. H. (1996). *Epidemiologia Clínica: elementos essenciais*, Artes Médicas.

Fletcher, S. W. & Elmore, J. G. (2005). False-positive mammograms - can the U.S.A. learn from Europe?, *Lancet* 1(365): 7–8.

Fowler, M. (2002). *Patterns of Enterprise Application Architecture*, Addison-Wesley Longman Publishing Co., Inc., Boston, MA, USA.

Giger, M. L., Chan, H.-P. & Boone, J. (2008). Anniversary paper: History and status of cad and quantitative image analysis: The role of medical physics and aapm, *Med. Phys.*.

Guadagnin, R., Santana, L., Brasil, L. M. & Neves, R. (2011). Visual modeling of skin wounds: A proposal to improve terapeutic processes and health management, *1.8-th Open German-Russian Workshop on PATTERN RECOGNITION and IMAGE UNDERSTANDING*.

Haus, A. G., Feig, S. A., Ehrlich, S. M. & others. others. others. others. (1990). Mammography screening: technology, radiation dose and risk, quality control and benefits to society, *Radiology* 1(No. 174): 627–656.

Heath, M., Bowyer, K., Kopans, D., Moore, R. & Kegelmeyer, W. P. (2001a). Anniversary paper: History and status of cad and quantitative image analysis: The role of medical physics and aapm, *Medical Physics Publishing* pp. 212–218.

Heath, M., Bowyer, K., Kopans, D., Moore, R. & Kegelmeyer, W. P. (2001b). The digital database for screening mammography, *Proceedings of the Fifth International Workshop on Digital Mammography* pp. 212–218.

Humphrey, L. L. et al. (2002). Breast cancer screening: a summary of the evidence for the u.s. preventive services task force, *Ann. Intern. Med.* 1(137): 347–360.

Koch, H. (1998). Projeto de detecção precoce do câncer de mama. in: Mamografia atual, *in* H. K. H. P. P. Pasquelete & C. Kemp (eds), *Comissão nacional especializada de diagnóstico por imagem da Febrasco*, Revinter, Rio de Janeiro, pp. 3–14.

Koenig, D. et al. (2007). *Groovy in Action*, Manning Publications.

Konofagou, E. (2004). *Ultrasonic Imaging*, CRC Press.

Kopans, D. (1995). Screening mammography and the controversy concerning women aged 40 - 49 years, *in* D. Kopans & E. Mendelson (eds), *Syllabus: a categorical course in breast imaging*, Oak Brook, lII: Radiological Society of North America, North America, pp. 39–49.

Kopans, D. B. et al. (1996). Positive predictive value of breast biopsy peformed as a result of mammography: There is no abrupt change at age 50 ages, *Radiology* 1(No. 200): 357–360.

Lamas, J. (2000). *Avaliação dos resultados de exames mamográficos para detecção precoce do câncer de mama, no* Distrito Federal, *segundo indicadores de qualidade.*, PhD thesis, UFRJ.

Lamas, J. & Pereira, M. G. (1998). *Prevalência de lesões malignas e pré-malignas subclínicas da mama em mulheres assintomáticas no* Distrito Federal., Master's thesis, UNB.

Liff, J. M. et al. (1991). Does increased detection account for the rising incidence of breast cancer?, *Am J Public Health* 1(No. 81): 462 – 465.

Lopes, E. R. et al. (1996). Câncer de mama: epidemiologia e grupos de risco, *Rev Bras Cancerol* Vol. 2(No. 42): 105–116.

Lux, M. P., Fasching, P. A. & Beckmann, M. W. (2006). Hereditary breast and ovarian cancer: Review and future perspectives, *1.Journal of Molecular Medicine* 1(84): 16–24.

MacPherson, K. et al. (1983). Oral contraceptives and breast cancer, *Lancet* pp. 1414–1415.

Maya, N. A. F. et al. (2006). Tendência de incidência e da mortalidade do cancer de mama em goiânia: Análise de 15 anos (1988-2002), *Rev Bras Mastol* 1(No. 1): 17–22.

Miller, A. B. et al. (1992). Canadian breast screening study: breast cancer detection and death rates among women aged 40 - 49 years, *Can Med. Assoc J.* 1(No. 147): 1459–1476.
Morrison, A. (1992). *Screening in chronic disease*, Oxford University Press.
Moskowitz, M. (1986). Breast cancer: age-specific growth rates and screening strategies, *Radiology* 1(No. 161): 37–41.
Pereira, M. G. (1996). Morbidade, *Epidemiologia:teoria e prática*, Guanabara Koogan, Rio de Janeiro, pp. 73–106.
Pereira, M. G. (2000a). Aferição dos eventos, *Epidemiologia: teoria e prática*, Guanabara Koogan, Rio de Janeiro, pp. 358–376.
Pereira, M. G. (2000b). *Epidemiologia: teoria e pratica*, Guanabara Koogan.
Roubidoux, M. A. et al. (1997). Women with breast cancer: histologic finding in the contralateral breast, *Radiology* 1(No. 203): 691–694.
Sickles, E. (1992). Quality assurance: how to audit your own mammography practice, *Radiol Clin North Arn* 1(No. 30): 265–275.
Sickles, E. (1995). Auditing your practice, *in* D. Kopans & E. Mendelson (eds), *Syllabus: a categorical course in breast imaging*, Oak Brook, lll: Radiological Society of North Arnerica, North Arnerica, pp. 81–91.
Sickles, E. A., Wolverton, D. E. & Dee, K. E. (2002). Performance parameters for screening and diagnostic mamography: specialist and general radiologists, *Radiology* 1(224): 861–869.
Smith, G. & Ledbrook, P. (2009). *Grails in Action*, Manning Publications.
Smith, R. (1993). Epidemiology ofbreast cancer, *in* A. Hans & M. Yaffe (eds), *Syllabus: categorical course in physics - technical aspects of breast imaging*, Oak Brook, lII: Radiological Society of North America, pp. 21–33.
Smith, R. (1995). The epidemiology of breast cancer, *in* D. Kopans & E. Mendelson (eds), *Syllabus: a categorical course in breast imaging*, Oak Brook, lII: Radiological Society of North America, North America, pp. 7–20.
Suckling, J. et al. (1994). The mammographic image analysis society digital mammogram database, *International Congress Series 1069* pp. 375–378.
Tabár, L. (1993). New swedish breast cancer detection results for women aged 40-49, *Cancer* 1(No. 72): 1437–1438.
Taplin, S. H., Ichikawa, L., Buist, D. et al. (2004). Evaluating organized breast cancer screening implementation: the prevention of late-state disease?, *Cancer Epidemiol Bio Prev* 1(No. 13): 225–234.
Thurfjell, E. & Lindgren, J. (1994). Population-based mammography screening in swedish clinical practice: prevalence and incidence screening in uppsala county, *Radiology* 1(No. 193): 351–357.
Vizcaíno, L. et al. (1998). Breast cancer screening: first round in the population-based program in valencia, spain, *Radiology* 1(No. 206): 253–260.
Warren-Burhenne, L. (1996). lmplications of international breast cancer screening of north american policies: The british columbia experience, *Supplement to Radiology*, Radiological Society of North Arnerica, North Arnerica, pp. 88–88.
Warren-Burhenne, L. H. T. & Burhenne, H. (1992). The british columbia mammography screening program: evaluation of the first 15 monrhs, *Am J Roentgenol* Vol. 1(No. 158): 45–49.
Zelen, M. (1976). Theory of early detection of breast cancer in the general population, *in* J. M. W. Heuson & M. Rozencweig (eds), *Breast Cancer: trends in research and treatment. New York*, Raven Press, pp. 287–300.

13

Fusion of Two-View Information: SVD Based Modeling for Computerized Classification of Breast Lesions on Mammograms

Rogério Daniel Dantas[1], Marcelo Zanchetta do Nascimento[2], Ricardo de Souza Jacomini[2], Danilo César Pereira[2] and Rodrigo Pereira Ramos[3]

[1]*Universidade do Grande ABC*
[2]*Universidade Federal do ABC*
[3]*Universidade Federal do Vale do Sao Francisco*
Brazil

1. Introduction

Over the past few years, the cancer has been one of the most responsible for the high number of deaths, and could become one of the main responsible for most deaths in the next decades. According to the World Health Organization, the number of deaths due to cancer, which was just 13% in 2008, is currently having a significant increase and one estimates that this number could reach approximately 12 million until 2030 (Tang et al., 2009).

Breast cancer is the second most common and leading cause of cancer death among women in Brazil. The National Cancer Institute (INCA) reports more than 50,000 new cases of the disease, with risk of 51 cases per 100,000 women. In the southeastern region of the country, this number is about 34% higher than the national average, with an estimate of 68 new cases per 100,000 women. For this reason, studies have shown that early detection is the key to improve breast cancer prognosis (Brasil, 2009).

Some works have shown that early detection of disease is a crucial factor for reducing mortality from breast cancer. Among the most important medical imaging methods (for example, MRI, ultrasonography and screen/film mammography), screen/film mammography is the method most easily accessible and has proved to be an effective aid for radiologists in the early detection of breast cancers and in the reduction of mortality rates. In this examination, four images are obtained, two corresponding to the right breast and two to the left breast of the projections cranio-caudal (CC) and medio-lateral oblique (MLO). The images acquisition improves visualization of breast tissue and increases the chances for detecting signs that characterize the presence of non-palpable lesions such as nodules, calcification, signs of bilateral asymmetry and architectural distortion (Rangayyan et al., 2007).

Retrospective evaluations of previous screening films of cancers, detected between screening rounds (interval cancers), show evidence of abnormality in 16% among 27% of cases. Missed cancers are due to many reasons: low disease prevalence, breast structure complexity, finding subtleties, and radiologist fatigue. To improve the accuracy of mammography, radiologists employed double reading of the same screening mammogram to increase the sensitivity rate

(Kinoshita et al., 2007). Second reading of the screening mammograms by a human reader can increase cancer detection rates (Thurfjell et al., 1994) (Warren & Duffy, 1995). Obviously, this procedure is too expensive, complex, and time consuming particularly in screening programs where a huge number of mammographic images have to be read (Mencattini et al., 2010).

The development of computerized systems as second readers represents an alternative. Computer-Aided Detection (CADe) and Computer-Aided Diagnosis (CADx) systems have been applied to mammographic images to assist radiologists on lesions analysis such as microcalcification, mass and architectural distortions. Algorithms for image processing together with artificial intelligence techniques, such as neural network and fuzzy logic, are used in order to enhance, segment, extract features and classify abnormalities (Jiang et al., 2007), (Balleyguier et al., 2007), (Doi et al., 1999). CADe schemes are systems that automatically detect suspicious lesions in mammograms, being used as a localization task. CADx systems extend the computer analysis to yield as output the characterization of a region or the estimated probability of lesion malignancy. The present chapter is focused on the classification task.

Although CADe and CADx systems have provided a large number of research and high rates of sensitivity, the majority of these works analyzes the MLO and CC views independently. In some situations, this system detects abnormalities in only one of the views. Radiologists believe that there is an inconsistency if a particular lesion is similar in both views and the system does not have the capability to find it. Studies have shown that these limitations have changed their impressions and radiologists are ignoring the results provided by these systems (Doi et al., 1999).

Several computer algorithms are used for identification of abnormalities in the breast by extracting features directly from digitized mammograms. Typically, two classes of features are extracted from mammograms with these algorithms, namely morphological and non-morphological features. Morphological features are intended to describe information related to the morphology of a lesion, such as lesion size and shape. Image texture analysis is an important class that represents gray level properties of images used to describe non-morphological features that are not easily interpreted by humans. This information can be obtained through a variety of image processing algorithms, calculated using a variety of statistical, structural and spectral techniques including co-occurrence matrices, fractal dimensions and multiresolution techniques. Using a different space by special data transform such as Fourier transform or wavelets transform could be helpful to separate a special data that contain specific characteristics. Multiresolution analysis allows for the preservation of an image according to certain level of resolution, i.e., it allows for the zooming in and out on the underlying texture structure. Therefore, the texture extraction is not affected by the size of the pixel neighborhood (Eltoukhy et al., 2010).

In this chapter, we present a method for extraction and selection of texture-related attributes and classification using the fusion of information from both CC and MLO visions. In the extraction stage, the wavelet transform method was applied to provide texture-related attributes for the considered images. Following, the singular value decomposition (SVD) technique was used to reduce the number of attributes. The application of analysis of variance (ANOVA) was also conducted for further reduction of the attributes after the SVD application. In the final step, we used the Random Forest and SVM classifiers to analyze mammogram lesions. The overall performance of the proposed method was evaluated by means of the area under the ROC curve.

2. Materials and methods

2.1 Data set

The database used in this work encompasses mammographic screen/film digitized images taken from the Digital Database for Screening Mammography (DDSM) (Balleyguier et al., 2007). The DDSM project is a joint effort of researchers from the Massachusetts General Hospital (D. Kopans, R Moore), the University of South Florida (K. Bowyer), and the Sandia National Laboratories – EUA (P. Kegelmeyer). The DDSM database has been widely used as a benchmark for numerous articles on the mammographic area, for being free of charge and having a vast and diverse quantity of cases. It is constituted of mammographic images and its corresponding technical and clinical information, including exam dates, age of patients, digitalization equipment (as well as resolution, number of rows, pixels per row and bits per pixel of the acquired images), lesion types (according to BIRADS®), and existent pathologies.

For the evaluation of the algorithms, a data set was used comprising 480 mammographic images from 160 patients (being 80 with no lesions and 80 with malignant lesion) which were randomly selected from DDSM dataset. These lesions have different sizes, densities, and margins types. For each case, we used four mammograms, taken from the left and the right breasts, obtained in CC and MLO views. We selected images digitized with a Lumisys laser film scanner at 50 mm pixel size. Each image has a resolution of 4096 gray level tones. The location and size of a mass, when it exists, were taken from the code-chain of the ".ics" file available at the DDSM project and were used to automatically extract square sub-images called regions of interest (ROIs) from the original image. The images used in the experiments were cuttings of size 128×128 pixels done in the sub-image, whose centers correspond to the centers of the presented abnormalities. An example of the cropping process that eliminates image label and background is given in Figure 1. To obtain subimages with no mass, we have followed the same procedure, except that the location was randomly taken from a healthy part of the mammogram. With this approach, a total of 480 sub-images were acquired, and each of these cropped images was used for texture feature extraction and subsequent classification.

2.2 Multiresolution analysis

Image analysis on multiple scales allows image resolution to be modified in order to process as little data as possible. This is accomplished by selecting relevant details for a given task (Mallat, 1996). The basic idea is to represent the image on several resolutions and analyse them on frequency domain, through the application of function transforms. In this chapter, we analyse the performance of wavelet transforms on a multiresolution environment. The basics of wavelet transforms are presented as follows.

2.2.1 Wavelet transforms

For a given function $f(x) \in \mathbb{R}$, the wavelet transform $Wf(a,b) \in \mathbb{R}$ is obtained from the inner product of $f(x)$ with a wavelet family, i.e.:

$$Wf(a,b) = \int_{-\infty}^{\infty} f(t)\psi_{a,b}(x)dx \tag{1}$$

where

$$\psi_{a,b}(x) = a^{-1/2}\psi\left(\frac{x-b}{a}\right) \tag{2}$$

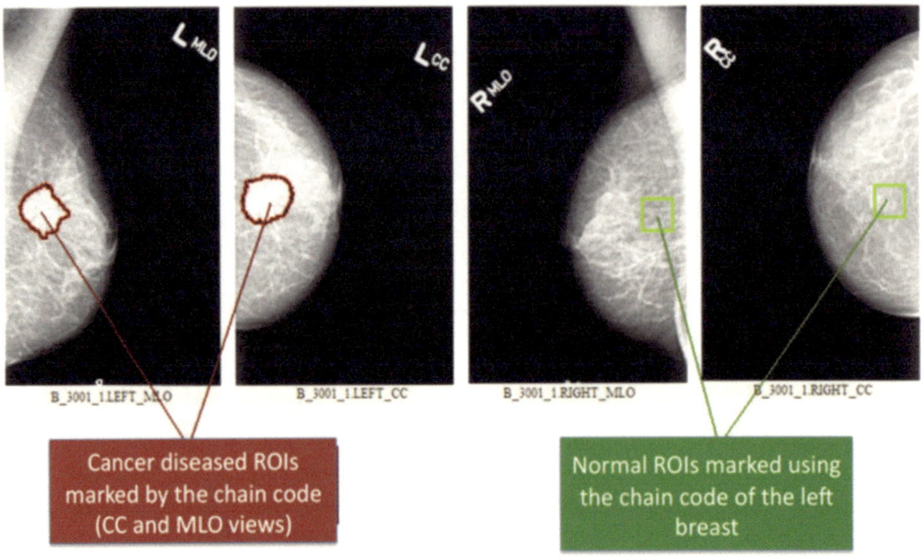

Fig. 1. Procedure applied for the selection of ROI's: images with malignant lesion and images no lesions.

are wavelets obtained from scaling and time shifting operations on a mother wavelet $\psi(x)$, with a and b being the scaling and translation factors, respectively. The mother wavelet $\psi(x)$ is an integrable function with zero mean, i.e.:

$$\int_{-\infty}^{\infty} \psi(x)dx = 0 \tag{3}$$

and centered in the neighborhood of $x = 0$. Examples of wavelets can be found on reference (Mallat, 1998). The scale parameter a is referred to as the transform resolution level. When $Wf(a,b)$ is known only for $a < a_0$, to recover $f(x)$ it is necessary a complement of information corresponding to $Wf(a,b)$ for $a > a_0$. This is obtained by introducing a scaling function $\phi(x)$, from which an approximation of $f(x)$ at scale a is achieved:

$$Lf(a,b) = \int_{-\infty}^{\infty} f(x) \frac{1}{\sqrt{a}} \phi \left(\frac{t-b}{a} \right) dx \tag{4}$$

In this way, $Wf(a,b)$ and $Lf(a,b)$ are defined as the detail and approximation coefficients of the wavelet transform, respectively.

To allow fast numerical implementations, it is common to impose that the scale and translation parameters vary only along discrete values, the most common being the dyadic wavelet decomposition, which is achieved when $a = 2^j$ and $b = k2^j$, for integers j and k. Therefore, one can construct wavelet and scaling families given, respectively, by:

$$\psi_{j,k}(x) = \frac{1}{\sqrt{2^j}} \psi \left(\frac{t - 2^j k}{2^j} \right) \tag{5}$$

$$\phi_{j,k}(x) = \frac{1}{\sqrt{2^j}} \phi \left(\frac{t - 2^j k}{2^j} \right) \tag{6}$$

which are orthonormal bases of some subspaces of $L^2(\mathbb{R})$ related to the resolution 2^j. Many families of wavelets have been developed, such as Haar, Daubechies, Coiflet, cubic splines, among others.

For discrete signals, the discrete wavelet transform (DWT) is obtained by the discretization of time as well as the translation and scale parameters. Mallat has proved that the dyadic DWT of a signal is equivalent to its decomposition through high-pass and low-pass filter banks, as many filters as is the desired resolution. The DWT achieves a multiresolution decomposition of a discrete signal $f[n]$ on J octaves (resolutions) labeled $j = 1, 2, \cdots, J$ and given by:

$$f[n] = \sum_{j=1}^{\infty} \sum_{k \in \mathbb{Z}} a_{j,k} \tilde{g}[n - 2^j k] + \sum_{k \in \mathbb{Z}} d_{J,k} \tilde{h}[n - 2^J k] \tag{7}$$

The sequences $\tilde{h}[n]$ and $\tilde{g}[n]$ are low-pass and high-pass synthesis filters, respectively. They are called reconstruction filters.

The wavelet coefficients, namely the approximation coefficients $a_{j,k}$ and the detail coefficients $d_{J,k}$, are obtained by the convolution operations:

$$a_{j,k} = \sum_n f[n] h_j[n - 2^j k] \tag{8}$$

$$d_{J,k} = \sum_n f[n] g_J[n - 2^J k] \tag{9}$$

where $h_j[n]$ and $g_J[n]$ are the analysis discrete filters, related to the approximation and detail coefficients, respectively. They are called decomposition filters. Considering two filters, a low-pass $h[n]$ and a high-pass $g[n]$, the analysis filters can be obtained iteratively as:

$$g_1[n] = g[n] \tag{10}$$

$$h_1[n] = h[n] \tag{11}$$

$$g_{j+1} = \sum_k g_j[k] h[n - 2k] \tag{12}$$

$$h_{j+1} = \sum_k h_j[k] h[n - 2k] \tag{13}$$

At each j-th resolution, the wavelet coefficients are obtained by convolving the previous one with $h_j[n]$ and $g_J[n]$ and taking every other sample of the convolution (downsampling the result by a factor of 2), as illustrated by Figure 2. If the decomposition filter $h[n]$ and the

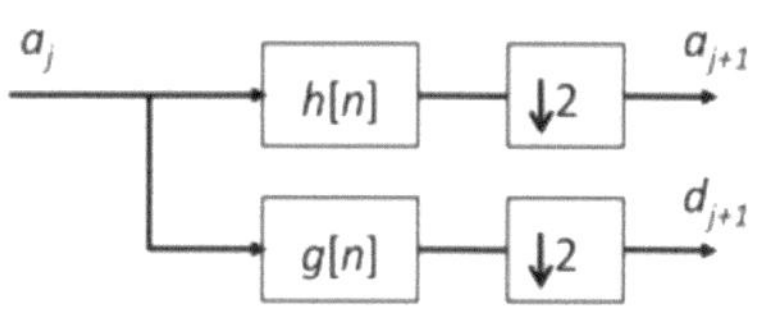

Fig. 2. DWT analysis filter bank.

reconstruction filter $\tilde{h}[n]$ are considered to be equal, this defines conjugate mirror filters and $h[n]$ and $g[n]$ completely characterizes the dyadic DWT, with $g[n] = (-1)^n h[N - 1 - n]$, where N is the number of filter coefficients. In this case, as it can be seen, the filter $h[n]$ plays an important role for wavelet transforms.

Different wavelet and scaling families can be constructed from the wavelet and scaling filters through:

$$\frac{1}{\sqrt{2}}\psi\left(\frac{t}{2}\right) = \sum_k g[k]\phi(t-k) \tag{14}$$

$$\frac{1}{\sqrt{2}}\phi\left(\frac{t}{2}\right) = \sum_k h[k]\phi(t-k) \tag{15}$$

As an example, the Daubechies wavelets are distinguished from each other by the number of vanishing moments. The Daubechies with 3 vanishing moments, referred to as Db3, was used in this work and has non-zero filter coefficients shown in Table 1.

n	$h[n]$
0	0.33267
1	0.80689
2	0.45988
3	−0.13501
4	−0.85441
5	0.35226

Table 1. Daubechies filter for a wavelet with 3 vanishing moments.

In what concerns images, which are bidimensional (2D) signals, the DWT can be computed as given by Figure 3, which shows an image decomposition from the j-th level to the $(j+1)$-th level of the DWT. The coefficients LL_j represent the pixel values of the original image. Firstly, the image is passed through a pair of filters on each row, followed by a downsampling of 2. The results are used as inputs of two filter banks, which are applied at the columns of the image, followed by downsampling. Four sub-images are generated in this process: the approximation LL_{j+1}, which represents the original image with a smaller resolution, and the details LH_{j+1}, HL_{j+1}, HH_{j+1}, which represent the horizontal, vertical and diagonal directions, respectively.

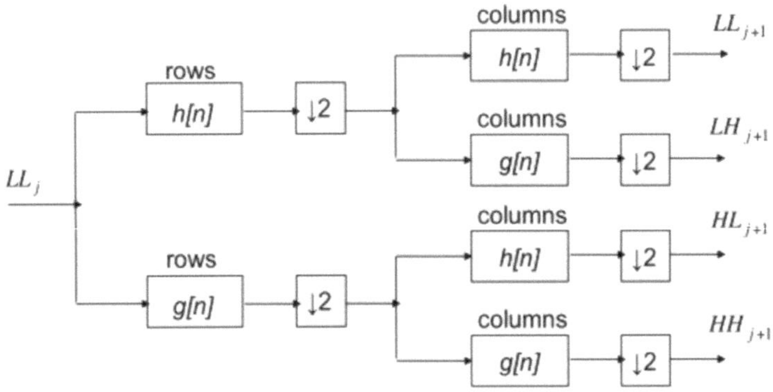

Fig. 3. Filter bank representing one DWT stage.

For each ROI, the 2D-DWT was applied using three different wavelet functions, Coiflet 5, Daubechies 3 e Symlet 4, with 2 resolution levels. The application of the first decomposition level yields the coefficient matrices LL_1 ,LH_1 ,HL_1 and HH_1. The second decompositon level applied in subband LL_1 resulted in the coefficient matrices LL_2 ,LH_2 ,HL_2 and HH_2, and so on. Once most of the information is contained in the detail coefficients, only the detail subimages are evaluated in this work.

2.2.2 Nonlinearity operator

Implementation of discrete wavelet transformation involves linear convolution of images with coefficients of filter meant for the wavelet basis function considered (Selvan & Ramakrishnan, 2007). However, linear convolution increases the size of subband images. This causes distortions at boundaries of the image, when the image is reconstructed.

To overcome this problem, we applied the method proposed by Selvan and Ramakrishnan to make the subband coefficients less sensitive to local variations (Selvan & Ramakrishnan, 2007). In this technique, each row and column of a $Q \times Q$ image is periodically extended by $R/2$ pixels on both sides, where R is the number of filter coefficients. That results in a $(Q+R) \times (Q+R)$ image. Addition of any value lower than $R/2$ will not yield the required core samples, after removing excess samples on the boundaries. An addition of any value higher than $R/2$ will lead to more number of samples than required. Hence, $R/2$ pixels are added on all four sides of the image. Convolution of the $(Q+R) \times (Q+R)$ image, with filter of length R, yields $((Q+R)+R-1)$ samples in one dimension. Out of these samples, core $(Q+2R-1-2(R-1)) = (Q+1)$ samples are considered for decimation, which results in $[(Q+1)/2]$ core samples after decimation. Hence, after one level of wavelet decomposition, a $Q \times Q$ image yields four $(Q/2) \times (Q/2)$ subbands, resulting in nonexpansive samples. In this case, the coefficient matrices were adjusted to the size 64×64 for one decomposition level. For two decompositon level, this method yieds subband matrices of size 32×32.

In order to make the subband coefficients less sensitive to local variations, nonlinearity and smoothing operators must be applied on wavelet transformation coefficients, before extracting the parameters. For nonlinearity and smoothing operations, the total energy of wavelet transformation coefficients in each sububand was calculated using the equation:

$$E_i = \frac{1}{PQ} \sum_{j=1}^{P} \sum_{k=1}^{Q} |w_i(j,k)|^2 \qquad (16)$$

where E_i is the overall energy in the i-th subband, $w_i(j,k)$ is the wavelet transformation coefficient at locations (j,k) in the i-th subband, and P and Q are the number of rows and columns of the i-th subband, respectively. Here, parameters P and Q have similar values.

In the present work, we also consider 3×3 neighborhoods, compute their average, and normalize the average, as proposed by (Selvan & Ramakrishnan, 2007). At each location $L_i(j,k)$, the local energy was computed in a 3×3 neighborhood using equation 17.

$$L_i(j,k) = \frac{1}{9} \sum_{u=0}^{2} \sum_{v=0}^{2} |w_i(j-1+u, k-1+v)|^2 \qquad (17)$$

where the local energies $L_i(j,k)$ were normalized by:

$$I_i(j,k) = \frac{L_i(j,k)}{E_i} \qquad (18)$$

The central wavelet coefficient from the 3×3 neighborhood was then replaced by the corresponding normalized energy.

Figure 4 represents the process of wavelet decomposition for each ROI to obtain the wavelet coefficient features.

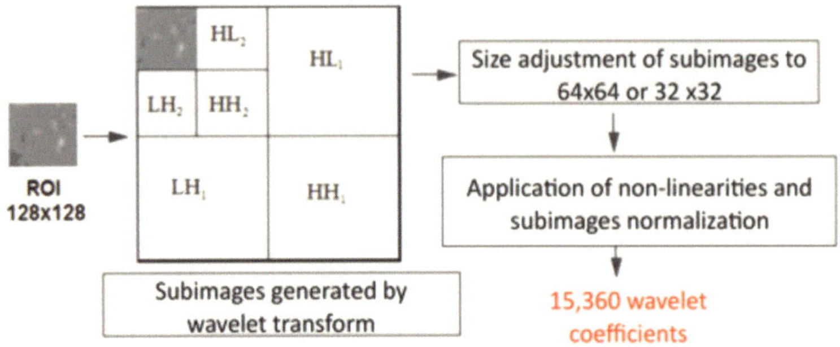

Fig. 4. Ilustration Wavelet decomposition of a mammographic image.

This process produced 12,288 wavelet coefficients for the first decomposition (64×64 in 3 subimages) and 3,072 coefficients for the second decomposition (32×32 in 3 subimages). Gathering together all detail coefficients from the subbands resulted on a feature vector of 15,360 attributes.

2.3 Singular value decomposition

In this work, the number of wavelet coefficients is very large and the estimation of model parameters is computationally demanding. Singular value decomposition (SVD) based method is a very powerful mathematical tool which is mainly used here to reduce a large dataset to a dataset with significantly fewer values, still containing a large fraction of the variability present in the original data. SVD is extraordinarily useful and has many applications such as data analysis, signal processing, pattern recognition and image compression (Pedrini & Schwartz, 2008). It is a linear algebra tool that allows for the decomposition of a matrix into the product of three more simple matrices (Selvan & Ramakrishnan, 2007) (Ramakrishnan & Selvan, 2007a) (Ramakrishnan & Selvan, 2007b).

To explain the aplication of SVD, consider the matrix $\mathbf{I_i}$ with size $P \times Q$, whose entries are the subband wavelet coefficients after the introduction of nonlinearity. The application of the SVD based method decomposes matrix $\mathbf{I}_i$ into the product of three matrices given by:

$$\mathbf{I}_i = \mathbf{U}_i \mathbf{S}_i \mathbf{V}_i^T \tag{19}$$

where $\mathbf{U}_i$, with size $P \times Q$, and $\mathbf{V}_i$, with size $Q \times Q$, are orthogonal matrices whose columns are the eigenvectors of matrices $\mathbf{I}_i \mathbf{I}_i^T$ and $\mathbf{I}_i^T \mathbf{I}_i$, respectively, and $\mathbf{S}_i$, with size $Q \times Q$, is a diagonal matrix whose non-zero entries are the singular values (square roots of the eigenvalues) of matrix $\mathbf{I}_i \mathbf{I}_i^T$, defined by:

$$\mathbf{S}_i = \begin{bmatrix} \sigma_1 & 0 & 0 & \cdots & 0 \\ 0 & \sigma_2 & 0 & \cdots & 0 \\ & & & \ddots & \\ 0 & 0 & \cdots & 0 & \sigma_Q \end{bmatrix} \tag{20}$$

where σ_i are the non-zero singular values, with $\sigma_1 \geq \sigma_2 \geq ... \geq \sigma_Q$. Once the SVD is unique for each matrix, the singular values completely represents the subband images.

A method of truncation of the lower singular values, which is equivalent to a filter based approach, was applied to matrix $\mathbf{S}_i$ for dimensionality reduction with images with noise. In (Selvan & Ramakrishnan, 2007), the authors have shown that the effect of noise is more intense on singular values with lower magnitudes. Therefore, the diagonal matrix can be truncated to a dimension $K \times K$, where K is given empirically by:

$$K = Q \frac{\sigma_1^2}{\sum\limits_n \sigma_n^2} \tag{21}$$

where σ_n is the n-th singular value and σ_1 is its highest value.

Since the wavelet transform in this work was considered for 2 resolution levels, there are subband images with sizes 64×64 and 32×32 pixels, what leads to a different number of truncated singular values (different K) for each mammogram. Therefore, Equation 21 was used to get a value of K_r for each resolution level, and the overall K was obtained by averaging the number of truncated singular values obtained. Having defined the average value K, singular values were extracted from each of the eight wavelet subimages, resulting in a feature vector of 6K elements representing texture characteristics of the original mammograms.

Figure 5 shows an example of the $\mathbf{S}_i$ diagonal matrix obtained from the subband LH_2 of a Coiflet wavelet mother used for texture analysis. The values of the diagonal matrix was truncated by the average value K, which corresponds to the attributes in the region marked in green, representing the texture features.

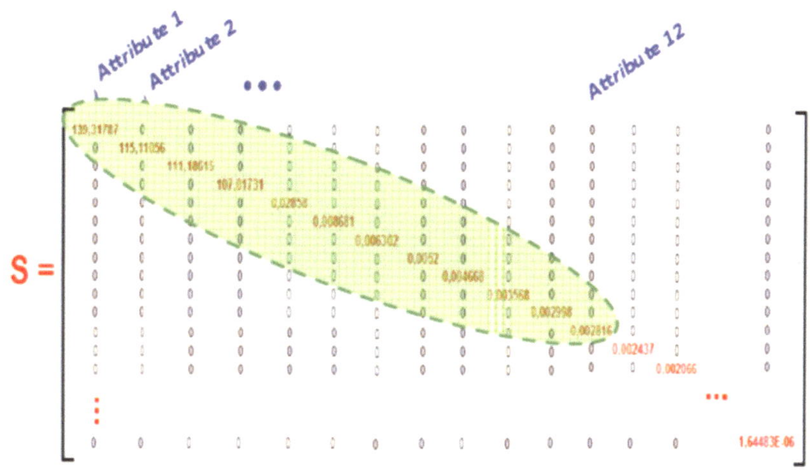

Fig. 5. Matrix $\mathbf{S}_i$ (32×32) of subband LH_2 obtained by SVD from wavelet transform.

2.4 Attributes reduction

In order to verify the relevance of the attributes obtained after the SVD procedure, we applied the technique of Analysis of Variance (ANOVA). This technique is a statistical model that compares the means of two or more experiments. This evaluation is performed to the extent that the observed differences between the means are significant for the comparison of two estimates Vieira (2006). For our experiments, this comparison was carried out on the mass and normal mammographic images. Then, mean and standard deviation were calculated for sets of texture data of the masses and normal images. This set was used to evaluate if each attribute belonged to a particular class. However, when there are differences between the attribute and these classes, this information was eliminated because they did not suit as a reference in the definition of classes in the classification stage Pedrini & Schwartz (2008) Susomboon et al. (2008).

The one-way ANOVA method was firstly applied on the singular values attributes generated by the SVD procedure to determine the statistical significance of these values. In this method, the null hypothesis is that all attribute means are the same. The alternative hypothesis is that at least two of them are different. An F-test is applied to generate this test with a confidence interval of $p = 5\%$. The set with singular values was tested to evaluate if each attribute is different from each other. If any two groups are statistically the same, both are discarded since they do not contribute to the classification step.

In many cases, the alternative hypothesis is quite general and one needs some information about which pairs of means are significantly different, and which are not. This is done with a test called multiple comparison procedure. The multiple comparison method was applied recurrently to determine a minimum value for the number of reduced attributes. This step occurred with the change in the p value down to the value $p = 1.10^{-16}$.

The selection of sets for ANOVA evaluation and a graphic with the analysis of the attributes are illustrated in Figure 6

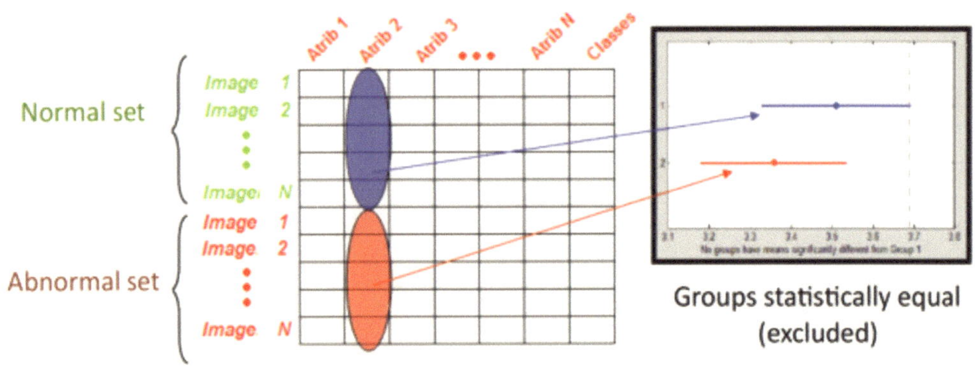

Fig. 6. Method of application of the ANOVA method on attribute 2.

2.5 Fusion of textural information

Several studies have demonstrated that the fusion of information extracted from two views, CC and MLO, allow for the reduction of false positive compared to the use of a single image Paquerault et al. (2002) Gupta et al. (2006).

For the process of fusion of information from two views, we applied the ANOVA technique to analyze the characteristics that are relevant in both images, i.e., information that was statistically different. The procedure resulted in an array of textural data with 50% of information from vision CC and 50% from MLO view. Only the common characteristics of the two views were used in the classification stage.

Figure 7 shows the block diagram of the algorithm to fusion information from the mammograms obtained in both CC and MLO view.

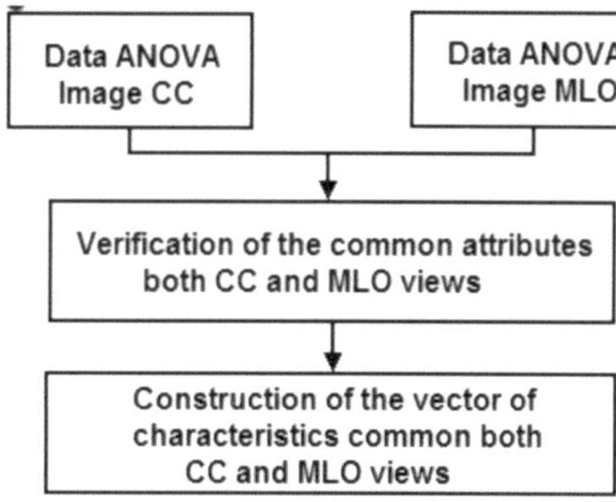

Fig. 7. Block diagram of the algorithm for obtaining the vector with the fusion of information from mammograms.

2.6 Classification stage

As a final stage of the computerized algorithm, after the information fusion step, a classification procedure was performed on the characteristic vectors outcome obtained from both views. In this work, we used the Random Forest and SVM classifiers, separately, to categorize the mammogram ROIs either as normal or abnomal tissues. These algorithms were implemented in WEKA (Waikato Environment for Knowledge Analysis) software (Vibha et al., 2006).

The Random Forest algorithm is built from a collection of classification trees. It is a concept of regression trees, bootstrap samples induced by a set of training data, using features selected in the random process of tree induction (Ramos & Nascimento, 2008).

The Support Vector Machine algorithm based on Sequential Minimal Optimization for implementation (SMO) is a machine learning technique based on statistical learning theory, which seeks to find a hyperplane with maximum separation between the classes, assuming that the data are linearly separable. If not, the SVM maps the data using a kernel function in a feature space of higher dimension, where the data becomes linearly separable (Osta et al., 2008).

To train and test the proposed computerized method, a cross validation procedure was performed on a dataset comprising 240 normal ROI (240 images) and 240 abnormal ROI (240 images). To obtain the performance for each classification we implemented a 10-fold cross validation procedure, in which the dataset were split into N parts. $N-1$ parts served as the training data to fit the classification model. The remaining part was used as the test data for the estimation of performance measures. Each of the N parts was used as test data in turn. The resulting N estimates were averaged to obtain the final expected value. Figure 8 presents the scheme of division into parts for the application of cross-validation procedure.

2.7 System evaluation

To give support to the performance evaluation of proposed method, we computed sensitivity (true positive rate), specificity (true negative rate) and accuracy for each of the confusion

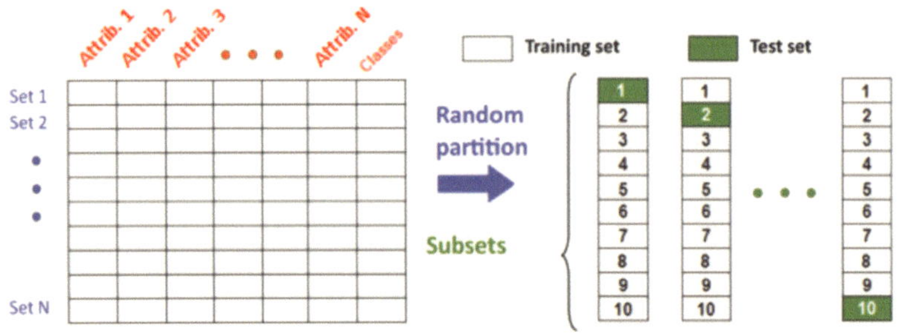

Fig. 8. Division scheme for the application of training and test classification step.

matrices (Tsai & Lee, 2002). A confusion matrix shows the predicted and actual classifications accomplished by a classifier. It has dimensions $L \times L$, where L is the number of classes evaluated by the classifier. In our case, $L = 2$ and the confusion matrix can be stated as shown in Table2. The parameters employed for performance evaluation can be summarized

Class	Positive	Negative
Positive	True Positive (TP)	False Negative (FN)
Negative	False Positive (FP)	True Negative (TN)

Table 2. Confusion matrix for $L = 2$ classes.

in Table 3, which shows the most commonly used formulas. Specificity measures the percentage of positive instances that were predicted as positives, while sensitivity measures the percentage of negative instances that were predicted as negatives. Overall accuracy is the probability that a diagnostic test is correctly performed.

Parameter	Definition
Sensitivity	TP / (TP + FN)
Specificity	TN / (TN + FP)
Accuracy	(TN + TP) / (TP + TN + FP + FN)

Table 3. Definition of performance evaluation parameters.

Performance evaluation was accomplished by means of the receiver operating characteristic (ROC) curves. An ROC curve is a two-dimensional graph of test sensitivity, plotted on the y-axis, versus its false positive rate (or $1 -$ specificity), plotted on the x-axis. An ROC graph depicts relative trade-offs between benefits (TP) and costs (FP), and is produced by varying the decision threshold of the classifier. Although it sometimes can lose some subtle information on classification results, the area under the ROC curve (AUC) is a good accurate measure of a given classifier performance. A test classification with an AUC of 1.0 is a perfect test and an AUC of 0.0 results in a perfectly inaccurate test.

3. Results

3.1 Extraction and reduction from wavelet transform

In the proposed method, texture information was extracted by wavelet tranform application and the SVD method was employed to reduce the number of coefficients before the classification stage. These methods were applied to each ROI obtained in the CC and MLO views. Table 4 shows the number of truncated singular values (K parameter) for the first and second levels of each subband image of each view, as well the resulting number of attributes after SVD application. The resulting number of coefficients is obtained multiplying the second and third rows of the table by 3 and summing the result, since it was employed a two level decomposition that results in 3 subimages for each level. Once the wavelet

Mother wavelet	**K (64×64)**	**K (32×32)**	**Number of Coefficients**
Coiflet 5	23	12	105
Daubechies 3	26	14	120
Symlets 4	23	13	108

Table 4. Value of truncated K parameter and resulting number of coefficients after reduction for each subband image of each CC and MLO views.

transform is a natural filtering process derived from distinct discrete filters, the use of different wavelet mothers conducted to a different number of coefficients, reflected in the truncated K parameter, for each analyzed image. As seen in the previous table, in summary, the SVD method can effectively reduce the number of coefficients obtained from wavelet subimages. As stated before, each wavelet transformed ROI initially encompassed a total of 15,360 wavelet coefficients extracted from a two-level decomposition procedure. The application of the SVD method provided an average reduction of 99.3% on the number of attributes necessary for evaluation of texture information. Comparing the different wavelet mothers evaluated, it can be observed that the Coiflet 5 wavelet provided the smaller number of coefficients.

To reduce the number of attributes and provide a better separation of diseased and normal classes, the method of analysis of variance (ANOVA) with significance level of 5% was applied on the coefficients resulting from the SVD method. Table 5 shows the number of coefficients resulting from the application of ANOVA method with a significance level of 0.05.

Type of Wavelet Mother	**CC**	**MLO**
Coiflet 5	51	48
Daubechies 3	62	48
Symlets 4	56	43

Table 5. Number of wavelet coefficients after application of ANOVA method with $p = 0.05$.

The procedure to determine the significance was applied again to determine a minimum value in reducing the number of attributes. Table 6 presents the obtained results in relation to the number of coefficients after the application of ANOVA method with the limiting value set to $p = 1.10^{-16}$ Applying the ANOVA method on the attributes resulting from the SVD method,

Type of Wavelet Mother	**CC**	**MLO**
Coiflet 5	7	14
Daubechies 3	5	11
Symlets 4	5	15

Table 6. Number of the wavelet coefficients after application of ANOVA method with $p = 1 \times 10^{-16}$.

it can be noticed that there is a significant reduction on the number of coefficients. These values are even more expressive when the ANOVA was applied recursively with the limiting significance level set to $p = 1 \times 10^{-16}$, which led to an average reduction of 81.34% compared to the first application of ANOVA.

3.2 Classification of CC and MLO views independently

Tables 7 and 8 show the mean values of sensitivity,specificity, accuracy and standard deviation (σ) for the Random Forest and SVM classifiers, respectively, for CC e MLO views independent after the reduction process of wavelet coefficients. Sensitivity and specificity are the basic

	Coiflet 5		*Daubechies 3*		*Symlet 4*	
	CC	**MLO**	**CC**	**MLO**	**CC**	**MLO**
Sensitivity	74,17	76,04	75,83	77,50	74,44	77,78
Specificity	75,83	77,29	77,08	77,83	75,00	78,06
Accuracy	75,00	76,67	76,46	77,67	74,72	77,92
σ	16,20	15,18	14,83	14,65	15,89	14,54

Table 7. Measurements obtained with the Random Forest classifier for each view of mammogram.

	Coiflet 5		*Daubechies 3*		*Symlet 4*	
	CC	**MLO**	**CC**	**MLO**	**CC**	**MLO**
Sensitivity	70,00	69,38	67,92	71,17	67,78	71,11
Specificity	81,67	85,63	83,33	86,33	84,44	87,22
Accuracy	75,83	77,50	75,63	78,75	76,11	79,17
σ	9,58	10,63	10,58	10,56	10,83	10,32

Table 8. Measurements obtained with the SVM classifier for each view of mammogram.

measures of the precision for a given diagnostic test. Observing the data on Tables 7 and 8 we can see a great variation on the results for the different wavelets considered. From Table 7, concerning the Random Forest classifier, it can be noticed that the MLO view provided the best results for all three wavelet mothers used. Among the wavelet functions considered, there is little difference on the results (approximately 1%), and the best results were obtained with the application of the Symlet 4 wavelet mother.

A similar result can be observed for the SVM classifier, as it can be seen on Table 8 that shows better results for the MLO views. Comparing the values for the MLO and CC views, the first one resulted on average values 3% superior than the latter. These results show that an inconsistency can occur if a particular lesion is similar in both views and the system does not have the capability to find it. As stated in (Doi et al., 1999), studies have shown that these limitations have been considered mistrusted and radiologists tend to ignoring the results provided by these systems.

When comparing both classifiers, this inconsistency can also be noted, since there is a large variability of results. The Random Forest presented better results for false positive rates than the SVM classifier, but the latter, on average, performed better for the false negative tests. Considering the accuracy results (overall system performace), the SVM classifier presented the better results on average.

Those results are corroborated when considering the AUC as a measure of the system performance. Figure 9 shows the results of AUC for the Random Forest classifier applied to the CC and MLO views independently, after the reduction procedure, parameterized by the different wavelet functions. In Figure 10, the same results of AUC are shown when applying the SVM classifier. As it can be noticed, SVM performed better for almost all cases, the exception being the Daubechies 3 wavelet on the CC view.

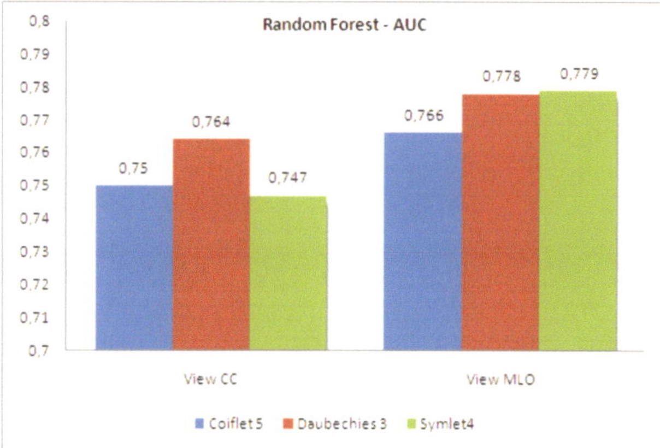

Fig. 9. Results of AUC after application of the reduction methods for different wavelets and Random Forest classifier.

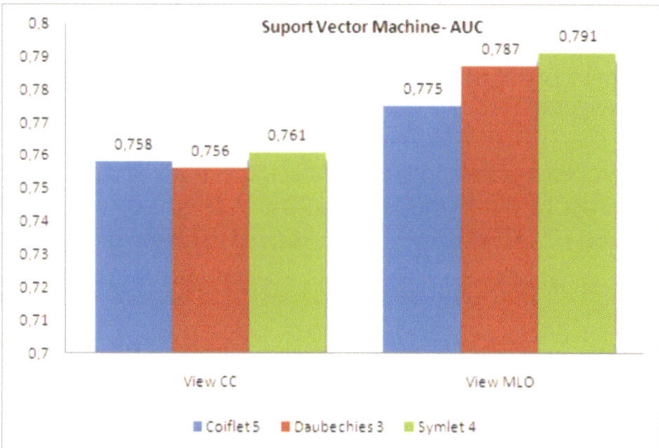

Fig. 10. Results of AUC after application of the reduction methods for different wavelets and SVM classifier.

3.3 Classification of two-view information fusion (CC and MLO)

Table 9 shows the number of texture data after application of the ANOVA technique in each view separately and the number of attributes after the two-view attributes fusion for each type of wavelet mother. Tables 10 and 11 show the mean values of sensitivity, specificity, accuracy

Type of Wavelet-Mother	CC	MLO	CC + MLO
Coiflet 5	7	14	14
Daubechies 3	5	11	10
Symlets 4	5	15	10

Table 9. Number of relevant textural information after application of the ANOVA technique with $p = 1 \times 10^{-16}$.

and standard deviation (σ) for the process of two-view information fusion, using the Random Forest and SVM classifiers, respectively.

	Coiflet 5	*Daubechies 3*	*Symlet 4*
	CC + MLO	**CC + MLO**	**CC + MLO**
Sensitivity	82,50	83,33	82,50
Specificity	81,67	82,92	80,83
Accuracy	82,08	83,13	81,67
σ	12,43	11,74	13,20

Table 10. Results for two-view fusion obtained using the Random Forest classifier.

	Coiflet 5	*Daubechies 3*	*Symlet 4*
	CC + MLO	**CC + MLO**	**CC + MLO**
Sensitivity	75,83	77,08	75,00
Specificity	88,33	89,17	88,61
Accuracy	82,08	83,13	81,81
σ	10,77	9,89	9,94

Table 11. Results for two-view fusion obtained using the SVM classifier.

As seen on Tables 10 and 11, the results for the two classifiers using two-view CC and MLO information fusion were increased for all wavelet functions considered. As an example, for the Coiflet 5 wavelet, the fusion procedure led the sensitivity (fraction of the number of regions detected as positive against those that actually have a mass) to be increased about 5% compared to the result of the same wavelet for individual visions. The same occurred to the other two wavelets. Furthermore, the results also show an increase in the specificity

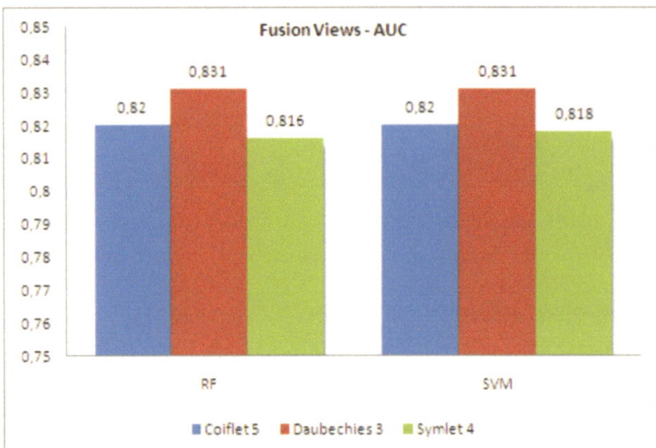

Fig. 11. Results of AUC after the two-view information fusion process for the Random Forest and SVM classifiers.

and accuracy parameters due to the two-view information fusion procedure. The results on the tables also show that the Daubechies 3 wavelet function have reached the best results compared to the other two applied wavelets. Since accuracy reflects the relation between sensitivity and specificity, that descriptor permited to note the similar overall performance between the two classifiers. This result is also visible when evaluating the AUC performance of the classifiers. Figure 11 shows the results of AUC after CC and MLO information fusion for the three different types of wavelet mother and the Random Forest and SVM classifiers.

4. Conclusion

In this work, we develop a method for extraction and selection of attributes using the information fusion from both CC and MLO views for breast cancer classification of mammogram images. Comparing the results of Tables 7 with 10 and 8 with 11, we observe that the use of textural information, obtained from the fusion of the CC and MLO views, might raise the rates of the descriptors evaluated.

Experimental results showed that the three types of wavelet mother had superior performance over the area under the ROC curve for the SVM classifier. Performance evaluation was conducted in relation to the AUC and the results obtained showed that the best classification rates were obtained using the Daubechies wavelel, giving an AUC = 0.831 for the Support Vector Machine classifiers. Future experiments may use other types of feature descriptors to evaluate possible improvements in image classification.

5. References

Balleyguier, C., Ayadi, S., Nguyen, K. V., Vanel, D., Dromain, C. & Sigal, R. (2007). Birads classification in mammography., *Eur J Radiol* 61(2): 192–194.
URL: *http://dx.doi.org/10.1016/j.ejrad.2006.08.033*

Brasil, Ministerio da Saude, I. N. d. C. I. (2009). Estimativa 2010: incidencia de cancer no brasil.
URL: *http://www.inca.gov.br/estimativa/2010/*

Doi, K., MacMahon, H., Katsuragawa, S., Nishikawa, R. M. & Jiang, Y. (1999). Computer-aided diagnosis in radiology: potential and pitfalls., *Eur J Radiol* 31(2): 97–109.

Eltoukhy, M. M., Faye, I. & Samir, B. B. (2010). Curvelet based feature extraction method for breast cancer diagnosis in digital mammogram, *Proc. Int Intelligent and Advanced Systems (ICIAS) Conf*, pp. 1–5.

Gupta, S., Chyn, P. F. & Markey, M. K. (2006). Breast cancer cadx based on bi-rads descriptors from two mammographic views., *Med Phys* 33(6): 1810–7.

Jiang, J., Yao, B. & Wason, A. (2007). A genetic algorithm design for microcalcification detection and classification in digital mammograms, *Computerized Medical Imaging and Graphics* 31(1): 49 – 61.
URL: *http://www.sciencedirect.com/science/article/pii/S0895611106001029*

Kinoshita, S., de Azevedo-Marques, P., Pereira, R., Rodrigues, J. & Rangayyan, R. (2007). Content-based retrieval of mammograms using visual features related to breast density patterns, *Journal of Digital Imaging* 20: 172–190. 10.1007/s10278-007-9004-0.
URL: *http://dx.doi.org/10.1007/s10278-007-9004-0*

Mallat, S. (1996). Wavelets for a vision, *Proceedings of the IEEE* 84(4): 604–614.

Mallat, S. (1998). *A wavelet tour of signal processing*, Academic Press.

Mencattini, A., Salmeri, M., Rabottino, G. & Salicone, S. (2010). Metrological characterization of a cadx system for the classification of breast masses in mammograms, *IEEE J IM* 59(11): 2792–2799.

Osta, H., Qahwaji, R. & Ipson, S. (2008). Comparisons of feature selection methods using discrete wavelet transforms and support vector machines for mammogram images, *Systems, Signals and Devices, 2008. IEEE SSD 2008. 5th International Multi-Conference on*, pp. 1 –6.

Paquerault, S., Petrick, N., Chan, H., Sahiner, B. & Helvie, M. (2002). Improvement of computerized mass detection on mammograms: Fusion of two-view information, *Medical Physics* 29: 238.

Pedrini, H. & Schwartz, W. (2008). Análise de imagens digitais: princípios, algoritmos e aplicações, *São Paulo: Thomson Learning* .

Ramakrishnan, S. & Selvan, S. (2007a). Image texture classification using wavelet based curve fitting and probabilistic neural network, *International Journal of Imaging Systems and Technology* 17(4): 266–275.

Ramakrishnan, S. & Selvan, S. (2007b). Multiwavelets domain singular value features for image texture classification, *Journal of Zhejiang University-Science A* 8(4): 538–549.

Ramos, R. & Nascimento, M. (2008). Comparação de extratores de características em imagens mamográficas., *XXI Congresso Brasileiro de Engenharia Biomédica* .

Rangayyan, R. M., Ayres, F. J. & Desautels, J. L. (2007). A review of computer-aided diagnosis of breast cancer: Toward the detection of subtle signs, *Journal of the Franklin Institute* 344(3-4): 312 – 348. Special Issue: Medical Applications of Signal Processing, Part I. URL: *http://www.sciencedirect.com/science/article/pii/S001600320600127X*

Selvan, S. & Ramakrishnan, S. (2007). SVD-based modeling for image texture classification using wavelet transformation, *Image Processing, IEEE Transactions on* 16(11): 2688–2696.

Susomboon, R., Raicu, D., Furst, J. & Johnson, T. (2008). A co-occurrence texture semi-invariance to direction, distance and patient size, *Proc. SPIE Medical Imaging*, Vol. 6914, Citeseer.

Tang, J., Rangayyan, R. M., Xu, J., El Naqa, I. & Yang, Y. (2009). Computer-aided detection and diagnosis of breast cancer with mammography: Recent advances, *IEEE Transactions on Information Technology in Biomedicine* 13(2): 236–251.

Thurfjell, E. L., Lernevall, K. A. & Taube, A. A. (1994). Benefit of independent double reading in a population-based mammography screening program., *Radiology* 191(1): 241–244.

Tsai, D. & Lee, Y. (2002). Fuzzy reasoning based computer-aided diagnosis for automated discrimination of myocardial heart disease from ultrasonic images., *Transactions* 84(12): 1431–1438.

Vibha, L., Harshavardhan, G. M., Pranaw, K., Shenoy, P. D., Venugopal, K. R. & Patnaik, L. M. (2006). Classification of mammograms using decision trees, *Proceedings of the 10th International Database Engineering and Applications Symposium*, IEEE Computer Society, Washington, DC, USA, pp. 263–266. URL: *http://portal.acm.org/citation.cfm?id=1193213.1193866*

Vieira, S. (2006). *Análise de variância: ANOVA*, Atlas.

Warren, R. M. L. & Duffy, W. (1995). Comparison of single reading with double reading of mammograms, and change in effectiveness with experience, *Br J Radiol* 68(813): 958–962. URL: *http://bjr.birjournals.org/cgi/content/abstract/68/813/958*

Part 4

Emerging Technologies – Computer Aided Detection, Diagnosis and Digital Mammography

14

Breast CAD (Computer Aided Detection) in FFDM (Full Field Digital Mammography)

Nachiko Uchiyama
Research Center for Cancer Prevention and Screening, National Cancer Center, Tsukiji, Chuo-Ku, Tokyo, Japan

1. Introduction

In this chapter, firstly, the author describes the differences between CAD for analog mammography and FFDM with reference to clinical workflow and physical characteristics, and secondly, addresses how the detection performance of CAD can differ in accordance with image quality utilizing different FFDM systems, including future possibilities of breast CAD.

2. Difference between CAD with analog mammography and with digital mammography in clinical workflow

With CAD and analog mammography the CAD device is a single, independent device (Figure 1). The quality and quantity of image data depends on the film and the digitizer. It is easy to collect and analyze digital data through a film digitizer and the CAD system is an independent machine mainly developed by a venture company.

On the other hand, with CAD and digital mammography, it is necessary to collect so-called raw digital data from an acquisition system. To develop CAD software, it is necessary to work in conjunction with acquisition systems. Furthermore, CAD is an independent instrument with analog mammography; on the other hand, with digital mammography, CAD will be one of the interpretation functions of the reading workstation. For the most effective utilization, it is necessary to integrate CAD well with the reading workstation workflow.

Therefore, to disseminate CAD with digital mammography, we should take into consideration how to organize complete systems, including acquisition systems, reading workstations, and network systems. If the acquisition system and the reading workstation are made by the same maker, we can transfer raw image data from the acquisition system to the CAD server, and indicate Structure Report (SR) on the monitors at the reading workstation without any problems. On the other hand, when the makers are different, it may be a problem (Figure 2). For most effective utilization, it is necessary to integrate CAD well into the reading workstation workflow [1].

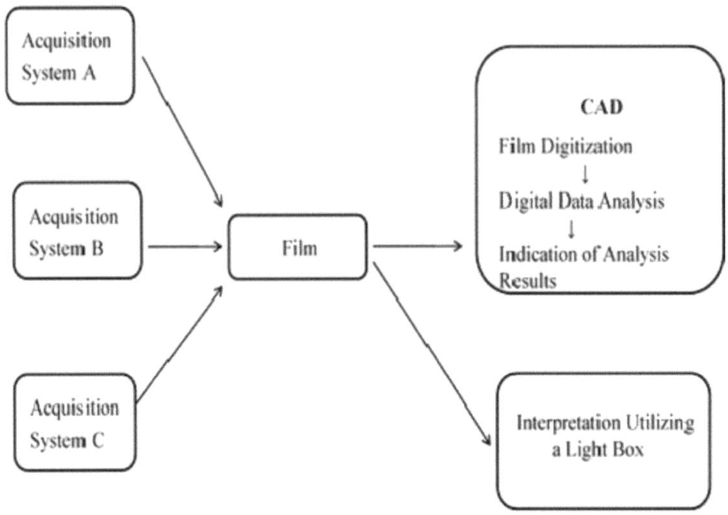

Fig. 1. Example of the Workflow of the CAD System Using Analog Mammography.

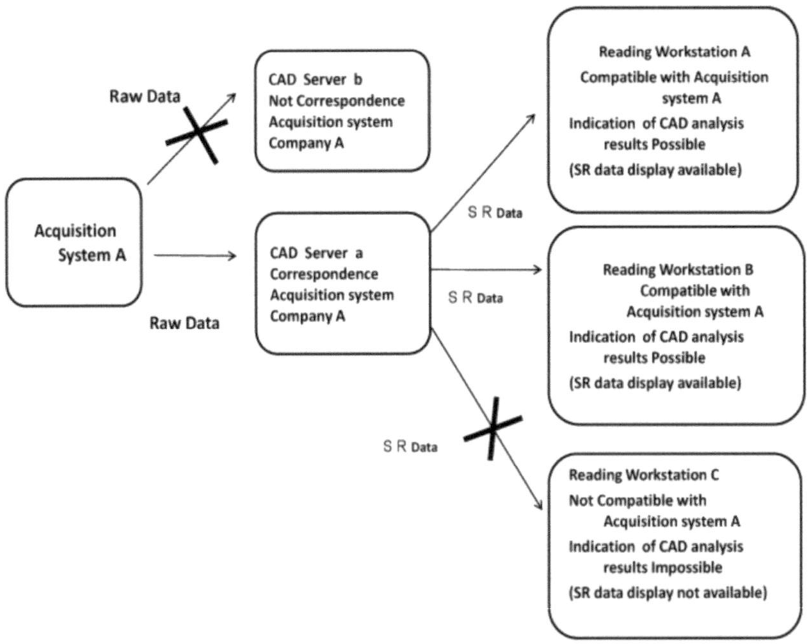

SR: Structure Report
CAD analyzes raw data from the acquisition system in a CAD server and refers the indication of CAD results to a reading workstation.
The quality and quantity of image data depends on the acquisition system. The operating system consists of three steps: (1) an acquisition system, (2) a CAD server, and (3) a reading work station. The number of makers of CAD systems that correspond to each acquisition system is limited. It is necessary to confirm before installation whether the reading workstation can display CAD analysis results.

Fig. 2. Example of the Workflow of the CAD System Using Digital Mammography.

3. How can image quality affect the detection performance of breast CAD in FFDM?

Purpose

At present, CAD, dedicated to digital mammography, analyzes the raw imaging data and detects candidate lesions including masses and microcalcifications. As for the physical characteristics, regarding the linear attenuation coefficient for breast tissue, the differential value between breast tissue and calcification is larger than the differential value between breast tissue and mass. In the raw imaging data, mass lesions have relatively localized large areas with a smaller number of photon counts compared to surrounding breast tissue. CAD analyzes the characteristics and detects the area as a candidate mass lesion. The raw imaging data is inverted and the mass lesion is recognized clinically as a localized high density area compared to background breast tissue density. In the raw imaging data, on the other hand, the images with microcalcification lesions have localized small and clustered areas with a smaller number of photon counts compared to the background breast tissue. CAD analyzes the characteristics and detects the area as a candidate microcalcification lesion. The raw imaging data is inverted and the microcalcification lesions are recognized clinically as small and clustered areas with higher density compared to the background breast tissue density. According to the background, CAD, dedicated to FFDM, can be directly affected by the physical characteristics of the raw imaging data. Unlike the raw imaging data on hard copy, utilizing digitizers for CAD processing in the analog system by groups, in units of 8-10 bits, the raw imaging data for CAD processing in FFDM are analyzed by groups, in units of 12-14 bits, which has a much more dynamic range compared to digitized hard copy data in the analog system. According to the background, in FFDM, there are more opportunities to apply a combination of anode/filters such as W/Rh that allows us to decrease the radiation dose while keeping higher image quality in CNR (Contrast to Noise Ratio), compared to the images using Mo/Mo and Mo/Rh in the analog system [2].The raw imaging data for CAD processing with FFDM can be more strongly influenced by the different contrast and image sharpness in clinical images, compared to the CAD dedicated to an analog system. Accordingly, the detection pattern in CAD can vary even in clinical cases. The author evaluated the variety of detection performance of CAD, utilizing two different FFDM systems with reference to analysis of physical characteristics such as CNR and spectral analysis of anode/filters. This study was conducted to retrospectively evaluate the variation of CAD performance according to different radiation exposure parameters [3,4]

4. Materials and methods

This study was conducted as part of research that was approved by the IRB at our institute on June 12th in 2007. All patients that were recruited for this study gave informed consent. The clinical cases in this study were selected from screening mammograms taken from June 12th in 2007 to December 24th in 2009. Clinical image data were acquired by two different FFDM systems. One was an a-Se FFDM system with a spatial resolution of 70ìm (System A) and imaging data were acquired from June 12th in 2007 to November 24th in 2008. Another was an a-Se FFDM system with a spatial resolution of 85ìm (System B) and imaging data were acquired from December 7th in 2008 to December 24th in 2009. Mammograms were diagnosed as BI-RADS category 1 or 2 by double-reading and breast ultrasound was performed in each case and diagnosed as a normal or a benign case. The total number of cases was 1140 cases in System A and 1178 cases in System B. The median patient age was 59.8 years old (range 40-75 years old) in System A and 60.0 years old (range 40-88 years old) in System B. To optimize radiation exposure parameters in clinical images, we measured CNR (Contrast to Noise Ratio) in accordance with EUREF (European Guidelines for Quality Assurance in Breast Cancer Screening and Diagnosis) guide lines simulating breast thickness, utilizing PMMA phantoms (20-70mm) and radiation exposure parameters, kV (24-34kV) and combinations of anode/filters (Mo/Mo, Mo/ Rh, and W/Rh). In addition, we performed spectral analysis of anode/filters (Mo/Mo, Mo/ Rh, and W/Rh) regarding both FFDM systems. A CAD dedicated to the FFDM systems was applied for the purpose of review and was verified, regarding detection areas, with reference to the diagnostic reports of the mammogram and ultrasound. The same CAD algorithm was utilized for the two FFDM systems.

5. Results

We optimized radiation exposure parameters in a clinical setting with reference to the results of the CNR analysis and dosimetry in accordance with EUREF Guidelines [5] (Fig.3.).

In System A, under 20mm breast thickness, the combination of 24kV with Mo/Mo was selected; from 21m to 30mm breast thickness, the combination of 26kV with Mo/Mo was selected; from 31mm to 40mm breast thickness, the combination of 28kV with Mo/Mo was selected; from 41to 60mm, the combination of 30kV with W/Rh was selected; from 61mm to 70mm, the combination of 32kV with W/Rh was selected; and above 70mm, the combination of 34kV with W/Rh was selected (Fig.4-5).

$$\text{CNR} = \frac{\text{mean pixel value (signal)} - \text{mean pixel value (background)}}{\sqrt{\dfrac{\text{SD (signal)}^2 + \text{SD (background)}^2}{2}}}$$

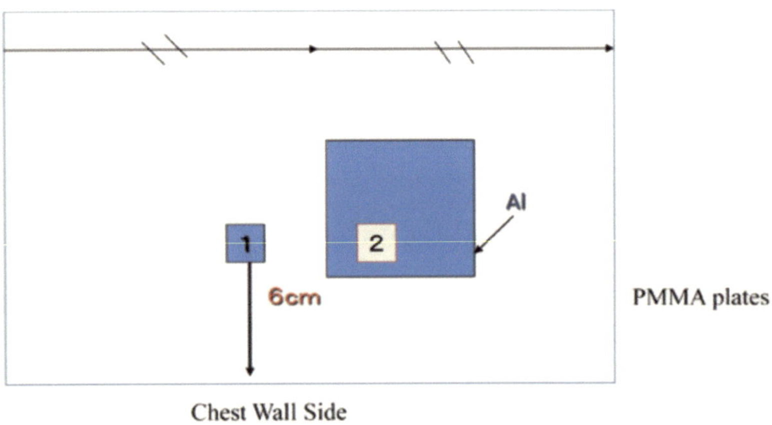

SD; Standard Deviation

Fig. 3. CNR Measurements in Accordance with EUREF.

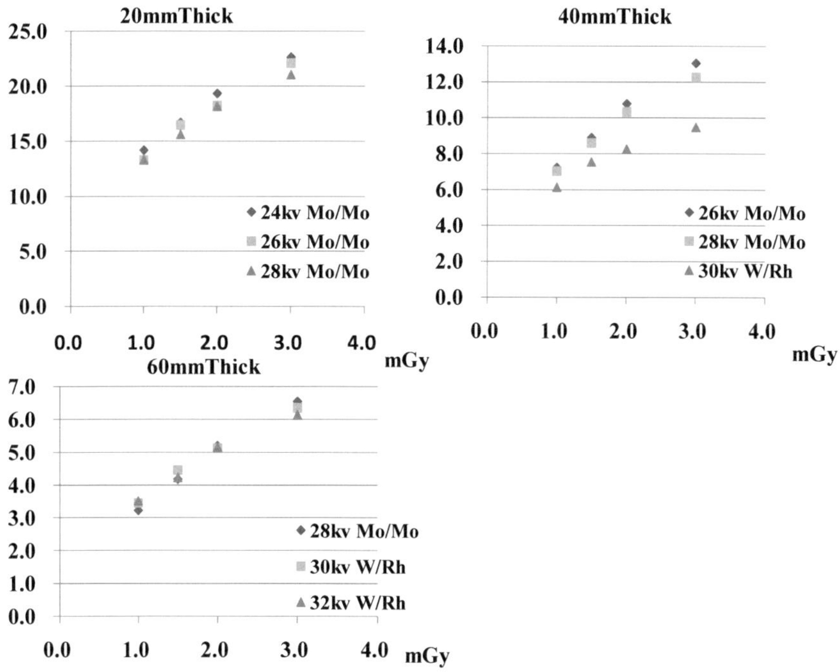

Fig. 4. CNR Analysis: 20mm, 40mm, and 60mmThick PMMA Phantoms in System A.

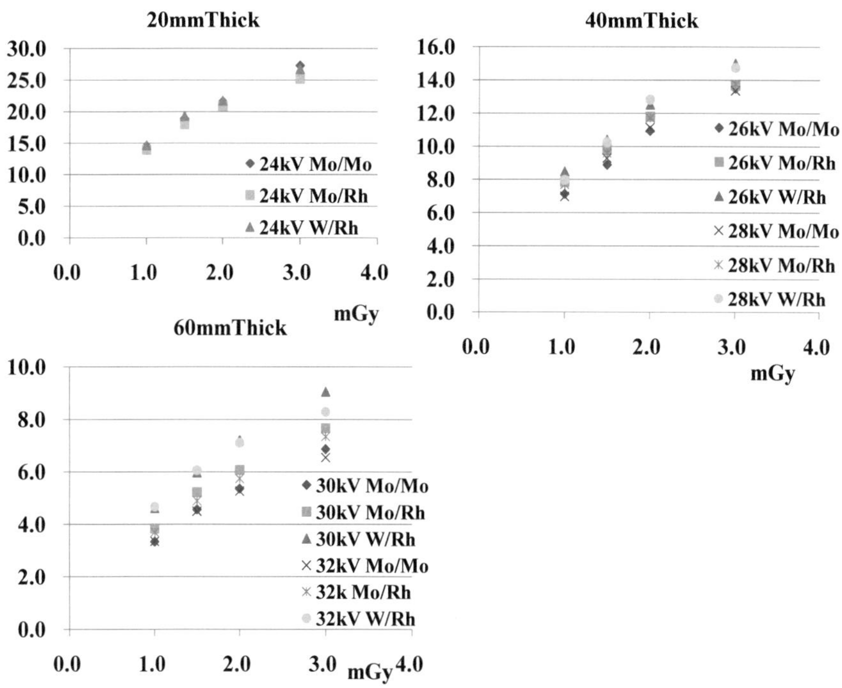

Fig. 5. CNR Analysis: 20mm,40mm,and 60mm Thick PMMA Phantoms in System B.

CAD detected relatively dense areas as false-positive masses at a rate of 9.8% (448/4560 images) and fibrous tissue as false-positive microcalcifications at a rate of 0.7% (34/4560 images).

In the cases utilizing 24-28kV Mo/Mo, CAD detected masses as false positives more frequently at a rate of 12.7% (279/2196 images), compared to the cases utilizing 30-34 kV W/Rh which detected false positives at a rate of 7.1% (169/2364 images). There was a statistically significant difference ($P=0.008<0.05$) between the two different combinations of anode/filters. CAD detected more false-positive masses in the cases utilizing the combinations with Mo/Mo in comparison with the cases utilizing the combinations with W/Rh. On the other hand, in the cases utilizing 30-34kV W/Rh, CAD detected false-positive microcalcifications more frequently at a rate of 1.1% (26/2364 images), compared to 0.4 % (8/2196 images) detected utilizing 24-28kV Mo/Mo. There was a statistically significant difference ($P=0.022<0.05$) between the two combinations with different anode/filters. CAD detected more false-positive calcifications in the cases utilizing W/Rh in comparison with the cases utilizing Mo/Mo (Table 1a.). In System B, under 25mm breast thickness, the combination of 24kV with W/Rh was selected; from 26m to 35mm breast thickness, the combination of 26kV with W/Rh was selected; from 36mm to 45mm breast thickness, the combination of 28kV with W/Rh was selected; from 46 to 55mm, the combination of 30kV with W/Rh was selected; and above 56mm, the combination of 32kV-34kV with W/Rh was selected. CAD detected false-positive masses at a rate of 2.7% (129/4712 images) and false-positive microcalcifications at a rate of 0.8% (37/4712 images) in total. With 24kV, CAD detected false-positive masses at a rate of 1.0% (5/500 images) and false-positive microcalcifications at a rate of 1.2% (6/500 images). With 26kV, CAD detected false-positive masses at a rate of 3.3% (32/960 images) and false-positive microcalcifications at a rate of 0.7% (7/960 images). With 28kV, CAD detected false-positive masses at a rate of 3.3% (48/1460 images) and false-positive microcalcifications at a rate of 1.2% (18/1460 images).With 30kV, CAD detected false-positive masses at a rate of 1.4% (16/1128 images) and false-positive microcalcifications at a rate of 0.5% (6/1128 images). With 32-34kV, CAD detected false-positive masses at a rate of 4.2% (28/664images) and 0% (0/664 images) false-positive microcalcifications. There was no significant difference among different kV levels with the same combination of anode/filters in System B ($P>0.05$) (Table 1b.).

Regarding spectral analysis of anode/filters, in System A, Mo/Mo and W/Rh demonstrated different spectrum characteristic curves. In addition, the two systems showed different spectrum characteristic curves with W/Rh and the peak value in System B with W/Rh was shown at a higher kV level compared to System A (Fig.6-7).

6. Discussion

At present, CAD dedicated to digital mammography analyzes the raw imaging data and detects the candidate lesions including masses and microcalcifications. As for the physical characteristics, regarding the linear attenuation coefficient for breast tissue [6], the differential value between breast tissue and calcification is larger than the differential value between breast tissue and mass (Table2).

Mass lesions have relatively localized large areas with a smaller number of photon counts compared to surrounding breast tissue in the raw imaging data. CAD analyzes the

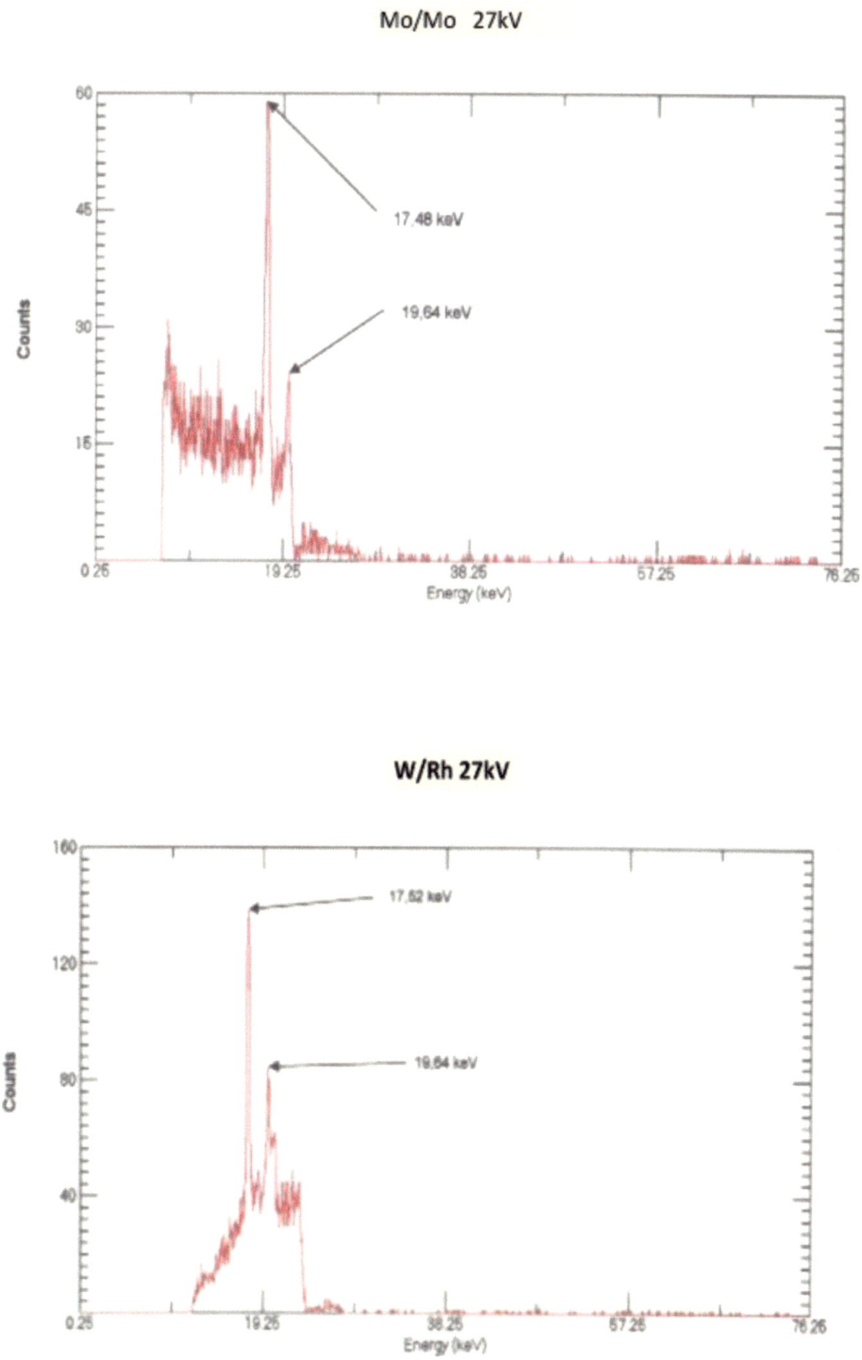

Fig. 6. Spectra of Mo/Mo and W/Rh in System A.

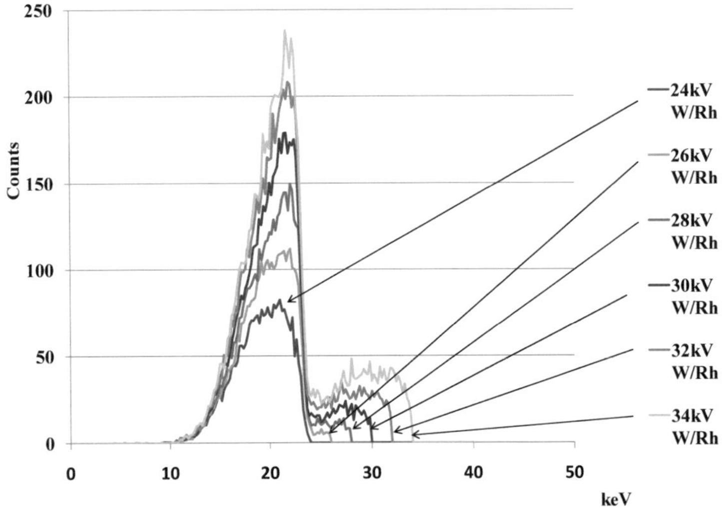

Fig. 7. Spectrum of W/Rh in System B.

Table1a.

	FP Mass		FP Microcalcifications	
24-28kV Mo/Mo	12.7% (279/2196)	P=0.008<0.05	0.4% (8/2196)	P=0.022<0.05
30-34kV W/Rh	7.1% (169/2364)		1.1% (26/2364)	
Total	9.8% (448/4560)		0.7% (34/4560)	

Table1b.

	FP Mass		FP Microcalcifications	
24kV W/Rh	1.0% (5/500)	P>0.05	1.2% (6/500)	P>0.05
26kV W/Rh	3.3% (32/960)		0.7% (7/960)	
28kV W/Rh	3.3% (48/1460)		1.2% (18/1460)	
30kV W/Rh	1.4% (16/1128)		0.5% (6/1128)	
32-34kV W/Rh	4.2% (28/664)		0% (0/664)	
Total	2.7% (129/4712)		0.8% (37/4712)	

Table 1. Clinical Radiation Exposure Setting of System A (Table 1a) and System B. (Table1b) regarding Frequency of False Positives (FPs) using CAD.

	Linear Attenuation Coefficient(cm^{-1})
Breast Tissue	0.8
Fatty Tissue	0.45
Skin	0.8
Mass	0.85
Calcification	12.5

Table 2. Linear Attenuation Coefficient of Breast Tissue at 20keV [6].

characteristics and detects the area as a candidate mass lesion. The raw imaging data is inverted and the mass lesion is recognized clinically as a localized high density area compared to background breast tissue density. On the other hand, the images with microcalcification lesions have localized small and clustered areas with a smaller number of photon counts compared to the background breast tissue in the raw imaging data. CAD analyzes the characteristics and detects the area as a candidate microcalcification lesion. The raw imaging data is inverted and the microcalcification lesions are recognized clinically as small and clustered areas with higher density compared to the background breast tissue density. According to the background, CAD dedicated to digital mammography can be directly affected by the physical characteristics of the raw imaging data. In this study, in System A, CAD detected more false positive masses with 24-28Kv Mo/Mo compared to those detected with 30-34Kv W/Rh. According to spectral analysis, Mo/Mo acquires a smaller number of photons compared to W/Rh . The raw imaging data with Mo/Mo has a relatively narrow range of photon counts and the differentials in the photon counts between background breast tissue and mass can be small. As a result, CAD can detect more false positive masses compared to imaging with W/Rh. On the other hand, CAD detected more false positive microcalcifications with 30-34Kv W/Rh compared to the number detected with 24-28Kv Mo/Mo (Fig.8-9).

This could be a result of the characteristics of W/Rh which can acquire a larger number of photons compared to Mo/Mo. Images with W/Rh have a much wider range of photon counts and the differential value of photon counts between background breast tissue and microcalcifications is large. As a result, imaging data with W/Rh can detect candidate microcalcification lesions with more sensitivity than imaging with Mo/Mo. Even with the same combination of anode/filters, the CAD in System A with 30-34kV W/Rh detected more false positive masses compared to System B with 30-34kV W/Rh.CAD results may differ even when the same system is used, according to which combination of anode/filter is used. On the other hand, CAD results may differ when different systems are used, even though the same combination of anode/filter is used. According to spectral analysis, the spectrum of W/Rh used in System A shows greater similarity to the spectrum of Mo/Mo than the spectrum of W/Rh used in System B. As a result, CAD detected more false positives using W/Rh with System A compared to System B. The CAD performance was

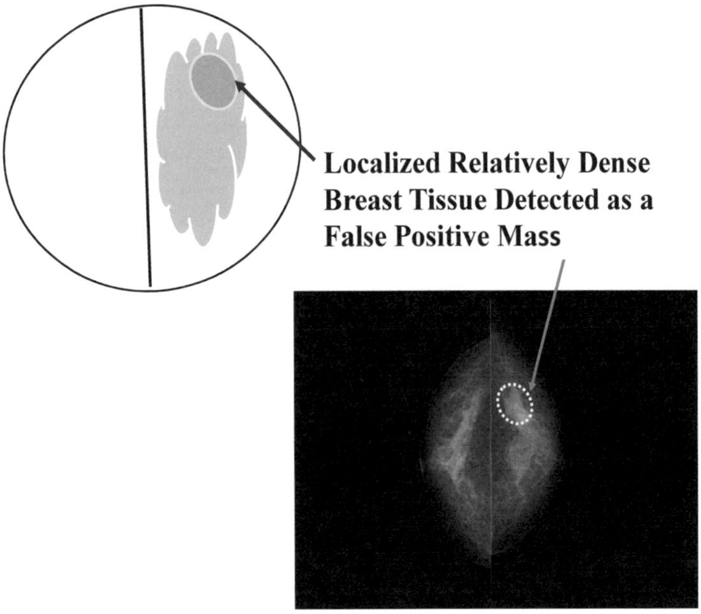

Fig. 8. Example Case with a False Positive Mass Marked by CAD.

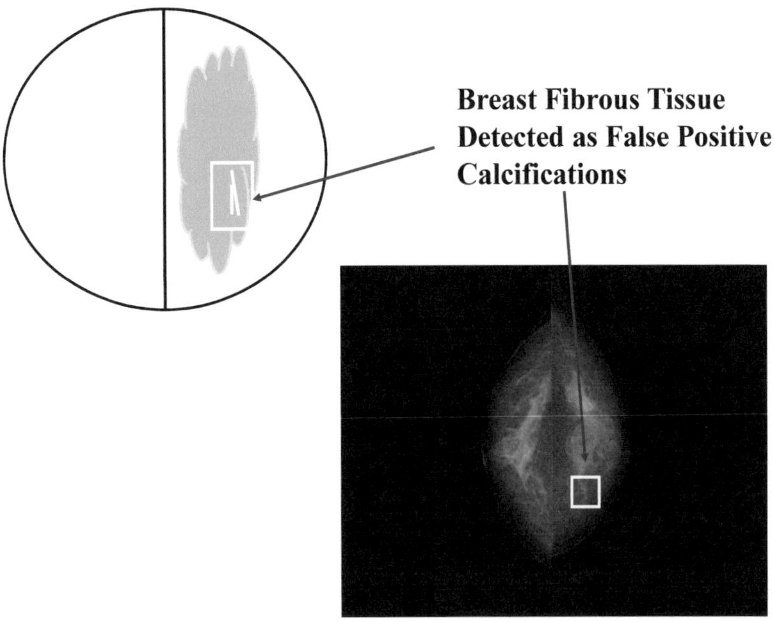

Fig. 9. An Example Case with False Positive Calcifications Marked by CAD.

affected by the difference in image quality produced by different radiation exposure parameters of the different anode/filters within one system and by differences in the two systems. In FFDM, CAD algorithms should be considered to vary depending on the image acquisition systems. In addition, recently, new breast image acquisition technologies, as well as digital breast tomosynthesis and dual-energy mammography, have been developed and have started to be acquired for breast diagnosis. These image acquisition approaches, utilizing new CAD techniques, will be capable of accurate volumetric measuring of breast density and microcalcifications, differently from conventional 2D images [7]-[9]. The results of this study imply that we should take into consideration the importance of analyzing physical characteristics with CAD, according to the different image quality with systems dedicated to new image acquisition technologies.

7. Conclusion

In this section, the author addresses the issue that CAD performance is affected by the difference in image quality produced by different radiation exposure parameters of the different anode/filters within one system and by differences in the two systems; also variations in CAD algorithms utilizing FFDM should be taken into account.

8. Acknowledgment

This study was supported by Grant-in-Aid for Scientific Research (C) (No. 23591810) in Japan.

9. References

[1] Uchiyama N.: Current status of CAD utilizing digital mammography in Japan. Breast Cancer. 2010; 17(3) 169-179.

[2] Toroi, P., Zanca, F., Young, K. C. et al.: Experimental Investigation on the Choice of the Tungsten/Rhodium Anode/Filter Combination for an Amorphous Selenium-Based Digital Mammography System. 2007.Eur. Radiol.17,2368-23752.

[3] Uchiyama N, Stoeckel J, Otsuka K, et al.:How Can Image Quality Affect the Detection Performance of Breast CAD (Computer Aided Detection) in FFDM (Full Field Digital Mammography)? A Comparative Study with Two Different FFDM Systems. Digital Mammography. 2010. 6136 288-295.

[4] Uchiyama N,Stoeckel J, Otsuka K. et al.:How Can Image Quality Affect the Detection Performances of Breast CAD (Computer Aided Detection) in FFDM (Full Field Digital Mammography)? 2009. Int J CARS;4:357-358.

[5] EUREF; European Guidelines for Quality Assurance in Breast Cancer Screening and Diagnosis 4th Edition 2006.

[6] Hammerstein, G.R., Miller, D.W., et al; Absorbed Radiation Dose in Mammography. Radiol. 1979. 130:485-491.

[7] Reiser I., Nishikawa R. M., Giger M. L. et.al. Computerized Detection of Mass Lesions in Digital Breast Tomosynthesis Images Using Two- and Three Dimensional Radial Gradient Index Segmentation.2004. Technol. Cancer Res. Treat. 3, 437–441

[8] Chan H.P., Wei J., Zhang Y., et.al. Computer-Aided Detection of Masses in Digital Tomosynthesis Mammography: Comparison of Three Approaches. 2008. Med. Phys. 35, 4087-4095.
[9] Ducote J. L. and Molloi S.. 2008. Quantification of Breast Density with Dual Energy Mammography: A Simulation Study.2008.Med. Phys. 35, 5411–5418.

15

Metrological Assessment of a CAD System for the Early Diagnosis of Breast Cancer in Digital Mammography

Arianna Mencattini and Marcello Salmeri
Dept. of Electronic Engineering, Univ. of Rome Tor Vergata
Italy

1. Introduction

Based on recent statistics from the International Agency for Research on Cancer (Ferlay et al., 2010), breast cancer account for 10.9% of all cancers diagnosed and ranks as the fifth cause of cancer death in the world. Although incidence rates are increasing, mortality rates are stable, representing an improved survival rate. This improvement can be attributed to effective means for the early detection as well as to significant improvement in treatment options, exposure, etc. Mammography is, at present, the only viable method for detecting most of tumors early enough for effective treatment, without unnecessary biopsies, or other invasive procedures. Therefore, screening mammography in women aged 40 to 70 years is currently the effective strategy to reduce breast cancer mortality. Early detection of invasive breast cancers is associated with better prognosis than waiting for women to become symptomatic. However, detecting the early signs of breast cancer is challenging because the cancerous structures have many features in common with normal breast tissue. Moreover, the accuracy of interpretation of screening mammograms is affected by several factors, such as image quality, the radiologist's level of expertise, and the high volume of cases. Recent statistics show that in current breast cancer screenings 10% − 25% of the tumors are missed by the radiologists (Burrell et al., 2001; Cheng, 2003; Nishikawa, 2007). Missed cancers are due to many reasons: low disease prevalence, breast structure complexity, finding subtleties, and radiologist fatigue. To accomplish with these difficulties, different methods have been analyzed: first of all, double reading, which provides either double perception or double interpretation of lesions. It has been demonstrated that a single radiologist is more accurate when reading mammograms methodically than quickly and that two observers achieve an improvement in detection rate of 5% − 15% (Mazzarella & Bazzocchi, 2007). Obviously, this procedure is too expensive, complex, and time consuming especially in screening programs where a huge number of mammographic images have to be read. The development of computerized systems as second readers represents an alternative. Researchers have been developing algorithms to detect mammographic abnormalities for more than 30 years with the aim of either automating mammographic interpretation or providing a tool that could enhance human film-reading accuracy. Computer-aided detection (CADe) and diagnosis (CADx) systems are widely used in mammography, where signs of breast cancer are often very subtle. Both systems involve the use of computer algorithms to detect patterns in images associated with signs of disease and to assign them a malignancy index. This result should attract the clinicians' attention to potentially abnormal regions in mammograms. In the recent years, the authors have developed a CADe-CADx system (CAD in the following), called Assisted Breast Cancer Diagnosis Environment (ABCDE) (Salmeri et al., 2009), to assist radiologists in the early detection of breast cancer. Beside the development of specific algorithms for the enhancement of abnormalities and the identification of pathological structures, the performance evaluation of each block of the whole CAD system has been also performed. In order to understand the actual complexity of the complete validation of a CAD system in mammography, consider the left-hand part of the flowchart reported in Fig. 1 where all the steps involved in the early breast cancer detection and diagnosis are considered.

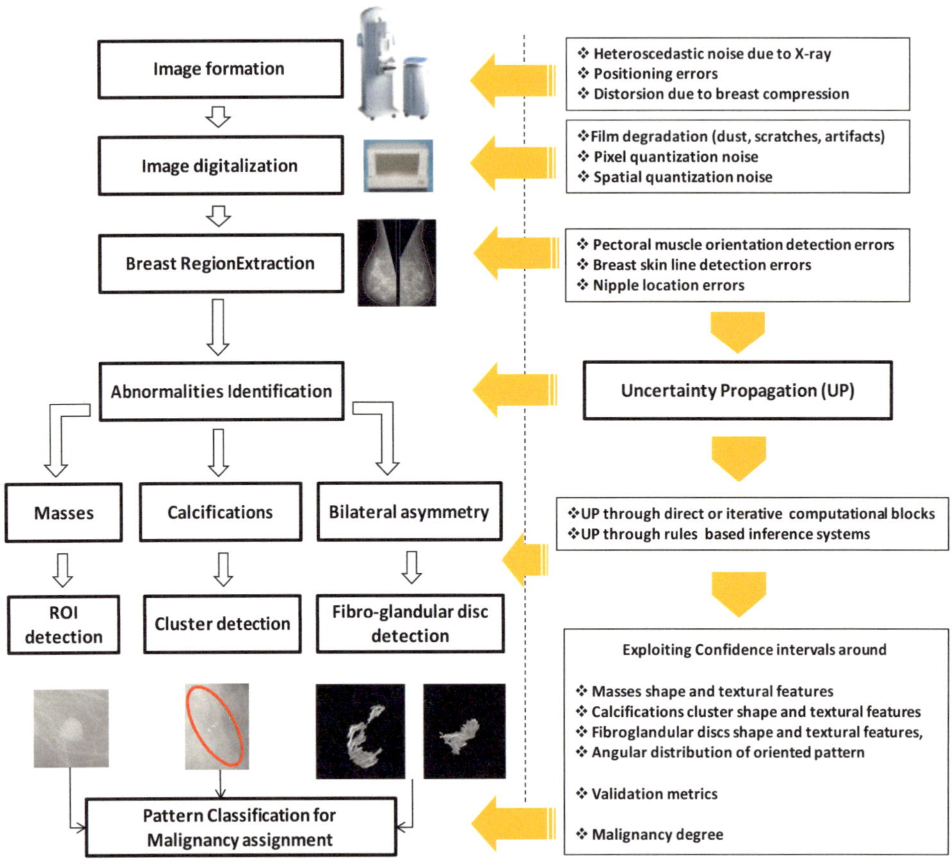

Fig. 1. Flowchart of the whole CAD ABCDE system. The right part shows the issues related to the uncertainty contributions handling and propagation through the blocks.

2. Motivations and objectives

This work stems from considerations of Wirth (Wirth, 2006) and Nishikawa (Nishikawa, 2007) regarding the performance evaluation of a CADe system. One of the major limitations in the design of novel computerized algorithms for breast cancer detection is related to the inherent difficulty of proving their effectiveness and improvement with respect to existing methods. In the context of performance evaluation a sequence of unresolved issues can be identified.

- The assessment of the whole CAD system does not coincide with the testing of individual components of the CAD system. The latter requires specific indicators according to each block and its functionalities, while the former coincides with testing classification ability of the system. In CADe systems, it means to test the capability of the system of discriminating between normal and pathological tissue, while in CADx systems, it is related to the ability of discriminating between malignant and benign abnormalities.
- In the literature, there are well-accepted characteristics needed to evaluate the performance of each algorithm in the CAD system: sensitivity, robustness, adaptability, accuracy and precision, reliability (or reproducibility), and efficiency. Each of them is defined in compliance with the definitions contained in reference documents such as (*International vocabulary of metrology. Basic and general concepts and associated terms (VIM)*, 2008). Unfortunately, exact limits beyond which the performance of the system is acceptable lack and are often verbally reported.
- Receiver Operating Characteristic (ROC) and Free-Response ROC (FROC) analysis are used to assess the classification performance of the whole CAD system. They plot sensitivity versus specificity or false positives per image/case. Optimal operating points can be derived based on the Youden-index, the distance from the ideal ROC curve, the optimal clinically acceptable false-detection rate. Unfortunately, often this is a subjective choice and depends on who is making the evaluation.
- Problems in the ROC analysis occur when more than two classes are used in the classification process, as for example in the classification of the lesion margins and shapes, or in algorithms used to automatically assess the breast tissue density.
- Standard ROC analysis does not implement the so called *failure assessment*, that is the analysis of the circumstances under which an algorithm fails and the correction of the failure causes. In some works, the authors verbally describe the specific cases where the algorithm fails, as for example in (Ferrari et al., 2004), examining in details the False Negatives produced by the algorithms and the possible causes.
- Datasets available is another important problem. Public databases such as MiniMIAS and DDSM are quite old and do not contain all the informations needed to evaluate the performance of a innovative CAD. In fact, modern issues in breast cancer detection involves important aspects such as bilateral asymmetry, architectural distortion, prior mammograms, interval cancers. The cited databases do not contain this kind of abnormalities, except for those reported in case there is also a lesion. Moreover, a few images are present with this kind of abnormalities and this limitation does not inspire full confidence in the final results produced by the CAD.
- The comparison of the various existing methods and possibly the introduction of improvements to one of them is extremely difficult if not impossible for two main reasons: the first one is that the algorithms are not completely described or documented so that it is not possible for authors to make a comparative analysis; secondly, the algorithms are often black-boxes so that testing involves only inputs and outputs, but not the internal decision-making process.

Many of the above mentioned problems can be partially solved or at least addressed considering a further important aspect in the CAD performance evaluation and algorithms testing, that is uncertainty sources modeling and propagation. In fact, considering all the uncertainty sources that can be present in the considered context of mammography, performing a detailed modelization of each of them, constructing a dedicated propagation procedure through each block of the CAD, according to the uncertainty nature, will allow us to address the following topics:

- An analysis of sensitivity could be performed in order to extract the influence of each uncertainty source on each algorithm parameter and on the final output value. In this way, both the design and the testing steps will be improved and completed, allowing to introduce corrective factors or change the algorithm, test the robustness of more systems.
- Extended ROC and FROC analysis could be performed, providing, for each decision point (corresponding to a pair of values for the sensitivity and the specificity in the ROC curve for example), a confidence interval given a certain coverage probability. In this way, a direct failure analysis can be guided by this kind of analysis as will be shown in the following sections.
- According to the context, screening programs or diagnostic mammography, requested coverage probabilities can be different. Moreover, it can be interesting to assign a confidence interval to each output of the CAD and of each block, for any coverage probability, from an high sensitive choice (95%) to a more specific or operating case (80%). The application of a Monte Carlo analysis, as that described in (JCGM, 2008), allows us to simulate every kind of sensitivity analysis, starting from very few assumptions on the nature of the uncertainty sources able to affect the CAD output. Specific estimation procedures should be implemented to preliminary provide accurate modeling of the uncertainty sources.
- Novel inference mechanisms, such as those based on fuzzy logic theory, would allow us to transform a black-box system into a white-box system, where interaction with the physician and with the developers is simple and constructive.

In light of this, we have already partially addressed some of the above cited issues: breast masses automatic segmentation (Mencattini et al., 2011d; Rabottino et al., 2008) and the uncertainty propagation through the algorithm (Mencattini et al., 2010b), microcalcifications classification (Ferrero et al., 2010), performance evaluation of an automatic tumoral masses identification algorithm (Mencattini et al., 2010a), uncertainty propagation through the classification of breast masses (considering also the features extraction and the feature selection procedures), the uncertainty propagation by Random Fuzzy Variables (RFVs) through a denoising and enhancement procedure for the detection of microcalcifications (Mencattini et al., 2009b), and the noise variance estimation results under the assumption of signal-dependent noise (.Mencattini et al., 2007; Salmeri et al., 2008).

3. Materials

The digital mammographic image can be obtained using Full-Field Digital Mammography (FFDM) or it can be obtained by digitizing a Screen Film Mammogram (SFM). The two kinds of images exhibit very different properties in linearity (relationship between pixel intensity and exposure to X-ray detector), contrast (contrast in SFM at low and high exposures is reduced with respect to FFDM), spatial resolution ($40-50$ μm in SFM, 100 μm in FFDM), and noise: in linear FFDM noise is proportional to the square root of the X-ray exposure, while at low exposures electronic noise is dominant; conversely, for logarithmic FFDM noise is proportional to the inverse of the square root of the X-ray exposure to the detector. The same holds for SFM, but changed according to the characteristic curve. Owing to these differences, robust validation and testing procedures should consider images either from SFM and from FFDM. In order to map gray-levels to optical density the calibration curve of each acquisition system is used. Each acquisition system In particular, in this work we will consider three databases: the Digital Database for Screening Mammography (DDSM) (Heath et al., 1998), the Mammographic Image Database (MIAS) (Suckling et al., 1994), and a FFDM database from the San Paolo Hospital in Bari (Mencattini et al., 2011d). In the following, we briefly describe the characteristics of the three databases.

3.1 MiniMIAS database

The Mammographic Image Analysis Society (MIAS) is an organization of UK research groups interested in the understanding of mammograms and has generated a public database of digital mammograms available via the Pilot European Image Processing Archive (PEIPA) of the University of Essex, at: *http://peipa.essex.ac.uk/info/mias.html*. Films taken from the UK National Breast screening Programme have been digitized to 50 μm pixel edge with a Joice-Loebl scanning microdensitometer, a device linear in the optical density range $[0 - 3.2]$ and representing each pixel with an 8-bit word. The original database has been reduced to a 200 μm pixel edge and padded/clipped so that all the images are 1024×1024 and the mammogram is centered in the matrix. Fig. 2 reports four examples of images taken from MiniMIAS database.

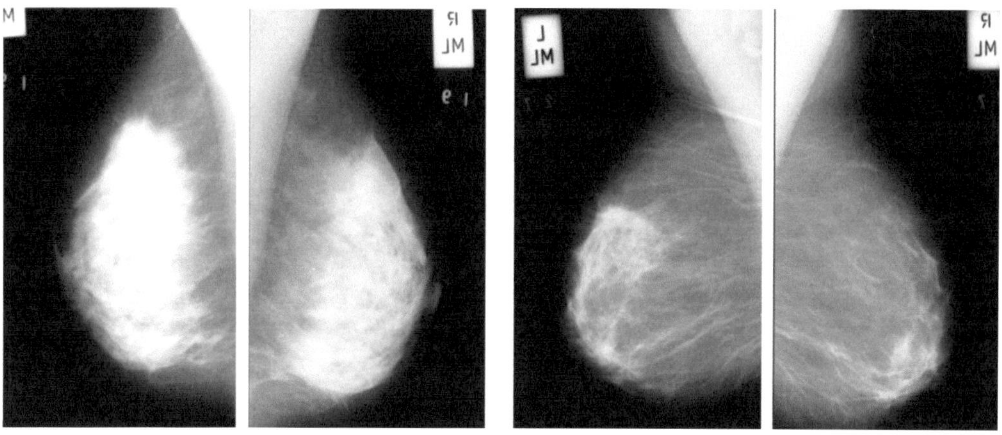

Fig. 2. Examples of mammographic images from the MiniMIAS database. (Figures-left) Normal case, right (mdb053) and left (mdb054) mammograms. (Figures-right) bilateral asymmetry case, right (mdb081) and left (mdb082) mammograms.

3.2 DDSM database

The Digital Database for Screening Mammography (DDSM) (Heath et al., 1998) was completed in 1999 and contains a total of 2620 cases. Primary support for this project was a grant from the Breast Cancer Research Program of the U.S. Army Medical Research and Materiel Command. The DDSM project is a collaborative effort involving co-p.i.s at the Massachusetts General Hospital (D. Kopans, R. Moore), the University of South Florida (K. Bowyer), and Sandia National Laboratories (P. Kegelmeyer). Additional cases from Washington University School of Medicine were provided by Peter E. Shile, MD,

Assistant Professor of Radiology and Internal Medicine. Additional collaborating institutions include Wake Forest University School of Medicine (Departments of Medical Engineering and Radiology), Sacred Heart Hospital and ISMD, Incorporated. Each study includes two images of each breast, along with some associated patient information (age at time of study, ACR breast density rating, subtlety rating for abnormalities, ACR keyword description of abnormalities) and image information (scanner, spatial resolution, bpp). Images containing suspicious areas have associated pixel-level "ground truth" information about the locations and types of suspicious regions. Unfortunately, lesion boundary drawn by radiologists are not always reliable and often include also pixels from normal tissue. The images are digitized by four different scanners (HOWTEK-A/D, LUMISYS, and DBA) using spatial resolution equal to [43.5, 50, 42] μm and a pixel resolution equal to 12 bpp for scanners (HOWTEK-A/D and LUMISYS) and equal to 16 bpp for scanner DBA. Each study contains four screening views, left and right mediolateral oblique (MLO) and cranio-caudal views (CC). Figure 3 reports three pairs of mammograms from DDSM, one for each scanner.

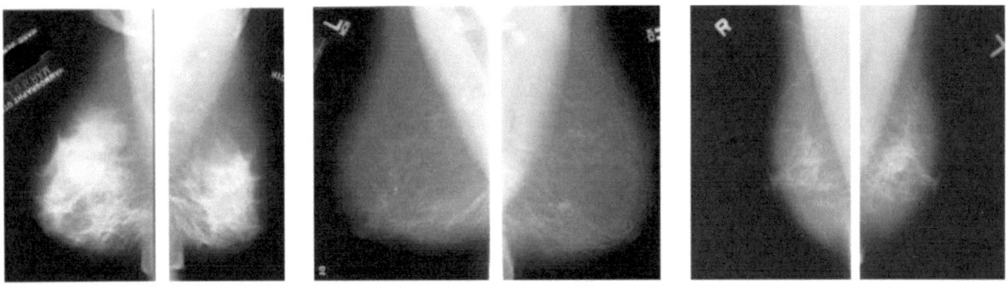

(a) (b) (c)

Fig. 3. Three pairs of DDSM images from three different scanners (a) DBA, (b) HOWTEK-A, (c) LUMISYS.

Images from scanner HOWTEK-D presents the same characteristics of scanner HOWTEK-A and are omitted.

3.3 FFDM database

Thanks to a collaboration with the San Paolo Hospital in Bari and with the Dept. of Mathematics at the University of Bari, we have access to Full Field Digital Mammographic (FFDM) images acquired using the Senograph 2000D ADS 17.3, GE Medical Systems, at a spatial resolution of 94 μm and a pixel resolution of 12 bpp. Each study contains two relevant series: a series including the four standard views (CC and MLO) for presentation state and a series including, if present, a screen save image reporting the lesion boundary manually drawn by radiologists. Currently, these images are used for the development and testing of an algorithm for the automatic extraction of the lesions boundary in order to assign a malignancy degree to each lesion detected by a radiologist. At the moment, the dataset includes 196 mammograms containing one or more benign or malignant massive lesions. The malignancy assessment is a part of the CADx section in ABCDE and is currently based on fractal analysis (Giuliato & Rangayyan, 2011; Mencattini et al., 2011d; Raguso et al., 2010). Figure 4 reports four FFDM images from San Paolo Hospital.

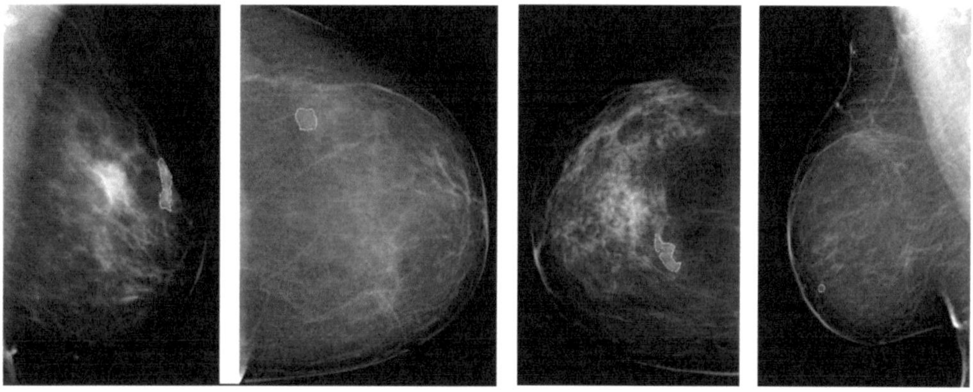

Fig. 4. Four FFDM images containing a massive lesion whose boundary has been drawn by a radiologist.

4. A Monte Carlo approach for CAD performance assessment

Recent reference documents (JCGM, 2008) revised almost totally the formal and practical definitions concerning measurement uncertainty, its modelization and propagation, as a part in the measurand estimation. There are two types of measurement error quantity that can occur during a measurement process: *systematic* and *random*. A systematic error (an estimate of which is known as a measurement bias) is associated with the fact that a measured quantity value contains an offset (that can be unpredictable and uncontrollable). A random error relies on the fact that when a measurement is repeated it will generally provide a measured quantity value that is different from the previous value. It is random in that the next measured quantity value cannot be predicted exactly from previous such values. The GUM (JCGM, 2008) provided a different way of thinking about measurement and in how to express the perceived quality of the result of a measurement. Rather than express the result of a measurement by providing a best estimate of the measurand, along with information about systematic and random error values (in the form of an "error analysis"), the GUM approach aims at expressing the result of a measurement as a best estimate of the measurand, along with an associated *measurement uncertainty*.

Let us denote with X_i any input quantities (measurands) and with Y the output quantity about which information is required. The output Y should be related to the inputs $X_1, \ldots, X_N$ by a measurement models that can be explicitly formulated $Y = f(X_1, \ldots, X_N)$ or implicitly defined $h(X_1, \ldots, X_N, Y) = 0$. Functions $f(\cdot)$ and $h(\cdot)$ should be estimated. The main stages of uncertainty evaluation are formulation, propagation, and summarizing.

- The *formulation* stage consists on defining the output quantity Y, identifying the input quantities on which Y depends (X_i), developing a measurement model relating Y to the input quantities (functions $f(\cdot)$ and $h(\cdot)$), and on the basis of available knowledge, assigning probability distributions to the input quantities (or a joint probability distribution to those input quantities that are not independent).
- The *propagation* stage consists of propagating the probability distributions for the input quantities through the measurement model to obtain the probability distribution for the output quantity Y. The propagation of distributions can be implemented in several ways: analytical methods, i.e. methods that provide a mathematical representation of the

probability density function (pdf) for Y; uncertainty propagation based on replacing the model by a first-order Taylor series approximation (also called the the law of propagation of uncertainty); numerical methods that implement the propagation of distributions, specifically using Monte Carlo method, that will be described in the following.

- The *summarizing* step is them performed to extract from the Y probability distribution the expectation of Y (the best estimation of Y), the standard deviation of Y (a measure of dispersion of Y), a confidence interval containing Y with a specified coverage probability.

Monte Carlo method provides a general approach to obtain an approximate numerical representation of the distribution function F_Y for Y. The heart of the approach is repeated sampling from the pdfs for the X_i. The implementation of the method is summarized below:

a) select the number M of Monte Carlo trials to be made;

b) generate M vectors, by sampling from the assigned pdfs, as realizations of the (set of N) input quantities X_i;

c) for each such vector, form the corresponding model value of Y, yielding M model values;

d) sort these M model values into strictly increasing order, using the sorted model values to provide the estimation G of F_Y;

e) use G to form an estimate y of Y and the standard uncertainty $u(y)$ associated with y.

f) use G to form an appropriate confidence interval for Y, for a stipulated coverage probability p.

Step f) is crucial because it can be formulated as a constrained minimization problem. In fact, given a coverage probability p, the associated confidence interval $[y_1, y_2]_p$ is obtained as the minimum interval $[a, b]$ such that $G^{-1}(b) - G^{-1}(a) = p$. When the pdf of Y is symmetric the solution is trivial an equal to $G^{-1}((1+p)/2) - G^{-1}((1-p)/2)$. Some relevant features of Monte Carlo method are: a reduction in the analysis effort required for complicated or non-linear models, especially since the partial derivatives of first- or higher-order of the model are not needed; generally improved estimate of Y for non-linear models; improved standard uncertainty associated with the estimate of Y for non-linear models, especially when the X_i are assigned non-Gaussian (e.g. asymmetric) pdfs, without the need to provide derivatives of higher order[1]; provision of a confidence interval corresponding to a stipulated coverage probability when the pdf for Y cannot adequately be approximated by a Gaussian distribution or a scaled and shifted t-distribution, i.e. when the central limit theorem does not apply.

Being the measurement uncertainty modeling a central part in the assessment of the CAD performance, in the following section, we will describe the major sources of uncertainty that can be identified in a CAD for mammography.

5. Uncertainty modeling in a CAD

Numerous sources of uncertainty have to be taken into account in a medical image processing system for breast cancer detection and diagnosis, both in the system development step and in the operating conditions. Keeping in mind the two different situations, here below, we recall the most relevant sources of uncertainty subdividing them into five groups: instrumental

[1] This point is crucial when an evident asymmetric pdf should be assigned to the input quantity such as for photon noise.

uncertainty, uncertainty sources related to the patient, model uncertainty related to the CAD parameters selection, uncertainty sources related to the input provided by the radiologist during the system development and validation steps (reference values etc.), the uncertainty sources related to the possible interaction among the CAD and the physician who is manually setting the algorithm parameters during the system operation.

- GROUP 1: image acquisition and digitalization process (i.e., spatial resolution, geometric distortion, noise, pixel quantization, film degradation, artifacts introduction, etc.);
- GROUP 2: biological and patient variability (related to both pathological or normal cases); intrinsic and unpredictable data variability (e.g., patient movement);
- GROUP 3: model uncertainty due to the unperfect or incomplete knowledge about algorithm parameters values and their influence on the final results. Major concern should be paid to algorithm with a random initialization, where some parameters are initially set to a value randomly selected in a certain interval.
- GROUP 4: human observer subjective interpretation of the image according to his/her experience, in providing reference boundary, malignancy degree, reference region of investigation, useful for the CAD validation.
- GROUP 5: interaction between the human observer and the image data, in manually enhancing the image contrast, selecting Region Of Interest, manually sectioning the breast region for inspection etc., during the operation of the system.

Some of these sources of uncertainty (GROUPS 1 and 3) can be reasonably modelled and considered in the uncertainty estimation process (Mazzarella & Bazzocchi, 2007), while some other (GROUPS 2, 4, and 5) have unknown nature and are difficult to be embedded, even if noteworthy. As a consequence of the large subjectivity in using the CAD system in this context, a metrological validation of medical image processing approaches is required to highlight the intrinsic characteristics and behavior of a method, to evaluate its performance and limitations, and to compare the method with different existing approaches.

In the following sections, we will describe with more details a possible modelization of the uncertainty contributions summarized above, providing examples taken from ABCDE's functionalities.

5.1 GROUP 1: Noise contribution in mammographic images

Each step that contributes to the final digital mammographic image influences the global uncertainty in a different way: the formation process, based on X-ray exposure, introduces a noise contribution that is intensity dependent (e.g., photon noise), the microscopic structure of the impressed film introduces the so-called *film grain noise*, finally the digitalization process when performed through scanner devices, introduces an uncertainty contribution that is related to the number of bit per pixel (bpp) used in the conversion, or an uncertainty term that presents systematic periodic patterns (Mencattini et al., 2009b) superimposed to the image. Photon noise is the dominant random contribution in this context, since the bpp is usually $12 - 16$, but other relevant noise contributions can be present at low and high exposures. Consequently, as suggested in (Jain, 1989), we consider an *heteroscedastic noise model* for the random contribution assuming that the noise variance depends on the intensity of each pixel, and it is not constant within the image. The noise model can be represented as follows:

$$\tilde{I}(n,m) = I(n,m) + \eta_1(n,m), \quad (1)$$

where $\tilde{I}(n,m)$ is the noisy image, $I(n,m)$ is the noise-free image, $\eta_1(n,m)$ is a zero mean non stationary random process given by $\eta_1(n,m) = \eta \cdot \sigma(n,m)$ with $\eta \sim \mathcal{N}(0,1)$ a normal random process with zero mean and unitary variance, and $\sigma^2(n,m)$ the spatial-dependent variance of the process $\eta_1(n,m)$.

The assumption of a normal random process with non constant variance is fully justified (Jain, 1989) for luminance values in the subrange $[0.2 - 0.8]$ that corresponds to what we are interested in; actually, dark or very bright pixels are corrupted by a saturated gaussian noise with cut tails. This problem could occasionally produce an underestimation of the noise variance we perform, but involving regions far from the regions of interest.

It is well known that the noise variance $\sigma^2(n,m)$ depends on the intensity $I(n,m)$. In particular, we get that $\sigma^2(n,m) = \alpha I(n,m)^\beta$ for scanner devices and $\sigma^2(n,m) = \gamma \cdot \log_{10}(I(n,m)) - d_0$ for photographic films. Consequently, an estimation procedure is needed in order to estimate the unknown dependence of the noise variance $\sigma^2(n,m)$ on the intensity $I(n,m)$. To do this, we implement the noise estimation introduced in (Gravel et al., 2004), later extended and improved in (.Mencattini et al., 2007; Salmeri et al., 2008). The strength of the estimation algorithm is that it can be applied to very different kind of medical images (MRI, ultrasound images, etc.) where noise is signal dependent following different probability distribution (Rician noise, Rayleigh, etc). In case of homoscedastic noise (where noise variance is constant through the image) the estimation algorithm still provides an accurate estimation of the noise variance, needed in many algorithms for image denoising and enhancement (Mencattini et al., 2010b; 2008). Here below, we only report a sketch of the whole estimation algorithm.

a) Extract low-frequency components from the image containing homogeneous regions. This step is performed by applying a low pass gaussian filter to the original noisy image obtaining a smoothed orignal image.

b) Evaluate the high frequency components of the image by the subtraction of the smoothed image to the original one. Obviously this image contains both small details, boundaries, and noise.

c) Eliminate edges by applying a robust edge detector to the original image. This further step is needed in order to eliminate edges from the estimation procedure, that would decrease noise variance estimation accuracy. Then, by thresholding we obtain a binary mask of principal edges.

d) Build an histogram of relating each bin to the intensity of image considering pixels at the same position in the smoothed image and in the noise image.

e) Evaluate the standard deviation of each bin by a Median Absolute Deviation (MAD) estimator.

f) Perform a robust regression analysis by Cubic Smoothing Spline in order to fit the data extracted at step (e).

A block diagram of the whole algorithm is reported in Fig. 5.

Unfortunately, uncertainty contribution do not embed only random effects, related to noise. In fact, in medical diagnosis, it is often crucial to take into account also non random contributions that can occur during the exposure, the acquisition and the digitalization of the image. We refer for example to physiological movements of the patient (a few

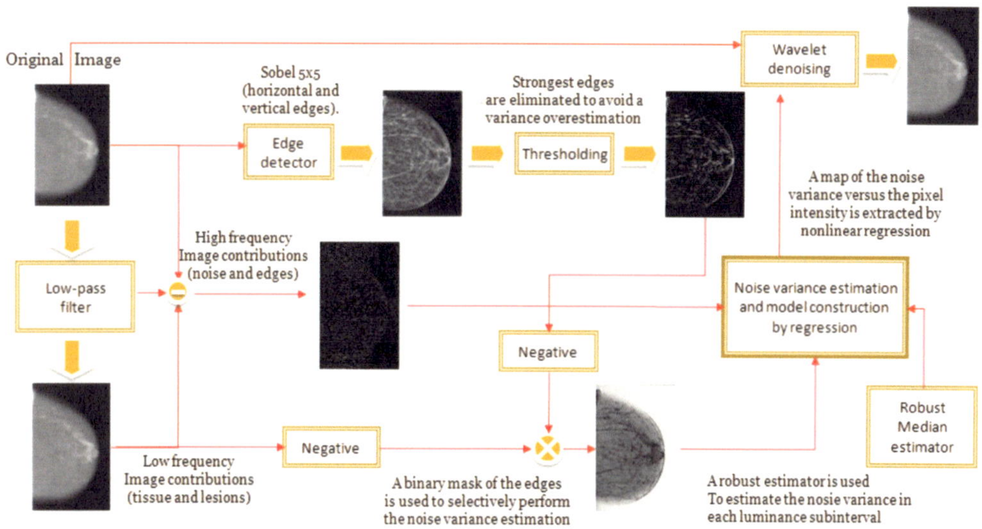

Fig. 5. The noise variance estimation algorithm.

seconds are needed in order to form a single mammographic image), to artifacts that can be present in the final image, due to dust, fingerprints, scratch, and to the non random contribution introduced by the scanner itself, such as the spatial non uniformity introduced in the luminance. For example, the images database we consider, e.g., the Digital Database for Screening Mammography (DDSM) (Heath et al., 1998) uses the three scanners DBA, HOWTEK, and LUMISYS to digitalize more than 4000 mammographic images. We can notice that the final images are corrupted by a periodic pattern contribution that we assumed to be systematic. An example is shown in Fig. 6(a)-(b) where two regions are extracted from the same mammographic image. Region A is dark and it is evident that there is an overlying periodic pattern that here is also emphasized by an histogram stretching. On the contrary, region B is corrupted by noise but the periodic pattern is much more subtle. In Fig. 6(c) the two-dimensional Fourier Transforms of the two regions are also shown proving that there is a unidirectional periodic pattern overlying region A and that the same does not hold for region B with the same evidence.

It is well known that systematic effects have to be corrected before performing a reliable uncertainty propagation of random effects (Santo et al., 2004). Unfortunately, as a consequence of the previous considerations, this kind of contributions is both luminance and spatial dependent so that it is very difficult to evaluate and correct it. Moreover, from both medical and visual viewpoints, it could be dangerous to preliminarily correct the images from non random contribution thus altering the final aspects of the images and falsifying the correct diagnosis of microcalcifications. In this regard, the new version of International Vocabulary of Metrology (VIM) (see (*International vocabulary of metrology. Basic and general concepts and associated terms (VIM)*, 2008) paragraph 2.26) states that *Sometimes, estimated systematic effects are not corrected for but, instead, associated measurement uncertainty components are incorporated.* Finally, scanner devices used in medical laboratories are not completely characterized from a metrological point of view thus making the exact evaluation of these effects for correction impossible. As a possible solution, we assume to treat non random contributions as systematic

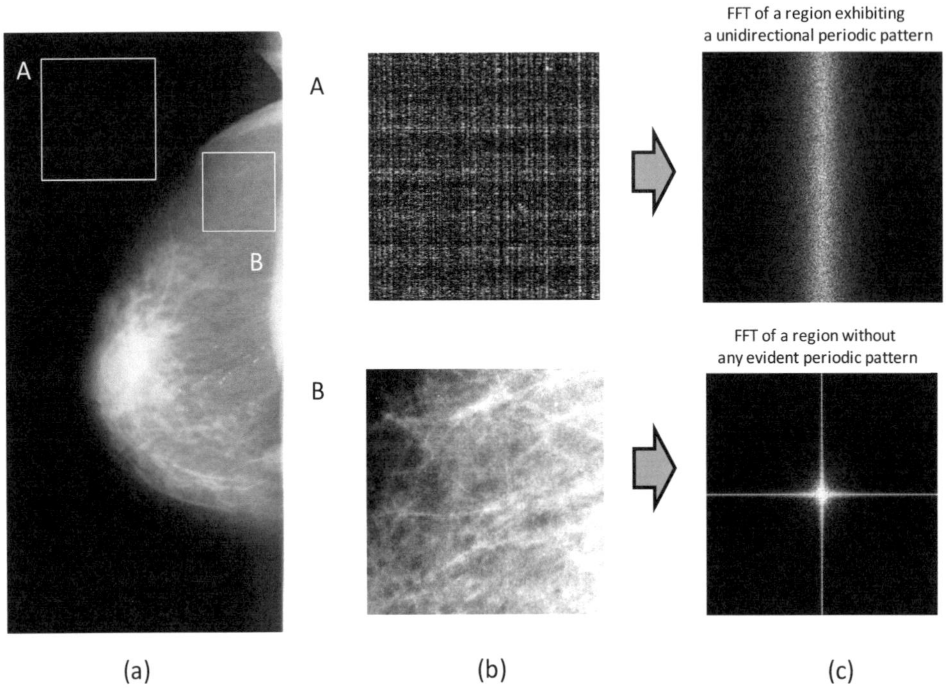

Fig. 6. (a) A mammographic image with a dark region (A) exhibiting a periodic pattern and a bright region (B) in which the same effect is much more subtle. (b) A zoom of the two regions A and B. (c) The 2D-FFT of the regions A and B respectively.

effects and to embed them in a unified uncertainty model, implementing an uncertainty propagation through a suitable method.

A viable solution is to use information extracted by the estimation procedure performed for the noise variance modeling. In this way, by merging different images coming from the same scanner or digitalization device, we are able to provide more accurate limits for the systematic contribution. In the following, we will provide an example for the whole noise estimation procedure considering the three different databases: MiniMIAS, DDSM, and San Paolo FFDM images.

Fig. 7 reports the noise variance modeling considering DDSM images for the three different scanners HOWTEK-A, LUMISYS, and DBA at different spatial and pixel resolution. Note that for low luminance values electronic noise in HOWTEK-A and in DBA is the dominant noise contribution, while photon noise due to X-ray exposure has a small variance at high and low exposure. Noise variance related to photon noise has a maximum value in the range $[0.4 - 0.6]$ for scanners LUMISYS, HOWTEK-A, and DBA. Fig. 8(a) shows the noise variance estimation for images from MiniMIAS database. Photon noise is low at high and low exposure and the noise variance has a maximum value in the same range as above. Both LUMISYS, HOWTEK-A, and MIAS scanning device have a linear characteristic curve. Conversely, scanner DBA has a logarithmic response. Finally, Fig. 8(b) reports the noise variance estimation performed on the FFDM images from the San Paolo Hospital. Also in

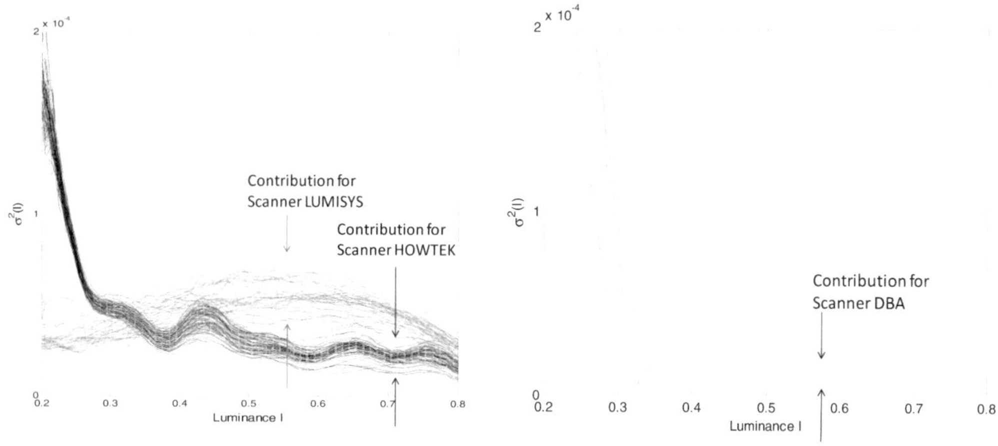

Fig. 7. Noise variance modeling for scanners HOWTEK-A and LUMISYS (left) and DBA (right). A Cubic Smoothing Spline regression is applied with a smoothing parameter equal to 0.9999 for scanners HOWTEK-A and LUMISYS and to 0.999 to scanner DBA. The systematic noise variation is marked by the arrows.

this case, photon noise is the dominant contribution. The digital mammography device has a logarithmic characteristic curve.

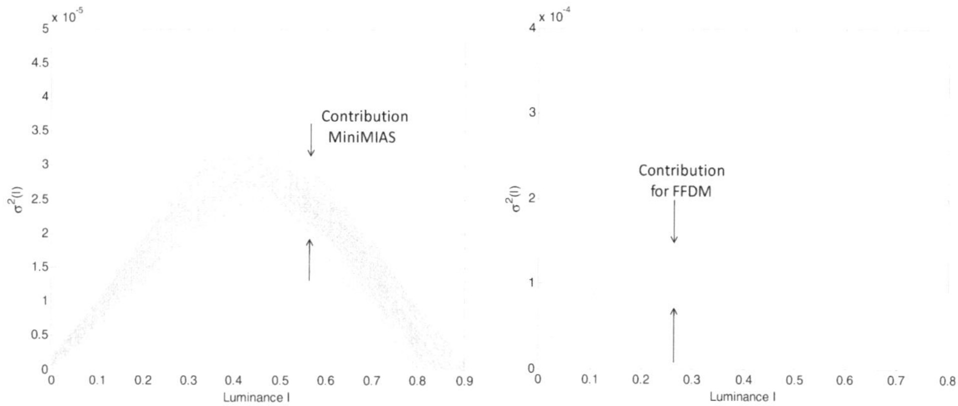

(a) (b)

Fig. 8. Noise variance modeling for Joice-Loebl scanning microdensitometer (a) and for GE Senograph 2000D ADS 17.3 (b). A Cubic Smoothing Spline regression is applied with a smoothing parameter equal to 0.999. The systematic noise variation is marked by the arrows.

It can be noted that the noise dependence from the pixel intensity strongly varies across different digitalization devices, according to pixel quantization, spatial resolution, scanner calibration curve, etc. Also, the systematic noise variation is different across the devices.

5.2 GROUP 2: biological and patient variability

Uncertainty sources due to biological and patient variability are probably the most difficult kind of uncertainty to consider because it groups together unpredictable variations in patient physiological status and position. Fortunately, the protocol that regulates mammography provides a set of rules that allow you to control many of these sources of uncertainty: the breast is compressed and locked during exposure to X-rays, reducing the possible involuntary movements also due to the simple respiratory motion; the hormonal changes that may occur during the patient's mammography are also controlled as much as possible through detailed recommendations about the optimal time to perform the examination in relation to the menstrual cycle. In any case, a complete and accurate CAD system should also provide the possibility to receive and process information relating to the phase of the woman's life: at puberty, lactation, or menopause, in order to adapt algorithm parameters such as for example those related to fibro-glandular disk extraction in bilateral asymmetry detection.

5.3 GROUP 3: model uncertainty

A CAD for mammography consists of several blocks, as already shown in the introduction. The correct functioning and adaptation of each block involve the use of inline tuned parameters that are initialized to a certain value (randomly or not) and can be changed during the system functioning, according to the image characteristics (adaptation) or according to pre-specified rules. The CAD developers identify these rules during the system development and validation steps, using large datasets of mammographic images, but a complete knowledge of the behavior of the selected parameters is not realistic. In light of this, a formal way to deal with this incomplete knowledge is to perform an analysis of sensitivity, that, considering a parameter at a time, introduces small perturbation of it and evaluate the final effect on the block output. By an iterative procedure, the developer can assign an interval of values to each block output with a dual effect: quantifying the most critical parameters that most influence the output and modify the block in order to improve the robustness of the whole system to unpredictable parameters variations.

The CAD elaboration units can be divided into three categories:

- direct computational blocks involving constant multiplicative coefficients and/or nonlinear operators;
- iterative blocks involving adaptive thresholds and signal-dependent parameters that change during the block functioning;
- conditional statements involving the comparison of input variables with thresholds (fixed or changing during the functioning).

According to the typology, different kind of uncertainty modelling should be performed. Here below, we provide some examples already investigated by the authors in previous works. In Section 6 will be described in more detail a recent study in the context of the identification of bilateral asymmetry.

5.3.1 Direct elaboration units

Context Handling and propagation of random and systematic uncertainty contributions due to image noise through a wavelet-based enhancement and denoising procedure for microcalcification detection (Mencattini et al., 2009b).
Materials DDSM Images containing malignant and benign calcifications.
Method Random Fuzzy Variables able to simultaneously represent and propagate through dedicated mathematical operators random and systematic terms. The method has been

developed by Ferrero and Salicone (Ferrero & Salicone, 2009; Salicone, 2007) and it is still under investigation the possible application of the method to iterative and more complex elaboration units.

5.3.2 Iterative elaboration units

Context Handling and propagation of random uncertainty contributions due to image noise through the automatic segmentation and classification of massive lesions in mammographic images (Mencattini et al., 2009a; 2010a; Rabottino et al., 2011).

Algorithm Segmentation is performed by an iris detection algorithm, an iterative region-growing procedure is applied to extract the mass boundary, geometric and textural (Haralick) features are computed for each segmented lesion, and finally a Bayes linear classifier is applied to assign a malignancy degree to each lesion (Mencattini et al., 2009a).

Materials DDSM Images containing malignant and benign massive lesions.

Method Monte Carlo simulations using 50 trials on ROIs 1000 $\times$ 1000. The AUC-based performance assessment has been performed. Fig. 9 reports the cumulative distribution function and the histogram of the AUC obtained after the trials. Note that the AUC parameter

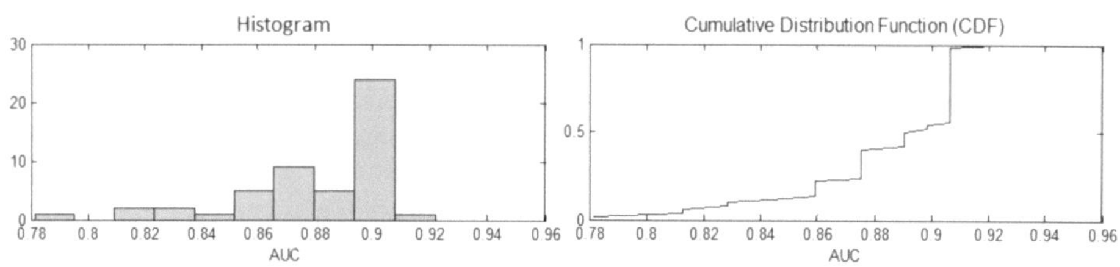

Fig. 9. AUC cumulative distribution function and histogram.

has a clear non-Gaussian probability distribution, such that the confidence interval for $p = 0.9$ is very different than the interval obtained under the assumption of normality.

Context and Algorithm An analogous study has been developed in collaboration with the San Paolo Hospital and the Dept. of Mathematics University of Bari, using the active contour algorithm developed by Chan and Vese (Chan & Vese, 2001) for the segmentation step, the fractal analysis and support vector machines for the malignancy assessment. Preliminary results can be found in (Mencattini et al., 2011d).

Materials San paolo FFDM Images and DDSM images containing malignant and benign massive lesions histologically proven.

Method Monte Carlo simulations using 100 trials.

5.3.3 Conditional elaboration units

Context Conditional statements in a fuzzy logic inference system for pattern classification (Ferrero et al., 2010; Mencattini & Salmeri, 2011a). The pattern classification step is an important section of a CAD because it is use in many functionalities: in the automatic identification of lesions a classifier is used to reduce false positive lesion candidates discriminating them from true lesions; in the malignancy assessment a classification step is used to assign the malignancy degree to each considered suspicious lesion; lastly, in the identification of bilateral asymmetry the classifier assigns the asymmetry degree to each pair of mammograms under test. Many different classifiers exist in the literature and have been used in developing a CAD for mammography: Bayesian classifier, decision trees, artificial neural networks, logistic regression, support vector machine, fuzzy logic inference systems are the most popular approaches. Each of them has its own peculiarity. For example, SVM is excellent for small training dataset, while artificial neural network has great flexibility to very large datasets. However, most of them can be considered as completely black boxes able to learn from examples and to produce a final class membership. None of them, excluding fuzzy inference systems and decision trees, produces simple classification rules that can be easily understood by physicians. Finally, only fuzzy inference systems can be directly modified by physicians who can add classification rules, according to his/her experience. *Algorithm* Since the method uses a non-standard fuzzy logic system, in the following we will provide a brief introduction of the method. A Fuzzy Inference System (FIS) for medical diagnosis is a nonstandard FIS firstly proposed by Andersson in (Andersson, 2007). The core of such a system is a simple structure composed of three agents: the patient (the mammogram in our context), the symptoms (in our context the features extracted to characterize the object to be classified), and finally the diagnosis (in our context the class, normal or abnormal tissue, benign or malignant lesions, normal or asymmetric breast, etc.). The architecture of such a FIS involves three kind or relations: two input relationships (the relation Mammogram-Features and the relation Features-Diagnosis) and a third relation (the Mammogram-Diagnosis relation) that is derived by the first two relations using a specific inference process. The first relation is built by physicians in the patient-history or anamnesis process, while is learnt by the CAD during the features extraction and training steps. The second relation is derived by the physician according to his/her experience, retrospective study and clinical trials in which a symptom has been confirmed to be significant for a certain diagnosis (e.g., spiculated margins of a mass represent the infiltrating properties of the lesion and a sign of possible malignancy). Finally, the third relation assigns a final class membership to a mammogram or simply to a region of interest (P in the following), according to the features extracted on it and on their significance for a certain class. Such a system has been already applied in different situations: the malignancy assessment of calcifications clusters (Ferrero et al., 2010), the false positive reduction in the automatic mass identification (Mencattini & Salmeri, 2011b), the development of a novel scoring system to measure the severity of illness of patients admitted in Intensive Care Units (Mencattini et al., 2011e). In this section, we will consider in details the malignancy assessment of calcifications.

A FIS rule has an IF-THEN structure, an example of two distinct rules is reported below.

IF *number of calcifications in a cluster is HIGH in mammogram P* AND *number of calcifications is HIGHLY significant for diagnosis MALIGNANT* THEN *mammogram P contains a MALIGNANT cluster of calcifications*

IF *mean entropy of calcifications is HIGH in mammogram P* AND *mean entropy of calcifications is HIGHLY significant for diagnosis BENIGN* THEN *mammogram P contains a BENIGN cluster of calcifications*

Each rule is preliminarily evaluated computing the two antecedents according to specific mathematical fuzzy operators and then the rules are aggregated through a weighted average operator (Ferrero et al., 2010). The evaluation of the two antecedents, *number of calcifications in a cluster is HIGH* and *number of calcifications in a cluster is HIGHLY significant for diagnosis MALIGNANT* involves the definition of the fuzzy variable *number of calcifications*, and consequently of the fuzzy sets *HIGH number of calcifications* and *LOW number of calcifications*. This definition consists in the construction of two trapezoidal Membership Functions (MFs) as those reported in Fig. 10 for the two symptoms *number of calcifications* (S_j) and *mean entropy of calcifications* (S_k). The two MFs are superimposed on the corresponding histograms. Note that,

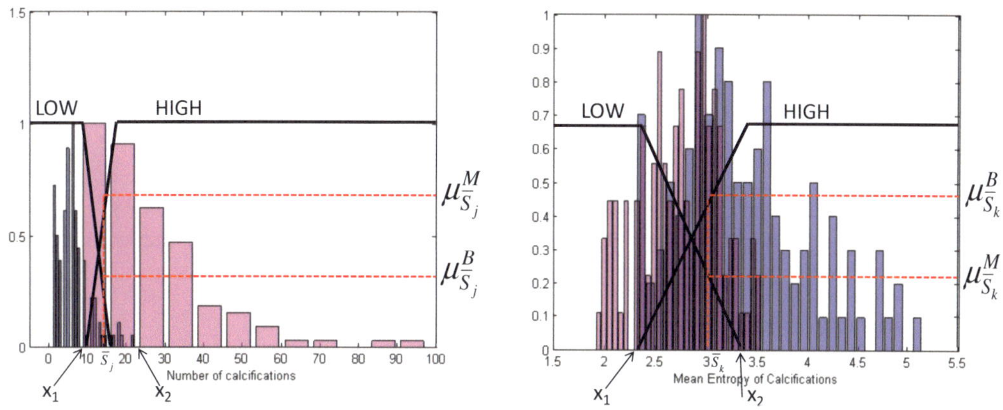

Fig. 10. Examples of MF construction for symptom S_j (number of calcifications) and S_k (mean entropy of calcifications). The magenta bars identify the class *M* while the blue bars represent the class *B*.

for a certain value $\bar{S}_J$ of the first symptom, the system assigns two degrees of membership $\mu^M_{\bar{S}_j}$ and $\mu^B_{\bar{S}_j}$ to the class MALIGNANT (M) and BENIGN (B) respectively. As long as the value of S_j increases from x_1 to x_2 then $\mu^M_{\bar{S}_j}$ increases toward the unity and $\mu^B_{\bar{S}_j}$ decreases toward zero. The opposite happens when S_j decreases from x_2 to x_1. It is evident that each of the two MFs depends on the two parameters x_1 and x_2 which are extracted from the distribution of the feature for the different classes. In particular, x_1 is the maximum value of S_j for benign cases such that all the S_j for malignant cases are greater than x_1. Conversely, x_2 is the minimum value of S_j for malignant cases such that all the S_j values for benign cases are smaller than x_2. The evaluation of x_1 and x_2 is performed after outliers elimination on each feature S_j. Parameters x_1 and x_2 influences the final class membership function and an analysis of sensitivity should be implemented for them.

The second antecedent *number of calcifications is HIGHLY significant for diagnosis MALIGNANT* involves the computation of what we called *Incidence Level* $IL^{D_i}_{S_j}$ of a symptom S_j for a diagnosis D_i, where in the considered example D_i is *M* or *B*. It represents the degree of influence that a symptom S_j can have on a certain diagnosis D_i and a degree of correlation among them. This correlation is evaluated according to physician's experience or again from the distribution of the symptom's values for each class. Two examples of this calculation are reported in Fig. 11 for the number of calcifications in a cluster and for the mean entropy of calcifications for the two classes Malignant and Benign. In particular, we get for symptom S_j

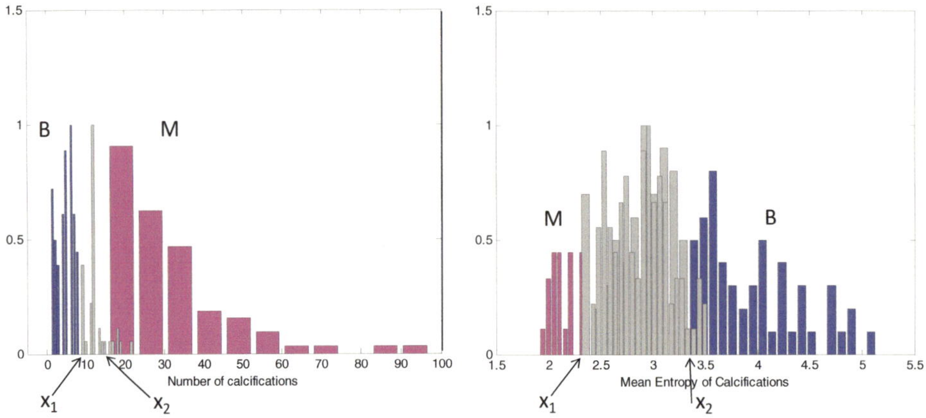

Fig. 11. Examples of evaluation of the incidence level IL for symptom S_j (number of calcifications) and S_k (mean entropy of calcifications). The gray bars identify those cases that do not contribute to the calculation of the incidence levels.

(number of calcifications) that

$$IL^M_{S_j} = \frac{\sharp\{S^M_j | S^M_j > S^B_j\}}{\sharp\{S^M_j\}}, \quad IL^B_{S_j} = \frac{\sharp\{S^B_j | S^B_j < S^M_j\}}{\sharp\{S^B_j\}} \tag{2}$$

From equations (2) it is fully justified that the incidence level has a strong influence on the final class membership and again a dedicated analysis of sensitivity should be performed. In the considered context, seven features are used to assess the malignancy of the calcifications: number of microcalcifications (S_1), minimum area of the microcalcifications (S_2), area of the convex hull containing microcalcifications (S_3), entropy of the cluster of microcalcifications (S_4), mean contrast of the microcalcifications (S_5), mean entropy of the microcalcifications (S_6), Haralick parameter H8 (Sum Entropy) (S_7).
Materials DDSM images, 119 benign and 122 malignant calcifications clusters.
Methods Recently, an innovative approach to propagate random and systematic uncertainty contributions through a FIS has been implemented (Ferrero et al., 2010). In light of this, within a collaboration with the Dept. of Electrical Engineering Politecnico of Milan, the method has been applied to our context. Basically, the method assigns a Random Fuzzy Variable (RFV) to each variable in order to model simultaneously random and systematic uncertainty terms. From Fig. 12 (figure top-left) it can be noted that an RFV is an extended Fuzzy Variable, whose Membership Function is composed of an inner and an outer standard MF. The inner MF represents the systematic uncertainty contribution, usually it is a rectangular MF, as in standard interval analysis; the outer part represents the random contribution and a direct approach can be implemented to derive it from the pdf of the variable (Dubois et al., 2004). Fig. 12 (figures right) reports the Random Fuzzy Variables (RFVs) for each feature used for calcifications malignancy assessment considering one of the images taken from DDSM. In this context, we assumed only systematic uncertainty contribution for discrete symptoms S_1, S_2, S_3 and only random contributions for symptom $S_4, \ldots, S_7$ [2]. The corresponding

[2] The random contributions in symptoms $S_1, \ldots, S_3$ are considered to be small and totally embedded in the systematic terms. On the contrary, we assumed that the systematic contribution in symptoms $S_4, \ldots, S_7$ was negligible with respect to random variations.

histograms for features $S_4, \ldots, S_7$ are reported on the left. Figure top-left reports the two RFVs representing the benign and the malignancy degrees associated to the considered cluster. The inner part results from the propagation of the systematic effects, while the outer part results from the propagation of the random effects through the FIS.

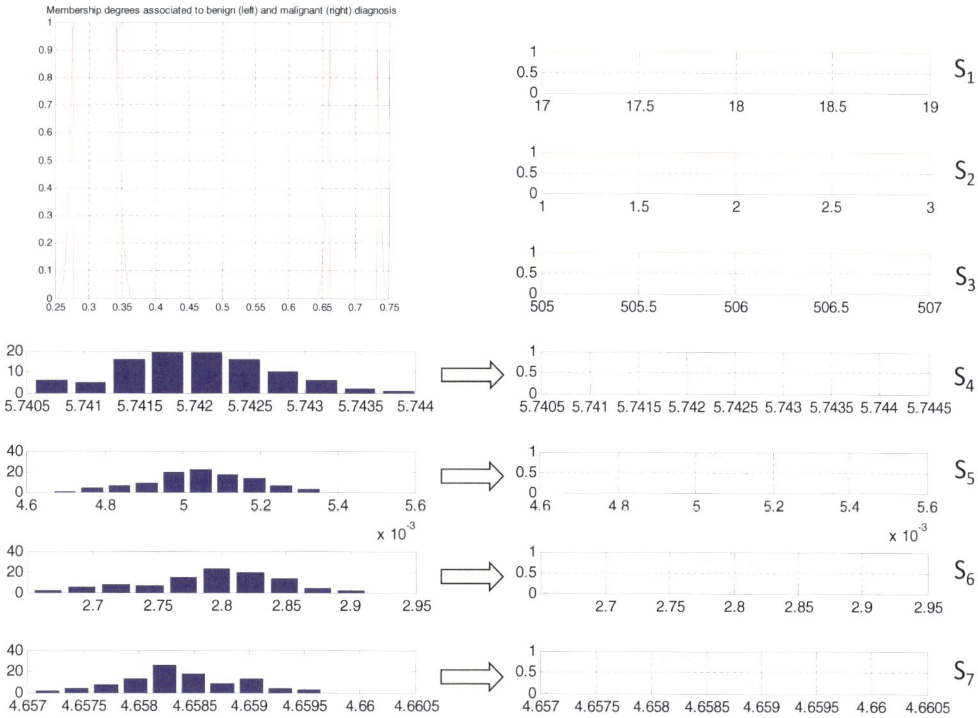

Fig. 12. Figure Top-left: RFVs of the malignancy and the benign degrees for one test image. Figure bottom-left: histogram of features $S_4 - S_7$. Figure right: RFVs of the features extracted. Red plot: inner MFs of the RFVs; blue plot: outer MFs of the RFVs.

5.4 GROUP 4: radiologist-dependent CAD inputs

During the development step and the CAD validation procedure, one or more radiologists should provide the ground truth needed as a reference to set the algorithm parameters.

i) During the validation of the breast region segmentation, radiologists provide the actual breast skin line, the nipple position, the pectoral muscle profile. In particular, in case of minoris, very obscure nipple, very dark uncompressed tissue, this reference strongly depends on radiologist experience and more than one radiologist should be interpelled using a voting procedure to select a final robust reference.

ii) During the validation of the automatic lesions identification, the radiologist is called to identify the possible lesion, whose position is then confirmed by biopsy.

iii) Also, the boundary of the lesion can be drawn by the radiologist, or, more rarely, a core and an external boundary are drawn, as in DDSM database. The core identifies the internal portion of the lesion, while the boundary includes also the spicules and the structures that radiate from the core.

iv) In some situations, the radiologist draws the boundary of a region representing a bilateral asymmetry or locate the center of an architectural distortion. This situation is much more radiologist's dependent, because there is not any histological test that can confirm this reference.

v) Finally, less frequently, the radiologist is called to provide additional information about the breast tissue such as ACR tissue density or ACR subtlety rating. Both these parameters are fundamental for the correct functioning of some algorithms such as bilateral asymmetry identification (Casti, 2011). A recent preliminary study proved the effectiveness of a procedure for the extraction of the fibro-glandular disk and of the oriented patterns in the breast, tuned according to the ACR tissue density.

All of the information provided by the radiologist influence both the CAD learning capability and the effectiveness of its operation. Each of them should be perturbated in order to evaluate the actual influence on the final results produced by the CAD. In particular, in Section 6 we will describe recent simulation results, obtained assuming a systematic perturbation of the ACR density rating assessed by a single radiologist. Using a leave one out cross-validation procedure, considering a pair of mammograms at a time, we assumed that the radiologist assessed a density rating higher than the actual density. Such a bias, is then propagated through the whole algorithm for the identification of bilateral asymmetry on a dataset including 23 pairs of normal mammograms and 23 pairs if asymmetric mammograms taken from MiniMIAS database. The same procedure has been implemented assuming that the radiologist assigns to the pair of mammograms under test a density rating smaller than the actual one. Doing so, the whole algorithm produces for each pair of mammograms an asymmetry degree in absence of perturbation and two asymmetry degrees in presence of a positive and a negative perturbation respectively. Further details will be provided later.

5.5 GROUP 5: CAD-radiologist interaction

A recent study by Nishikawa (Nishikawa, 2007) reports important considerations on the evaluation of a CADe system. He recalls that a CADe system does not need to detect cancers, but it needs to assist radiologist in doing this. This means that the real help is in detecting tumors missed by the radiologist increasing the overall sensitivity of the radiologist-CADe system. It is possible to have a CADe scheme with a sensitivity lower than 50% and still be a useful aid. So, one of the crucial point is the interaction CADe-radiologist. If cancers missed by the computer is too high then the radiologist will lose confidence in the ability of the computer to detect cancers. On the other hand, false detections reduce radiologist's productivity because the radiologists must spend time reviewing all computer detections.

Conversely, a CAD could over-learn from available samples produced by the same apparatus and reported by the same radiologist. Nishikawa observes that a positive bias can occur even if training and test set are the same or if the dataset used for features selection and the training set are the same. To reduce this bias and to reduce over-learning, more than one radiologist should report the images used for development, validation, training, and test, using a voting procedure to select one report for each case. Moreover, a separate dataset for each of the above phase should be used, preferably extracted from different databases.

6. A numerical example of uncertainty propagation through ABCDE: bilateral asymmetry identification

For almost thirty years, methods have been developed to try to use computers as second readers to make up for this potential loss of reliability. Almost all fields of image processing and analysis have been explored but little attention has been paid to the identification of bilateral asymmetry on mammograms. Asymmetric breast tissue is usually benign, but an asymmetric area may indicate a developing mass or an underlying cancer. Thus, the American College of Radiology (ACR) Breast Imaging Reporting and Data System (BI-RADS), which has developed a standardized method for breast imaging reporting, describes bilateral asymmetry as one of the four signs of breast cancer that radiologists have to detect. Some commercial CAD systems have obtained the Food and Drug Administration (FDA) approval and are beginning to be applied widely for the detection of masses and microcalcification on mammograms, but none of them has been developed for bilateral asymmetry identification. The paucity of works related to this topic may be due to the fact that bilateral asymmetries are difficult to be identified for the following reasons:

1. it needs a comparison between the left and right views which is a difficult task owing to the natural asymmetry of the breasts, and to the absence of good corresponding points to perform matching;
2. distortion inherent to the manual position of the breast during X-ray exposure;
3. the wide range of appearance associated with differences between women in the amount and distribution of fibroglandular tissue, which is also influenced by age and hormonal status and whose asymmetry could also represents simply a physiological sign.

The authors are currently working on the development of an automatic bilateral asymmetry identification procedure, one of the most innovative part of ABCDE (Casti, 2011; Mencattini et al., 2011c). The aim is to improve the early diagnosis of breast cancer, especially in screening test, providing clues about the presence of early signs of tumors like parenchymal distortion, small asymmetric bright spots and contrast, that are not detected by other methods. Asymmetric breasts could be reliable indicators of future breast disease in women and this factor should be considered in a woman's risk profile. The Breast Imaging Reporting and Data System (BIRADS) defines bilateral asymmetry as an area of fibroglandular tissue that is more extensive in one breast as compared to the contralateral one. Thus an asymmetric finding can be represented by a difference in shape and distribution of the fibroglandular tissues of the two breasts but also by a difference in the oriented pattern of the two disks. The oriented features detectors used in this work is a set of real Gabor filters oriented at different angles (spaced at angles of 18 degrees) (Rangayyan et al., 2008). Real Gabor filters, in fact, yield good performances in terms of capability to detect the presence of oriented features as well as in terms of accuracy in the estimation of the angle of the directional components and are fundamental tools in image understanding where the information of interest is displayed in the form of oriented features. The foregoing considerations guided the choice to segment the fibroglandular tissue from the rest of the breast parenchyma using Gaussian mixture modelling (Ferrari et al., 2004). Differences between the left and right breasts in terms of directional and morphological features are then extracted and used to assess the asymmetry degree of the patient. The idea is that the integration of measures of shape and distribution of the fibroglandular tissue with measures of the oriented pattern through a Gabor filtering analysis, can provide a better and accurate characterization of the tissue, allowing the detection of the asymmetric abnormalities eventually present on the mammographic images. Once a numerical representation of the pairs of mammographic images has been obtained, bilateral asymmetry identification has been performed by pattern classification, based on a Support Vector Machine (SVM) classifier. Fig. 13 shows the flowchart of the whole procedure. The highlighted block denotes the most innovative part of the algorithm. It involves the tuning of the parameters of the algorithm according to the ACR breast tissue density. In particular, the thickness parameter in the Gabor filters and the

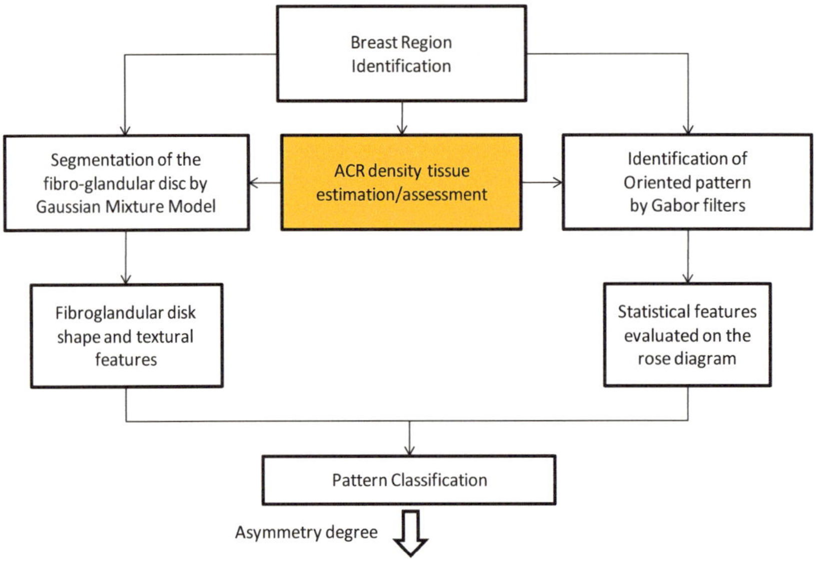

Fig. 13. A flowchart of the whole algorithm for the identification of bilateral asymmetry.

clustering procedure inside the gaussian mixture model estimation depend on the tissue density. This approach leads inevitably to a strong dependence on the density assigned to the final result, i.e. the degree of asymmetry. Fig. 14 reports two examples taken from DDSM images for an asymmetric and a normal pair of mammograms. The fibroglandular disks are also included along with the oriented pattern derived using Gabor filters. Finally, the rose diagram of the angular distribution of the left and right breast is reported. The considered asymmetric case has a density equal to 4 (at least 90% of the breast is composed of dense tissue), while the normal case has an assigned density equal to 3 (a portion in the range of 49% – 90% of the whole breast region is occupied by heterogeneously dense tissue).

The recent work has been devoted to the identification of the most relevant sources of uncertainty in the described algorithm. Two uncertainty contributions, respectively random and systematic, have been investigated:

1) the image power noise, estimated as described in previous sections;
2) subjective radiologist's bias in assessing the ACR density category, simulated by the assignment of a density value higher or lower than that assigned by the first radiologist.

The two different sources of uncertainty have to be separately considered and simulated, in order to avoid the interactions of them, possible compensation effects, in order to perform an individual failure analysis.

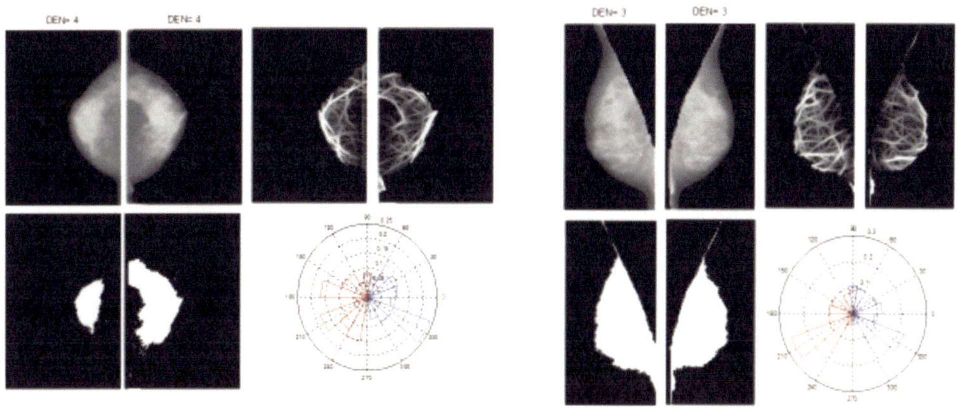

Fig. 14. Figure left: a pair of mammograms from DDSM with an assigned bilateral asymmetry ($B - 3056$ CC views). Figure right: a pair of normal symmetric mammograms from DDSM ($A - 0048$ MLO views).

6.1 Random uncertainty contribution: image noise

The Monte Carlo Method (MCM) has been implemented to evaluate and propagate the uncertainty contribution due to noise on the mammographic images. The implemented procedure is described as follows:

i) represent the luminance of each pixel by a pdf of a normal random variable with mean value taken from a smoothed version of the given image and standard deviation given by the noise variance estimation;

ii) select the number M of Monte Carlo trials;

iii) generate M different noisy images, by sampling from the assigned pdf using the model in (1), thus producing M realizations of the input mammographic image;

iv) apply the CADe algorithm to each of M image realizations and form the corresponding M different asymmetry degrees for each image;

v) sort these M values into strictly increasing order and construct a discrete representation G of the cumulative distribution function for the asymmetry degree;

vi) use G to derive an appropriate confidence interval for the asymmetry degree, for a given coverage probability p.

vii)Repeat steps i)-vi) for any image in the test set, considering a smoothed version of the remaining $N - 1$ original images for training, in a leave one out cross-validation testing procedure, thus producing $N \times M$ different asymmetry degrees.

viii)Using the values in vii) compute two vectors of M sensitivities and M specificities, thus producing extended ROC curves for each coverage probability.

Fig. 15 reports the asymmetry degrees for the asymmetric and normal cases taken from MiniMIAS database. The confidence interval associated is for a coverage probability equal to $p = 0.90$. The green circles identify the most critical pair of mammograms in terms of noise influence among the asymmetric and the normal cases. Fig. 16(a) reports the extended ROC curve accounting for the confidence intervals around the sensitivity and the specificity computed by steps: i)-viii).

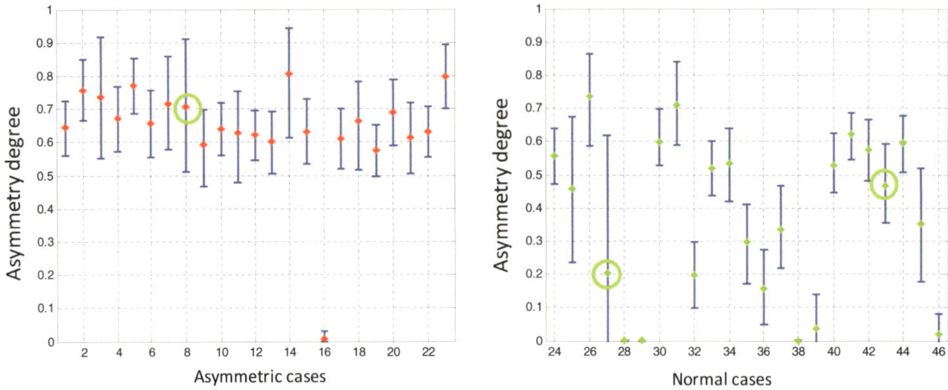

Fig. 15. Asymmetry degree for each case in the data set and the relative confidence interval, due to the noise uncertainty contribution, with 90% coverage probability. (a) Asymmetric cases. (b) Normal cases.

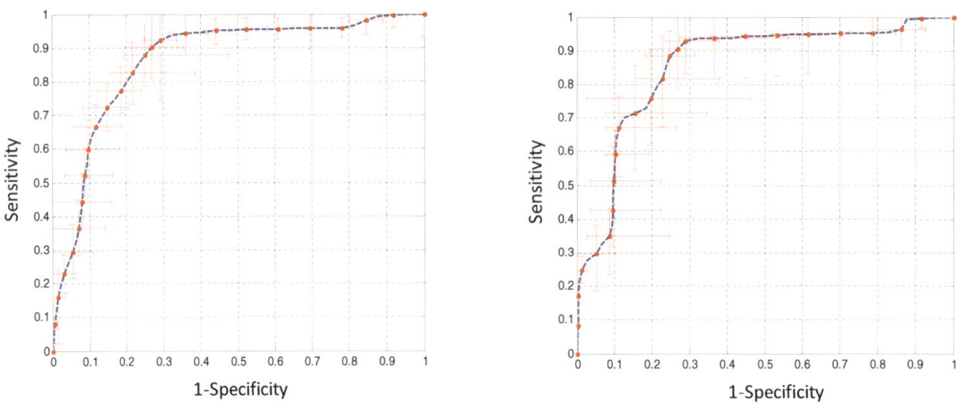

(a) (b)

Fig. 16. ROC curve of the classifier (mean value in blue) with the uncertainty contribution due to (a) image noise and (b) ACR density assessment bias propagated to the False Positive Rate and to the True Positive Rate.

6.2 Systematic uncertainty contribution: density category assessment

As seen before, the assessment of the density ACR category plays an important role in the whole algorithm. As a consequence, a different value assessed to the test image by the radiolgist could lead to changes in the system performance, which instead was calibrated using tree expert radiologists criterions and their experience. This kind of uncertainty contribution however is not random but systematic. In fact, a radiologist can introduce a subjective bias in assessing the ACR category to the mammographic image, which depends on his/her personal experience or on the particular mammographic equipment he/she is using. Therefore the CADe system has been tested using to different kind of bias:

1) a negative bias modeled as [3]: $ACR_{biased} = ACR_{unbiased} - 1$;

[3] Obviously, in this case density rating equal to 1 remains unchanged.

2) a positive bias modeled as [4]: $ACR_{biased} = ACR_{unbiased} + 1$.

The following procedure has been implemented to perform the uncertainty propagation of the two kinds of bias:

i) for each image of the dataset add a negative bias;

ii) test the CADe algorithm on each image obtained in i) and form the corresponding model value of the output, yielding N output values (where N is again the number of images of the dataset);

iii) for each image of the dataset add a positive bias;

iv) test the CADe algorithm on each image obtained in iii) and form the corresponding model value of the output, yielding other N output values;

v) sort these $2N$ values into strictly increasing order, using the sorted values to provide a discrete representation G of the distribution function for the asymmetry degree;

vi) use G to form an appropriate confidence interval for the asymmetry degree, for a given coverage probability p.

Fig. 17 reports the asymmetry degrees for the asymmetric and normal cases taken from MiniMIAS database. The confidence interval associated is for a coverage probability equal to $p = 0.90$. The green circles identify the most critical pair of mammograms in terms of density bias influence among the asymmetric and the normal cases. Fig. 16(b) shows the extended

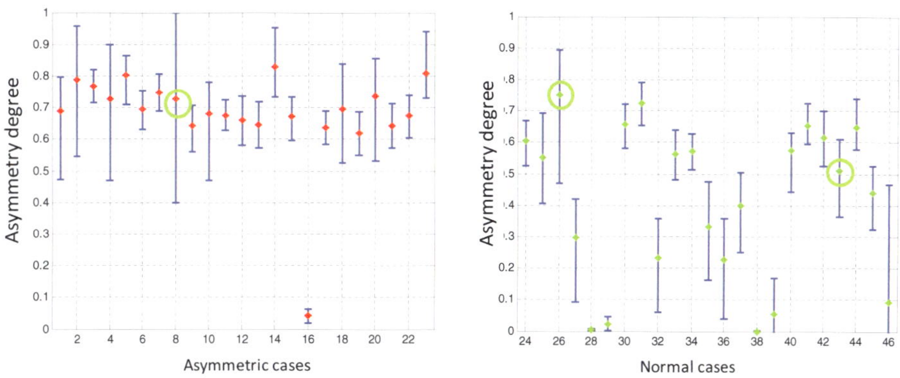

Fig. 17. Asymmetry degree for each case in the data set and the relative confidence interval, due to the noise uncertainty contribution, with 90% coverage probability. (a) Asymmetric cases. (b) Normal cases.

ROC curve accounting for the propagation of the ACR density assessment bias through the whole identification algorithm. A failure analysis could be guided from this kind of validation procedure.

7. Conclusions

This chapter has addressed the problem of metrological validation of a CAD system (both CADe-CADx) in mammography. Guided by the work of Wirth and that of Nishikawa, we

[4] Obviously, in this case density rating equal to 4 remains unchanged.

realized that there are still several open issues concerning the validation of CAD in this context. Based on the experience gained in the context of modeling and propagation of measurement uncertainty in the medical field, we have prepared this review providing some guidelines to expand and improve the validation and performance evaluation of CAD. Several examples have been inserted drawing inspiration from the CAD ABCDE that our research team is developing, especially showing those points that are distinctive compared to other commercial CAD already on the market. These points relate mainly to the metrological assessment, to the adaptability to different databases (either analog and digital), to the presence of new functional blocks relating to the identification of bilateral asymmetry, and last but not least to the ability to interact with the radiologist who can add rules in the CAD decision making process. This last functionality is allowed by the use of Fuzzy Inference Systems. Finally, taking a cue from the considerations of Wirth, we have also provided some hints on how to implement a failure assessment of the resulting False Negatives/Positives produced by a CAD.

8. References

Andersson, E. (2007). *Fuzzy and rough techniques in Medical Diagnosis and Medication*, Studies in Fuzziness and soft computing, Springer.

Burrell, H., Evans, A., Wilson, A. & Pinder, S. (2001). False-negative breast screening assessment: What lessons we can learn?, *Clin. Radiol.* 56(5): 385 – 388.

Casti, P. (2011). *Development and validation of a computer-aided detection system for the identification of bilateral asymmetry in mammographic images*, Master's thesis, Medical Engineering, Faculty of Engineering, University of Rome Tor Vergata.

Chan, T. & Vese, L. (2001). Active contours without edges, *IEEE Trans. Image Proc.* 10(2).

Cheng, H. (2003). Computer-aided detection and classification of microcalcifications in mammograms: a survey, *Pattern Recognition* 36(12): 2967 – 2991.

Dubois, D., Foulloy, L., Mauris, G. & Prade, H. (2004). Probability-possibility transformations, triangular fuzzy sets, and probabilistic inequalities, *Reliable Computing* 10(4): 273 – 297.

Ferlay, J., Shin, H.-R., Bray, F., Forman, D., Mathers, C. & Parkin, D. (2010). Estimates of worldwide burden of cancer in 2008: Globocan 2008, *Int. J. of Cancer* 127: 2893 – 2917.

Ferrari, R., Rangayyan, R., Borges, R. & Frere, A. (2004). Segmentation of the fibro-glandular disc in mammograms using gaussian mixture modeling, *Med. Biol. Eng. Comp.* 42: 378 – 387.

Ferrero, A. & Salicone, S. (2009). The construction of random-fuzzy variables from the available relevant metrological information, *IEEE Trans. on Instr. and Meas.* 58(2): 365 – 374.

Ferrero, A., Salicone, S., Mencattini, A., Rabottino, G. & Salmeri, M. (2010). Uncertainty evaluation in a fuzzy classifier for microcalcifications in digital mammography, *IEEE Inst. and Meas. Tech. Conf. (IMTC '10)*, Austin, TX, USA.

Giuliato, D. & Rangayyan, R. (2011). Modeling and analysis of shape with applications in computer-aided diagnosis of breast cancer, *Synthesis Lect. on Biom. Eng.* .

Gravel, P., Beaudoin, G. & Guise, J. (2004). A method for modeling noise in medical images, *IEEE Trans. on Medical Imaging* 23(10): 1221 – 1232.

Heath, M., Bowyer, K., Kopans, D., Kegelmeyer, W., Moore, R., Chang, K. & MunishKumaran, S. (1998). *Digital Mammography*, Kluwer, chapter Current status of the Digital Database for Screening Mammography, pp. 457 – 460.

International vocabulary of metrology. Basic and general concepts and associated terms (VIM) (2008). *Technical report.*

Jain, A. (1989). *Fundamentals of digital image processing*, Prentice Hall.

JCGM (2008). Evaluation of measurement data - an introduction to the guide to the expression of uncertainty in measurement 104:2009 and supplement 1 to the guide to the expression of uncertainty in measurement - propagation of distributions using a monte carlo method, *Technical Report 100:2008*, JCGM.

Mazzarella, F. & Bazzocchi, M. (2007). Cad systems for mammography: a real opportunity? a review of the literature, *La radiologia Medica* 112(3): 329 – 353.

Mencattini, A., Rabottino, G., Salicone, S. & Salmeri, M. (2009). Uncertainty modeling and propagation through RFVs for the assessment of CADx systems in digital mammography, *IEEE Trans. on Instr. and Meas.* 58(11).

Mencattini, A., Rabottino, G., Salmeri, M. & Lojacono, R. (2009). An iris detector for tumoral masses identification in mammograms, *IEEE Int. Work. on Med. Meas. and App. (MEMEA '09)*, Cetraro, Cosenza, Italy.

Mencattini, A., Rabottino, G., Salmeri, M. & Lojacono, R. (2010). Assessment of a breast masses identification procedure using an iris detector, *IEEE Trans. on Instr. and Meas.* 59(10): 2505 – 2512.

Mencattini, A., Rabottino, G., Salmeri, M., Sciunzi, B. & Lojacono, R. (2010). Denoising and enhancement of mammographic images under the assumption of heteroscedastic additive noise by an optimal subband thresholding, *Int. J. of Wavelets, Mult. Inf. Proc.* 8(5).

Mencattini, A. & Salmeri, M. (2011a). Breast masses detection using phase portrait analysis and fuzzy inference systems, *International Journal of Computer Assisted Radiology and Surgery* . DOI: 10.1007/s11548-011-0659-0.

Mencattini, A. & Salmeri, M. (2011b). Breast masses detection using phase portrait analysis, intrinsic coherence, *Computer Assisted Radiology and Surgey (CARS '11)*, Berlin, Germany.

Mencattini, A., Salmeri, M., Caselli, F., Sciunzi, B. & Lojacono, R. (2008). Subband variance computation of homoscedastic additive noise in discrete dyadic wavelet transform, *Int. J. of Wavelets, Mult. and Inf. Proc.* 6(6): 895–906.

Mencattini, A., Salmeri, M. & Casti, P. (2011). Bilateral asymmetry identification for the early detection of breast cancer, *IEEE Int. Work. on Med. Meas. and App. (MEMEA '11)*, Bari, Italy.

Mencattini, A., Salmeri, M., Casti, P., Raguso, G., L'Abbate, S., Chieppa, L., Ancona, A., Mangieri, F. & Pepe, M. (2011). Automatic breast masses boundary extraction in digital mammography using spatial fuzzy c-means clustering and active contour models, *IEEE Int. Work. on Med. Meas. and App. (MEMEA '11)*, Bari, Italy.

.Mencattini, A., Salmeri, M., Lojacono, R. & Arnò, M. (2007). Noise estimation in mammographic images for adaptive denoising, *EFOMP Eur. Conf. on Med. Phys. (EFOMP '07)*, Castelvecchio Pascoli, Italy.

Mencattini, A., Salmeri, M., Lordi, A., Casti, P., Ferrero, A., Salicone, S., Natoli, S., Leonardis, F. & P.David (2011). A study on a novel scoring system for the evaluation of expected mortality in icu-patients, *IEEE Int. Work. on Med. Meas. and App. (MEMEA '11)*, Bari, Italy.

Mencattini, A., Salmeri, M., Rabottino, G. & Salicone, S. (2010). Metrological characterization of a CADx system for the classification of breast masses in mammograms, *IEEE Trans. on Instr. and Meas.* 59(11): 2792 – 2799.

Nishikawa, R. (2007). Current status and future directions of computer-aided diagnosis in mammography, *Comp. Med. Imag. and Graph.* 31: 224 – 235.

Rabottino, G., Mencattini, A., Salmeri, M., Caselli, F. & Lojacono, R. (2008). Mass contour extraction in mammographic images for breast cancer identification, *IMEKO TC4 Symposium (IMEKOTC4 '08)*, Firenze, Italy.

Rabottino, G., Mencattini, A., Salmeri, M., Caselli, F. & Lojacono, R. (2011). Performance evaluation of a region growing procedure for mammographic breast lesion identification, *Computer Standard and Interfaces (Elsevier)* 33(2): 128 – 135.

Raguso, G., Ancona, A., Chieppa, L., L'abbate, S., Pepe, M., Mangieri, F., Palo, M. D. & Rangayyan, R. (2010). Application of fractal analysis to mammography, *IEEE Int. Conf. of the IEEE Engineering in Med. and Biol.*

Rangayyan, R., Prajna, S. & Ayres, F. (2008). Detection of architectural distortion in mammograms acquired prior to the detection of breast cancer using gabor filters, phase portraits, fractal dimension, and texture analysis, *Int. J. Comput. Assist. Radiol. Surg.* 2(6): 347 – 361.

Salicone, S. (2007). *Measurement uncertainty. An approach via the mathematical theory of evidence*, Springer, NY, USA.

Salmeri, M., Mencattini, A., Rabottino, G., Accattatis, A. & Lojacono, R. (2009). Assisted breast cancer diagnosis environment: A tool for DICOM mammographic images analysis, *IEEE Int. Work. on Med. Meas. and App. (MEMEA '09)*, Cetraro, Cosenza, Italy.

Salmeri, M., Mencattini, A., Rabottino, G. & Lojacono, R. (2008). Signal-dependent noise characterization for mammographic images denoising, *IMEKO TC4 Symposium (IMEKOTC4 '08)*, Firenze, Italy.

Santo, M. D., Liguori, C., Paolillo, A. & Pietrosanto, A. (2004). Standard uncertainty evaluation in image-based measurements, *Measurements* 36(3/4): 347 – 358.

Suckling, J., Parker, J., Dance, D., Astley, S., Hutt, I., Boggis, C., Ricketts, I., Stamatakis, E., Cerneaz, N., Kok, S., Taylor, P., Betal, D. & Savage, J. (1994). The mammographic image analysis society digital mammogram database, *in* E. A. G. Gale et al. (ed.), *Proc. 2nd Int. Workshop Digital Mammography*, York, U.K., pp. 375 – 378.

Wirth, M. (2006). *Recent Advances in Breast Imaging, Mammography, and Computer Aided Diagnosis of Breast cancer*, SPIE Press, Bellingham, Washington USA, chapter Performance Evaluation of CADe algorithms in Mammography, pp. 639 – 699.

16

Computerized Image Analysis of Mammographic Microcalcifications: Diagnosis and Prognosis

Anna N. Karahaliou, Nikolaos S. Arikidis, Spyros G. Skiadopoulos, George S. Panayiotakis and Lena I. Costaridou
Department of Medical Physics, Faculty of Medicine, University of Patras, Rio, Greece

1. Introduction

Breast cancer is the second leading cause of cancer deaths in women today (after lung cancer) and is the most frequently diagnosed cancer among women, excluding skin cancers. According to the American Cancer Society, an estimated of 230,480 new cancer cases are expected to be diagnosed in 2011; about 2,140 new cases are expected in men. In addition to invasive breast cancer, 57,650 new cases of in situ breast cancer are expected to occur among women in 2011. Of these, approximately 85% will be ductal carcinoma in situ (DCIS). An estimated 39,970 breast cancer deaths (39,520 women, 450 men) are expected in 2011. Death rates for breast cancer have steadily decreased in women since 1990, with larger decreases in women younger than 50 (a decrease of 3.2% per year) than in those 50 and older (2.0% per year), representing progress in both earlier detection and improved treatment.

Breast imaging has a key role in the early detection of breast cancer, which in conjunction with increased public awareness (prompting for monthly self-breast examination and annual examination by physician) yields the reduction in mortality from breast cancer.

Screen-film (SF) mammography is currently the most effective imaging modality for the early detection of breast cancer, challenged however by the presence of dense breast parenchyma. Furthermore, radiologist accuracy in diagnostic task (discrimination of malignant from benign lesions) is relatively low and is also differentiated with respect to lesion type (masses versus microcalcifications) (Cole et al., 2003). Despite the advantages offered by digital mammography the diagnosis of indeterminate lesions is still a challenging task. Breast ultrasound and Dynamic Contrast Enhanced Magnetic Resonance Imaging (DCE-MRI) are significant adjuncts to mammography providing additional diagnostic information by exploiting 3D structural and functional tissue properties related to lesion angiogenesis.

Computer-Aided Detection (CADe) and Computer-Aided Diagnosis (CADx) schemes have been proposed across breast imaging modalities to improve radiologist performance in detection and diagnosis tasks (Bassett, 2000; Cheng et al., 2003; Sampat et al., 2005; Chan et al., 2005; Giger et al., 2008; Costaridou et al., 2008; Elter & Horsch, 2009). These schemes also aim to reduce intra- and inter-observer variability by quantifying information that the human observer can perceive but in an objective and reproducible way ("mimic the human eye"), or to further quantify any information that may not be readily perceived by human eyes. The challenges of the CADx approaches are differentiated across breast imaging modalities and lesion types.

The American College of Radiology (ACR) Breast Imaging Reporting and Data System (BI-RADS) lexicon (ACR BIRADS 2003) defines masses, microcalcification (MC) clusters, architectural distortion and bilateral asymmetry as the major breast cancer signs in X-ray mammography. A mass is a space occupying lesion seen at least in two different mammographic projections. If a mass is seen only in a single projection is called asymmetric density. When a focal area of breast tissue appears distorted with spiculations radiating from a common point and focal retraction at the edge of the parenchyma, while no central mass is definable, it is called architectural distortion.

Calcifications are small deposits of calcium within the breast tissue and as masses are associated with both malignant and benign underlying biological processes (Kopans, 2007). Calcifications appear as high Signal-to-noise-ratio (SNR) bright structures, due to the high attenuation coefficient of calcium (higher than other breast constituents such as water, fat and glandular tissue). Calcifications can be large (>1mm) referred to as macro-calcifications and are commonly associated with benign conditions. MCs are tiny deposits of calcium in the breast with size ranging from 0.1mm to 1mm. A number of MCs grouped together is termed as a cluster and it may be a strong indication of cancer. A cluster is defined as at least three MCs within a 1 cm^2 area. Benign MCs are usually larger and coarser with round and smooth contours. Malignant MCs tend to be numerous, clustered, small, varying in size and shape, angular, irregularly shaped and branching in orientation.

In x-ray mammography, the automated interpretation of MCs is an open issue and more difficult than the corresponding task for masses (Cheng et al., 2003; Sampat et al., 2005). Difficulty in automated MCs interpretation is attributed to MCs fuzzy nature (varying size and shape), low contrast and low distinguishability from their surroundings (Cheng et al., 2003) rendering the accurate segmentation of MCs a challenging task. CADx schemes for MC clusters can be categorized into two major approaches: morphology-based and texture-based approaches. The morphology-based CADx schemes are highly dependent on the robustness of the employed segmentation algorithm. Texture-based CADx schemes assume that the presence of MCs alters the texture of the background tissue that MCs are embedded in; focused on extracting texture features from Regions of Interest (ROI) containing the cluster, these approaches do not depend on the robustness of a segmentation algorithm (i.e. the segmentation step is omitted). Since it is the breast tissue surrounding MCs that is subjected to histopathological analysis, to derive a malignant or a benign outcome, mammographic image texture analysis seems a more natural choice, while the bias induced by the presence of MCs on the texture pattern of the ROI being analyzed should also be considered (Thiele et al., 1996).

The following sections provide the current state-of-the-art approaches towards computer-aided diagnosis of MC clusters. Specifically, morphology-based and texture-based approaches are reviewed and an application paradigm focusing on their inter-comparison is provided.

2. Computer-aided detection and diagnosis of breast lesions in x-ray mammography

While SF mammography is currently the most effective breast imaging modality for the early detection of breast cancer (detection of breast abnormalities/lesions), its specificity in differentiating malignant from benign lesions is relatively low resulting in a high number of unnecessary biopsies.

Digital mammography allows the separation of image acquisition, processing, and display and represents a solution to many of the inherent limitations of SF mammography (Pissano, 2000). The digital detector has a linear response to x-ray intensity, in contrast to the sigmoidal response of screen-film systems. As a result, use of a digital detector provides a broader dynamic range of densities and higher contrast resolution. Through image processing, display parameters may be chosen independently from image acquisition factors. Small differences in attenuation between normal and abnormal breast tissue can be amplified, rendering digital mammography most suitable for screening of dense breast.

Despite the advantages offered by digital mammography, the radiologic interpretation of MCs still remains a major issue and is more challenging than the interpretation of breast masses. Studies have shown that the performance of radiologists in interpreting breast lesions is highly dependent on lesion type (masses vs. MCs) even with the use of image post-processing techniques (Cole et al., 2003). Specifically, it has been shown that radiologist performance in MCs interpretation is reduced as compared to masses interpretation, independent of the post-processing method used (Cole et al., 2003). Furthermore, inter- and intra-observer variability is higher in MCs interpretation as compared to masses interpretation (Skaane et al., 2008), and is also similar to observer variability in SF mammography (Baker et al., 1996; Skaane et al., 2008).

CADe and CADx schemes have a key role in detection and diagnosis of breast lesions aiming to improve radiologist performance, reduce observer variability and quantify lesion properties (Bassett, 2000; Cheng et al., 2003; Sampat et al., 2005; Chan et al., 2005; Costaridou et al., 2008; Costaridou, 2011). They were originally proposed and applied on digitized images with proven benefits, but as being better suited to digitally acquired images they are expected to cast further insights towards breast cancer detection and management. These systems act only as "second readers" and the final decision is made by the radiologist. The term "CADe/x" refers to formulating the clinical detection or diagnosis problem into the context of quantitative image feature extraction and pattern classification with the goal of solving it automatically (Duncan &Ayache, 2000).

CADe schemes have been developed to improve radiologists' performance in detecting breast lesions, by identifying suspicious regions of masses and MC clusters in an image (i.e. by placing prompts over areas of concern). The input to a CADe scheme is an image and the output is a location of a possible abnormality. Recent CADe schemes also provide the lesion boundary. CADx schemes in breast imaging aim to assist radiologists in the diagnostic task of lesion characterization (malignancy vs. benignity), thus affecting patient management (follow-up vs. biopsy). The input to a CADx scheme is a ROI indicating a breast lesion/abnormality. The output of a CADx scheme is a probability of malignancy for the lesion considered. Both CADe and CADx schemes share similar processing stages, such as segmentation, feature extraction and classification adjusted however to the specific task at hand. Figure 1 depicts the typical architecture of a CADe and a CADx scheme.

The high performances achieved by CADe schemes for breast lesions in x-ray mammography have led to their incorporation in commercially available FDA approved systems. These systems have shown to improve the performance of radiologists in detecting breast lesions, however, the high rate of false positives reported by some studies arise controversies concerning their exact impact on radiologist interpretation (Gur et al., 2004, Fenton et al., 2007). On the other hand, the development of commercially available CADx systems is still ongoing (Sampat et al., 2005).

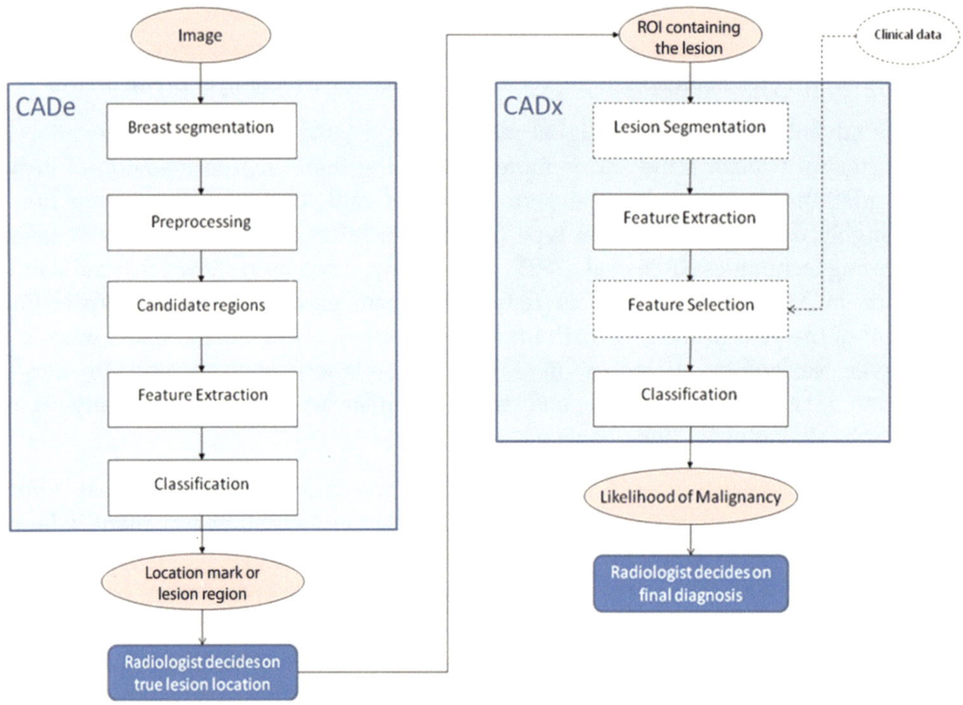

Fig. 1. Flowchart depicting the typical architecture of a CADe and a CADx scheme. Optional steps are indicated with dashed line

3. CADx schemes for MC clusters

3.1 Morphology-based CADx schemes

In the clinical practice the diagnosis of MC clusters in based on morphology (shape, size and intensity) properties and distribution properties of individual particles within a MC cluster, thus, most CADx schemes are also focused on the automated quantification of such properties (Cheng et al., 2003; Sampat et al., 2005; Costaridou et al., 2008; Elter & Horsch, 2009; Costaridou, 2011).

A number of authors have utilized a wide range of quantitative individual MC morphology properties (Patrick et al., 1991; Shen et al., 1994; Papadopoulos et al., 2008; Sklansky et al., 2000; Jiang et al., 1996). Specifically, size and shape features (area, perimeter, elongation, circularity, compactness, eccentricity, moment ratio, axis ratio, concavity index, effective thickness and volume as well as, shape signature) and MC intensity features (mean intensity, background intensity, contrast and edge strength) have been exploited.

CADx schemes that classify MC clusters are based on two categories of cluster features:

- Category I: Cluster features based on descriptive statistics (e.g. average, standard deviation, coefficient of variation, maximum, median, range) of individual MC morphology properties.
- Category II: Cluster features describing cluster morphology considering the cluster as an entire object (cluster area, diameter, perimeter, circularity, eccentricity, elongation, solidity and cluster background intensity). In this category the spatial distribution of individual MC particles within a cluster is also considered (number of MCs, structural index, proximity to the nearest MC, cluster density, as well as distance to pectoral and breast edge).

Table 1. summarizes morphology-based CADx schemes for MCs in terms of discriminant features (derived from Category I and/or Category II) including feature selection and classification techniques employed. Classification performance is also provided in terms of area under Receiver Operating Characteristic - ROC curve (A_z index) on patient and cluster-basis. Performance in patient-basis is derived by considering decision scores by both mammographic views (mediolateral oblique and craciocaudal). A disadvantage of these methods is that their performance is dependent on the accuracy of the segmentation method used. Specifically, the segmentation accuracy of less robust segmentation methods reduces the performance of morphology-based CADx schemes (Paquerault et al., 2004; Arikidis et al., 2008; Arikidis et al., 2009).

3.2 Texture-based CADx schemes

Another approach that overcomes limitations associated to segmentation issues is texture analysis applied on ROIs containing the MC cluster. This approach is based on the hypothesis that a malignancy (e.g. the MC) would cause changes in the texture of tissue surrounding it. Aiming at capturing such tissue texture alterations, CADx schemes have exploited various texture feature sets as well as feature selection and classification algorithms (Cheng et al., 2003; Sampat et al., 2005; Elter & Horsch, 2009), summarized in Table 2. Table 2 also provides classification performance of reported CADx schemes in a cluster-basis. Since a direct comparison of the reported CADx methodologies is not feasible, mainly due to the heterogeneous datasets analyzed, the attempted comparisons in the following paragraphs are only indicative of existing trends in texture analysis.

The grey level co-occurrence matrix (GLCM) characterizes the spatial distribution of grey levels in an image (Haralick et al., 1973). Features extracted from GLCMs provide information concerning image texture heterogeneity and coarseness, which is not necessarily visually perceived. The discriminating ability of GLCMs features, as extracted from original image ROIs containing MCs, has been demonstrated by most studies (Dhawan et al., 1996; Kocur et al., 1996; Kramer & Aghdasi 1999; Chan et al., 1997; Chan et al., 1998; Soltanian-Zadeh et al., 2004), with specific GLCMs feature combinations achieving an

Study	Discriminant Features	Feature selection / Classification	Performance (A_z index)
Jiang, et al. 1996	[I]Mean area and effective volume, Standard Deviation (SD) of effective thickness and effective volume, 2nd highest MC-shape-irregularity measure. [II]Number of MCs, circularity, area.	Qualitative correlation with radiologist's experience / Artificial Neural Network (ANN)	0.92 (patient) 0.83 (cluster)
Betal, et al. 1997	[I]Percentage of irregular and round MCs, inter-quartile range of MC area. [II]Number of MCs.	Exhaustive search / k-nearest-neighbour	0.84 (patient)
Chan, et al. 1998	[I]Coefficient of mean density variation, moment ratio variation and area variation, maximum moment ratio and area.	Genetic algorithm and stepwise discriminant analysis / Linear Discriminant Analysis (LDA)	0.79 (cluster)
Veldkamp, et al. 2000	[I]SD of individual MC area, orientation and contrast, mean of individual MC area and orientation, cluster area. [II]Number of MCs, distance to pectoral edge and breast edge.	Sequential forward feature selection based on A_z value / k-nearest-neighbour	0.83 (patient) 0.73 (cluster)
Sklansky, et al. 2000	[I]Mean area, aspect ratio and irregularity. [II]Number of MCs.	Genetic algorithm / ANN	0.75 (cluster)
Leichter, et al. 2000	[I]Mean shape factor, SD of shape factor, brightness and area [II]Mean number of neighbours, mean distance to the nearest MC.	Stepwise discriminant analysis / LDA	0.98 (cluster)
Buchbinder, et al. 2002	[I]Average of length extreme values.	Stepwise discriminant analysis / LDA	0.81 (cluster)
Paquerault, et al. 2004	[I]Mean area and effective volume, relative SD of effective thickness and effective volume, 2nd highest MC-shape-irregularity. [II]Number of MCs, circularity, area.	Qualitative correlation with radiologist's experience / LDA and Bayesian ANN	0.86 (patient) 0.82 (cluster)
Arikidis, et al. 2008	[I]SD of length extreme values.	Exhaustive search / LDA	0.86 (patient) 0.81 (cluster)

Table 1. Morphology-based CADx schemes for MC clusters

A_z of 0.88 in discriminating malignant from benign MC clusters (Chan et al., 1997). In addition, GLCMs feature have shown to be more effective than morphology-based features (Chan et al., 1998), while their combination can provide an even higher classification performance. Soltanian-Zadeh et al. (2004) demonstrated that GLCMs extracted from ROIs containing the MCs were superior to GLCMs extracted from segmented MCs and suggested that "there may be valuable texture information concerning the benignity or malignancy of the cluster in those areas that lie outside the MCs".

Aiming at capturing tissue texture alterations in multiscale representation, studies have also exploited first order statistics (FOS) (i.e. energy, entropy and square root of the coefficients norm) extracted from wavelet (Dhawan et al., 1996; Kocur et al., 1996; Soltanian-Zadeh et al., 2004) or multi-wavelet (Soltanian-Zadeh et al., 2004 transform subimages. Wavelet/

Study	Features	Feature selection / Classification	Performance (A_z±SE)
Dhawan et al., 1996	• GLCMs features • Entropy, Energy (wavelet packets; Daubechies 6/20) • Cluster features	Genetic Algorithm-based method / Backpropagation Neural Network, Linear classifier, k-Nearest Neighbor	Combined: 0.86±0.05 (cluster)
Kocur et al., 1996	• SRN (DWT; \Daubechies4 & Biorthogonal 9.7) • GLCMs feature (angular second moment). • Eigenimages (Karhunen-Loeve coefficients)	ANN, Decision Boundary Analysis / Multilayer Perceptron Neural Network	Wavelet: 88%* (cluster)
Chan et al., 1997	• GLCMs features	Stepwise Discriminant Analysis / Artificial Neural Network	0.88 (cluster)
Chan et al., 1998	• GLCMs features • Cluster features (Morphological)	Genetic Algorithm, Stepwise Discriminant Analysis / Linear Discriminant Analysis	Combined: 0.89±0.03 (cluster) 0.93±0.03 (patient)
Kramer & Aghdasi, 1999	• GLCMs features • Entropy, Energy (DWT; Daubechies 4/6/20 & Biorthogonal 2.8) • Co-occurrence-based (DWT; Daubechies 4/6/20 & Biorthogonal 2.8)	Sequential Forward Selection/ ANN, k-Nearest Neighbor	Combined: 94.8%* (cluster)
Soltanian-Zadeh et al., 2004	• GLCMs features from segmented MCs and from ROIs containing the MCs • Entropy, Energy (wavelet packets; Daubechies 6/10/12) • Entropy, Energy (multi-wavelet, 3 Filters) • Cluster features (shape)	Genetic Algorithm / k-Nearest Neighbor	Multi-wavelet: 0.89 (cluster)
Karahaliou et al., 2008	• First order statistics • GLCMs features • Laws' texture energy measures • Energy, Entropy (redundant DWT; B-spline) • Co-occurrence based (Decomposition: redundant DWT; Filter: B-spline; Levels: 1-3)	Exhaustive search/ Probabilistic Neural Network	0.98±0.01 (cluster)

*Performance provided in % classification accuracy; GLCMs: Grey-level co-occurrence matrices; SRN: Square Root of the Norm of coefficients; DWT: Discrete Wavelet Transform.

Table 2. Texture-based CADx schemes for MC clusters

multiwavelet FOS have shown to be more effective than GLCMs features (Kocur et al., 1996; Soltanian-Zadeh et al., 2004) and shape features (Soltanian-Zadeh et al., 2004) suggesting the advantages offered by the multiscale representation of the tissue analyzed. Dhawan et al. (1996) demonstrated that the combination of GLCMs with FOS wavelet features, representing global and local texture respectively, is superior to cluster features; however, best performance was achieved by a selected feature set including GLCMs, wavelet and cluster features. An obvious extension of wavelet FOS is the computation of co-occurrence matrix features from wavelet decomposed subimages, to describe coefficients second order statistics (Van de Wouwer et al., 1998). Kramer and Aghdasi (1999) demonstrated that co-occurrence matrices features extracted from wavelet decomposed subimages were superior to GLCMs and wavelet FOS in discriminating malignant from benign MC clusters.

3.2.1 Texture analysis of the tissue surrounding MCs

As opposed to the previously described CADx approaches which analyze the texture pattern of ROIs containing the MC cluster, the MCs surrounding tissue analysis approach focuses on the investigation of the "net texture pattern" of the underlying breast tissue removing any bias induced by the presence of MCs.

The biological basis of the hypothesis is that as the tissue surrounding MCs is the one sampled and subjected to histopathological analysis to decide on benignity or malignancy, this tissue area should be subjected to texture analysis. The hypothesis was introduced by Thiele et al. (1996) who investigated texture properties of the tissue surrounding MCs on digital scout views acquired during the stereotactic biopsy procedure. The hypothesis was tested on a dataset of 54 cases (18 malignant/36 benign) exploiting GLCMs and fractal geometry based features and achieved a classification performance 85% (sensitivity 89%, specificity 83%) employing Linear and Logistic Discriminant analysis. Since its introduction on digital scout views, the feasibility of the MCs surrounding tissue analysis hypothesis has been further investigated on screening mammograms (Karahaliou et al., 2007a, 2007b, 2008).

In the following sections (4.1, 4.2 and 4.3) the potential contribution of this approach in CADx of MC clusters is investigated and compared to current state-of-the-art approaches, by means of a meta-analysis application paradigm of the sample analysed in (Karahaliou et al., 2007a, 2008; Arikidis et al., 2008).

4. Application paradigm

4.1 Texture vs. morphology analysis for MC cluster diagnosis

Methods performance inter-comparison is tested on a pilot dataset of 92 MC clusters. 49 MC clusters were malignant (as proven by biopsy) while 43 MC clusters were benign (either biopsy proven or without call-back). Mammograms were originated from the Digital Database for Screening Mammography (DDSM) (Heath et al., 2000) and correspond to digitization with a single laser scanner (LUMISIS) at a pixel depth of 12 bits and 50 μm pixel resolution. Mammograms correspond to extremely dense and heterogeneously dense breast parenchyma (density 3 and 4 according to ACR BIRADS lexicon). Figure 2 depicts the distribution of the 92 MC clusters with respect to malignancy assessment.

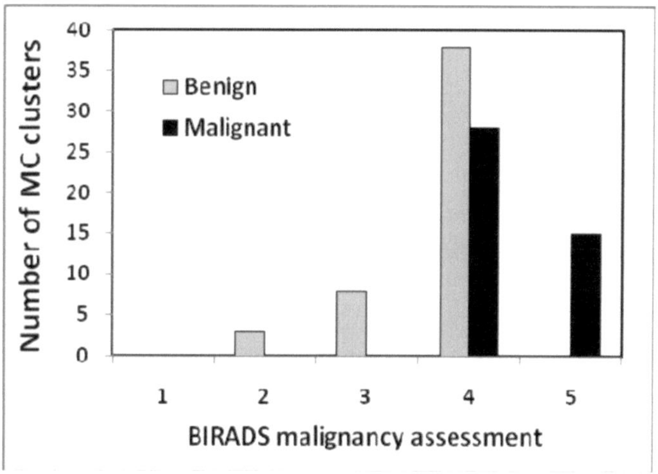

Fig. 2. Distribution of the dataset of 92 MC clusters with respect to malignancy rating provided in the DDSM. 1: negative, 2: benign, 3: probably benign, 4: suspicious abnormality, 5: highly suggestive of malignancy

a. Texture analysis of tissue surrounding MCs

The "MCs surrounding tissue" area is provided by MC segmentation and subsequent "exclusion" of the segmented MC areas from the ROI containing the cluster (Figure 3). As the approach requires only a "coarse" MC segmentation, requirements for accurate segmentation are relaxed, as compared to the corresponding ones of morphology-based CADx schemes. Wavelet based signatures (Van de Wouwer et al., 1998) were employed for quantification of the "net texture pattern" of the breast tissue. The specific texture feature category was selected due to its improved discriminating ability over three robust texture feature categories (first order statistics features (Gonzalez & Woods, 2000), Laws' texture energy measures (Laws, 1979)) and grey level co-occurrence matrices (Haralick et al., 1973) previously adopted in CADx approaches for the differentiation of malignant form benign MC clusters.

Wavelet coefficient co-occurrence matrices (WCCMs) (Van de Wouwer et al., 1998) features were generated employing the redundant dyadic wavelet transform whose wavelet filter is the first-order derivative of a cubic B-spline (Mallat & Zhong, 1992). The transform was implemented using the 'algorithme `a trous' (algorithm with holes), which does not involve down-sampling. The gradient magnitude coefficients of the 2nd and 3rd dyadic scale were considered for co-occurrence matrices feature extraction. Co-occurrence matrices were generated for 4 angles (0°, 45°, 90°,135°) and for various displacement vector values *d*. From each co-occurrence matrix 16 features were extracted. For each *d*, the mean and range value of each feature over the four co-occurrence matrices were calculated. In order to define the "MCs surrounding tissue" area, wavelet decomposition was performed on original mammogram ROIs (513x513 pixels) containing the MC clusters. To deal with contaminated pixels adjacent to MC areas, the "coarsely" segmented MC areas were dilated in proportion to the filter lengths used to derive wavelet gradient magnitude coefficients. Figure 4 illustrates ST-ROIs on original mammogram and on gradient magnitude coefficients of the 2nd and 3rd dyadic scale of the wavelet transform employed.

The Stepwise Discriminant Analysis (SDA) was then employed to select one single feature subset from extracted WCCMs features. The selected subset referred here in as WCCMs*, is comprised of 3 WCCMs features corresponding to: Mean of Shade (d=18, scale 2), Range of Difference Variance (d=14, scale 3) and Mean of Information Measure of Correlation 1 (d=18, scale 3).

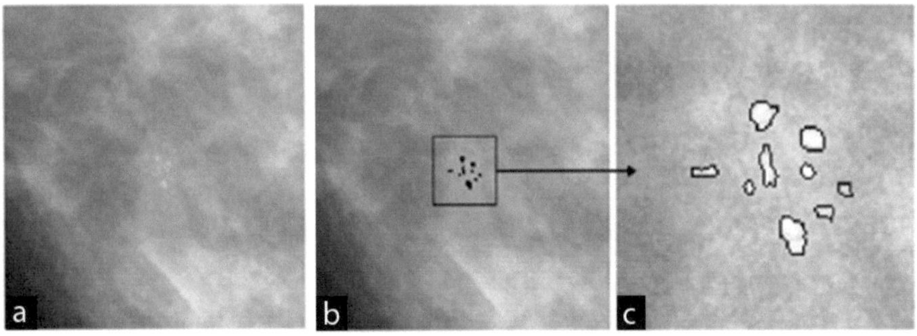

Fig. 3. Illustrative example of ST-ROI definition. (a) 513x513 pixel part of original mammogram containing a MC cluster (DDSM: volume cancer_09, case B_3406, RIGHT_CC). (b) Segmented MC areas (in black) of the cluster and 129x129 pixel ROI (black rectangle) containing the cluster. (c) Magnified ROI of figure (b). Surrounding tissue ROI (i.e. ST-ROI) corresponds to the area resulting from exclusion of segmented MC areas from the 129x129 pixel ROI. Borders of excluded MC areas are indicated with solid line

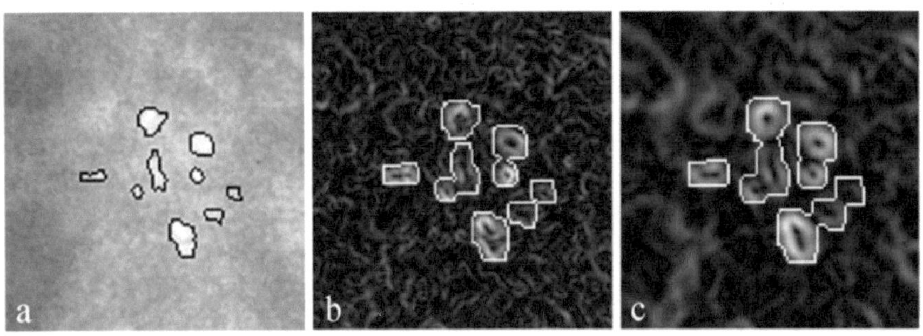

Fig. 4. ST-ROIs (129x129 pixels) on original (a) and wavelet gradient magnitude coefficients of the 2nd (b) and 3rd (c) dyadic scale. Borders of excluded MC areas are indicated with solid line

b. Texture analysis of ROIs containing the MCs

This approach is similar to the "MCs surrounding tissue" one with respect to texture feature extraction and classification without however requiring the "coarse" MC segmentation step. Specifically, 129x129 pixel ROIs centered at each cluster, identical to the ones employed in the "MC surrounding tissue" apporach, were subjected to texture feature extraction by means of wavelet based signatures. The SDA was then employed to select one single feature subset. The selected subset referred here in as WCCMs**, is comprised of 4 WCCMs features corresponding to: Range of Inverse Difference Moment (d=1, scale 2), Mean of Difference Variance (d=6, scale 2), Range of Prominence (d=6, scale 2) and Mean of Contrast (d=18, scale 2).

c. **Morphology analysis of MCs**

A recently proposed segmentation algorithm was employed to segment individual MCs within each cluster, details of which can be found elsewhere (Arikidis et al., 2008). Briefly, the method is based on implementation of active rays on B-spline wavelet representation to identify MC contour point estimates in a coarse-to-fine strategy at two levels of analysis. An iterative region growing method is then used to delineate the final MC contour curve, with pixel aggregation constrained by the MC contour point estimates.

Ten (10) individual MC features were extracted from each segmented MC corresponding to: area, length, eccentricity, compactness, radial standard deviation, relative contrast, 2 regional moments (one related to the spread and one related to the eccentricity of object mass), one moment of region boundary and a shape roughness measure provided by Fourier descriptors. Twenty (20) MC cluster features were then generated by computing the mean and range of the above feature values over the entire cluster. The SDA was then employed to select one single feature subset from the 20 cluster features. The selected subset comprised of 3 cluster features corresponding to: mean of relative contrast, range of relative contrast and the regional moment related to object mass eccentricity.

The discriminating ability of the three selected feature subsets was investigated using a least squares minimum distance (LSMD) classifier, using the Leave-One-Out (LOO) (Theodoridis & Koutroumbas 1999) training-testing methodology. Classification performance of the three feature subsets (morphology, WCCMs* and WCMMs**) was evaluated by means of the A_z index (area under ROC curve).

The morphology-based feature subset achieved an A_z±standard error (SE) of 0.809±0.046 with lower and upper 95% Confidence Interval (CI) values of 0.698 and 0.882, respectively. On the same dataset (of 92 MC clusters) the "MCs surrounding tissue texture analysis" approach achieved A_z±SE of 0.882±0.036 (95% CI values: 0.788, 0.936) employing the WCCMs* subset. The commonly adopted approach of analysing tissue ROIs containing the MCs achieved A_z±SE of 0.803±0.048 (95% CI values: 0.688, 0.879) employing the WCCMs** subset. ROC curves corresponding to the three feature subsets are provided in Fig. 5. Table 3 provides classification performance comparison among the three selected feature subsets.

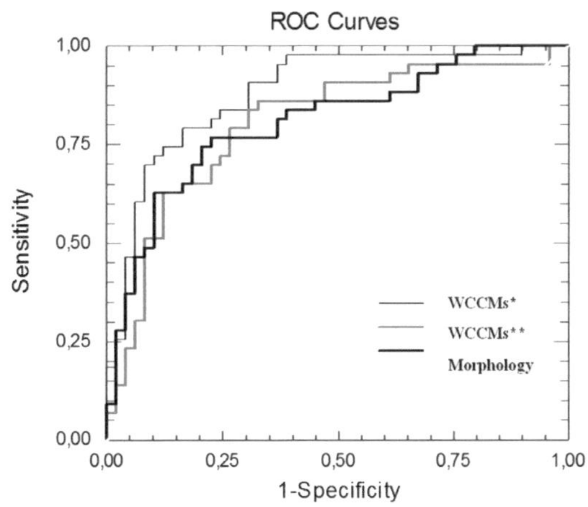

Fig. 5. ROC curves corresponding to the morphology, the WCCMs* (MCs surrounding tissue) and the WCCMs** (tissue containing the MCs) selected feature subsets

	A_z ± SE	p-value
Morphology vs. WCCMs*	0.809±0.046 vs. 0.881±0.036	0.15
Morphology vs. WCCMs**	0.809±0.046 vs. 0.803±0.048	0.92
WCCMs* vs. WCCMs**	0.881±0.036 vs. 0.803±0.048	0.11

Table 3. p-values (z-test) for classification performance comparison among selected subsets from the three approaches

4.2 Texture plus morphology analysis for MC cluster diagnosis

In order to investigate the combined performance of texture- and morphology-based analysis two additional feature sets were generated by (a) merging the morphology-based selected subset with the WCCMs* subset and (b) merging the morphology-based selected subset with the WCCMs** subset.

From each merged feature set one subset was generated by means of an exhaustive search procedure. Specifically, the LSMD classifier was designed with all possible feature combinations, from 2 up to 6 features, and for each combination the classifier performance was evaluated by means of the LOO training-testing methodology. The feature combination with the highest classification performance (by means of A_z index) and the minimum number of features was selected.

Table 4 summarizes classification performance of the two selected subsets by means of A_z ± SE and 95% asymmetric CI values. No statistically significant difference was observed in classification performance of the two approaches (p>0.05).

	Features included in subset	A_z ± SE	[Lower, Upper] 95% asymmetric CI
Morphology and WCCMs*	Regional Moment (eccentricity) Mean of Shade (*d*=18, scale 2) Range of Difference Variance (*d*=14, scale 3) Mean of Information Measure of Correlation 1 (*d*=18, scale 3)	0.899±0.035	[0.802, 0.950]
Morphology and WCCMs**	Mean of Relative Contrast Range of Relative Contrast Regional Moment (eccentricity) Mean of Difference Variance (*d*=6, scale 2) Mean of Contrast (*d*=18, scale 2)	0.868±0.038	[0.771, 0.926]

Table 4. Classification performance of the two combined (texture and morphology) selected subsets by means A_z ± SE and 95% asymmetric Confidence Interval (CI) values. WCCMs*: selected texture feature subset employing the "MCs surrounding tissue" approach. WCCMs**: selected texture feature subset employing the commonly adopted approach of analysing tissue ROIs containing the MCs

4.3 Discussion

Texture analysis is ultimately concerned with automated methods that can derive image information from a purely computational point of view. As such, is nothing than numeric manipulation of digital or digitized images to get quantitative measurements (Tourassi, 1999). However, in contrast to morphology analysis, texture analysis can potentially improve decision making by capturing clues "beyond the human eye". Morphology analysis based schemes quantify visually perceived properties, mimicking radiologist decision making in an objective and reproducible way. Texture analysis has a divergent role when considered in decision making. It can mimic radiologist perception of image texture (when texture differences are visually perceived) or it can augment the visual skills of the radiologists by extracting/quantifying image features that may be relevant to the diagnostic problem, but are not visually extractable.

In case of CADx schemes based on morphology analysis of MCs the first approach is applicable. Specifically, image analysis approaches are employed to quantify individual MCs properties that are commonly assessed by the radiologist to provide a final decision concerning diagnosis and patient management. In case of CADx schemes based on texture analysis of ROIs including MCs the second approach is applicable. Specifically, image analysis approaches are employed to quantify the texture properties of ROIs, e.g. to capture the increased heterogeneity, due to presence of large number of MCs within ROI, but also capture texture alterations of tissue surrounding MCs. The first is visually perceived, and in a sense is also one of the diagnostic criteria adopted in clinical practice for MCs. The second (i.e. the MCs surrounding tissue heterogeneity) is not currently evaluated in the clinical practice but accounts for an approach worthy of being further exploited.

Nonetheless, texture analysis is not a panacea for the diagnostic interpretation of radiographic images. As the pursuit of texture analysis is based on the hypothesis that the texture signature of an image is relevant to the diagnostic task at hand, the hypothesis should always be tested (Tourassi, 1999).

In the current application paradigm, we tested the hypothesis that wavelet texture signatures of tissue surrounding MCs as depicted on screening mammograms is relevant to the diagnostic task. Results have demonstrated the feasibility of the "MCs surrounding tissue" texture analysis approach in the differentiation of malignant from benign MC clusters on screening mammograms, in support of the hypothesis originally formulated by (Thiele et al., 1996) on stereotactic scout views. While a direct comparison with the results of this study (Thiele et al., 1996) is not feasible, due to the different nature of the datasets analyzed, comparable performance is achieved.

As compared to other texture-based CADx schemes analyzing ROIs containing the cluster (Dhawan et al., 1996; Kocur et al., 1996; Chan et al., 1997; Chan et al., 1998; Kramer & Aghdasi 1999; Soltanian-Zadeh et al., 2004), the performance achieved by the wavelet texture signatures, employing the MCs surrounding tissue approach, is also comparable. However, heterogeneity of the datasets analyzed renders direct comparison not feasible.

As compared to the morphology-based CADx schemes, the "MCs surrounding tissue" texture analysis approach has the advantage of relaxing segmentation accuracy requirements. However, the current study demonstrated the advantages of combining wavelet texture signatures derived from the tissue surrounding MCs with morphology features of MC clusters, in accordance to Chan et al. (1998) who combined GLCMs features (from ROIs containing the cluster) with morphology-based ones.

While no statistically significant difference between the two texture-based approaches was observed, the results of this study demonstrate a trend in favour of the "MCs surrounding tissue" texture analysis approach over the commonly adopted one of analysing ROIs containing the MCs. We attribute this trend to the fact that the "MCs surrounding tissue texture analysis" allows an investigation of the net texture pattern of the underlying tissue, which is the one that generates the MCs, removing bias due to the number and distribution of MCs within the depicted tissue.

Additional research efforts are required for validating/establishing the computer-extracted image features (morphology-based or texture-based) of MC clusters as diagnostic image-based biomarkers for breast cancer. Specifically, research should be focused on investigating the relationship between quantitatively extracted features and histopathological indices.

5. Migration to computer-aided prognosis

Computer-aided diagnosis of mammographic MCs has also been extended from the task of differentiating malignant from benign MC clusters to prognostic tasks towards the identification of potential mammographic image-based prognostic markers.

Specifically, morphology-based analysis of MC clusters applied on magnification mammograms has been exploited for the classification of 58 MC clusters into fibroadenoma, mastopathy, noninvasive carcinoma of the noncomedo type, noninvasive carcinoma of the comedo type and invasive carcinoma (Nakayama et al., 2004). Features considered are (i) the variation in the size of microcalcifications within a cluster, (ii) the variation in pixel values of microcalcifications within a cluster, (iii) the shape irregularity of microcalcifications within a cluster, (iv) the extent of the linear and branching distribution of microcalcifications, and (v) the distribution of microcalcifications in the direction toward the nipple. The Bayes decision rule was employed for distinguishing between five histological categories demonstrating promising results.

The potential contribution of follow-up mammograms in this specific prognostic task (i.e. in identifying the histological classification of clustered MCs) was also evaluated (Nakayama et al., 2006). Specifically, the previously defined five morphology features were extracted from previous and current magnification mammograms. The ten features were merged by means of a Modified Bayes discriminant function for the histological classification of 93 MC clusters (55 malignant and 38 benign).

Classification results were improved by employing a nearest neighbor criterion and by augmenting the feature set (i.e. adding the number of microcalcifications within the cluster) (Nakayama et al., 2007).

The identification of potential image-based prognostic markers for breast cancer, i.e. quantitative image features capable of predicting biological behaviour and disease aggressiveness, accounts for an emerging research area, expected to have a significant impact on patient management and treatment response assessment.

6. Conclusions

Only a few research efforts (Chan et al., 1998; Soltanian-Zadeh et al., 2004) have focused on comparing state-of-the-art approaches for computer-aided diagnosis of breast cancer, including the presented application paradigm which considered a pilot dataset. Thus, the systematic evaluation of proposed methods performance utilizing large and publicly available datasets is a necessity. Furthermore, method inter-comparison should consider testing on datasets generated by multicenter studies to ensure a large size, inclusion of varying case subsets with respect to lesion types (e.g. MCs of varying morphology and distribution) and image acquisition systems (i.e. digitized vs. FFDM).

It is important to investigate the effect of reported CADx schemes on radiologist performance in breast cancer diagnosis task, by considering a radiologist's diagnosis task aided by a specific CADx scheme and an un-aided corresponding one, also taking into account issues related to interaction of radiologist with a CADx scheme. The contribution of CADx schemes in reducing intra- and inter-observer variability should also be investigated.

Advances in breast imaging have broadened the role of computer-based approaches in breast cancer diagnosis further suggesting multimodality and multi-parametric approaches. Multi-modality CADx schemes that combine features extracted from different imaging modalities, each one capturing additional tissue properties, may be advantageous to single-modality CADx in the task of differentiating between malignant and benign lesions (Yuan et al., 2010), especially in the case of benign and malignant lesions with overlapping imaging features on a single imaging modality. Finally, the multi-modality approach has an increased potential towards identification of potential new diagnostic and prognostic biomarkers for breast cancer.

7. Acknowledgments

Part of this work is supported by the Caratheodory Programme (C.183) of the University of Patras, Greece.

8. References

American College of Radiology (ACR) Breast Imaging Reporting and Data System Atlas (BI-RADS Atlas): Mammography, Ultrasound, and Magnetic Resonance Imaging, 4th ed. Reston, VA: ACR, 2003

Arikidis, N.S.; Skiadopoulos, S.; Karahaliou, A.; Likaki, E.; Panayiotakis, G.; & Costaridou, L. (2008). B-spline active rays segmentation of microcalcifications in mammography. *Medical Physics*, Vol. 3, No. 11, (November 2008), pp. 5161-5171, ISSN 0094-2405

Arikidis, N.; Karahaliou, A.; Skiadopoulos, S.; Likaki, E.; Panayiotakis, G.; & Costaridou, L.(2009). Integrating multiscale polar active contours and region growing for microcalcifications segmentation in mammography. *Journal of Instrumentation*, JINST 4, P07009, (July 2009), pp. 12-16, ISSN 1748-0221

Baker, J.A.; Kornguth, P.J & Floyd, C.E. (1996). Breast imaging reporting and data system standardized mammography lexicon: observer variability in lesion description. *American Journal of Roentgenology*, Vol. 166, No. 4, (April 1996), pp. 773-778, ISSN 0361-803X

Bassett, L.W. (2000). Digital and Computer-Aided Mammography. *The Breast Journal*, Vol. 6, No. 5, pp. 291-293, ISSN 1075-122X

Betal, D.; Roberts, N. & Whitehouse, G.H. (1997). Segmentation and numerical analysis of microcalcifications on mammograms using mathematical morphology. *The British Journal of Radiology*, Vol. 70, No. 837 , (September 1997), pp. 903-917, ISSN 0007-1285

Buchbinder, S.S.; Leichter, I.; Lederman, R.; Novak, B.; Bamberger, P.; Coopersmith, H. & Fields. S.I. (2002). Can the size of microcalcifications predict malignacy of clusters at mammograpgy? *Academic Radiology*, Vol. 9, No.1 , (January 2002), pp. 18-25, ISSN 1076-6332

Chan, H.P.; Sahiner, B.; Petrick, N.; Helvie, M.A.; Lam, K.L.; Adler, D.D. & Goodsitt, M.M. (1997). Computerized classification of malignant and benign microcalcifications on mammograms: Texture analysis using an artificial neural network. *Physics in Medicine and Biology*, Vol. 42, No. 3, pp. 549-567, ISSN 0031-9155

Chan, H.P.; Sahiner, B.; Lam, K.L.; Petrick, N.; Helvie, M.A.; Goodsitt, M. & Addler D.D. (1998). Computerized analysis of mammographic microcalcifications in morphological and texture feature spaces. *Medical Physics*, Vol. 25, No. 10, (October 1998), pp. 2007-2019, ISSN 0094-2405

Chan, H.P.; Sahiner, B.; Petrick, N.; Hadjiiski, L.; Paquerault, S. (2005). Computer-Aided Diagnosis of Breast Cancer. In: *Medical Image Analysis Methods*, Costaridou, L. (Ed.), CRC Press, Taylor & Francis Group, ISBN 0-8493-2089-5, Boca Raton, FL, US

Cheng, H.D.; Cai, X.; Chen, X.; Hu, L.; Lou, X. (2003). Computer-aided detection and classification of microcalcifications in mammograms: a survey. *Pattern Recognition*, Vol. 36, No. 12, (December 2003), pp.2967-2991, ISSN 0031-3203

Cole, E.B.; Pisano, E.D.; Kistner, E.O.; Muller, K.E.; Brown, M.E.; Feig, S.A. et al. (2003). Diagnostic Accuracy of Digital Mammography in Patients with Dense Breasts Who Underwent Problem-solving Mammography: Effects of Image Processing and Lesion Type. *Radiology*, Vol. 226, (January 2003),pp.153-160, ISSN 0033-8419

Costaridou, L.; Skiadopoulos, S.; Karahaliou, A.; Arikidis, N.; Panayiotakis, G. (2008). Computer-Aided Diagnosis in Breast Imaging: Trends and Challenges, In: *Handbook of Research on Advanced Techniques in Diagnostic Imaging and Biomedical Applications*. Exarchos, T.P.; Papadopoulos, A. & Fotiadis, D .I. (Eds), IGI Global., ISBN 9781605663142

Costaridou, L. (2011). CADx Mammography. In: Biomedical Image Processing, Biological and Medical Physics, Biomedical Engineering, T.M. Deserno (Ed.), Springer-Verlag, ISBN 978-3-642-15815-5, Berlin Heidelberg

Dhawan, A.P.; Chitre, Y.; Kaiser-Bonasso, C. (2000) Analysis of mammographic microcalcifications using gray-level image structure features. *IEEE Transactions on Medical Imaging*, Vol. 15, No. 3, (June 1996), pp. 246–259, ISSN 0278-0062

Duncan, J.S. & Ayache, N. (2000). Medical Image Analysis:Progress over two decades and the challenges ahead. *IEEE Transactions on Pattern Analysis and Machine Intelligence*, Vol. 22, No. 1, (January 2000), pp. 85-106, ISSN 0162-8828

Elter, M. & Horsch, A. (2009). CADx of mammographic masses and clustered microcalcifications: A review. *Medical Physics*; Vol. 36, No. 6, (June 2009), pp. 2052-2068, ISSN 0094-2405

Fenton, J.J.; Taplin, S.H.; Carney, P.A.; Abraham, A.; Sickles, E.A.; D'Orsi, C.B. et al. (2007). Influence of computer-aided detection on performance of screening mammography. *The New England Journal of Medicine*, Vol. 356, No. 14, (April 2007), pp. 1399-1409, ISSN 0028-4793

Giger, M.L.; Chan, H.P. & Boone, J. (2008). Anniversary paper: History and status of CAD and quantitative image analysis: the role of Medical Physics and AAPM. *Medical Physics*, Vol. 35, No. 12, (November 2008), pp. 5799-5820, ISSN 0094-2405

Gonzalez, R.C. & Woods, R.E. (Eds). (2002). *Digital image processing*, Prentice-Hall, Inc., ISBN: 0201180758, New Jersey, USA

Gur, D.; Sumkin, J.H.; Rockette, H.E.; Ganott, M.; Hakim, C.; Hardesty, L.; Poller, W.R.; Shah, R. & Wallace, L. (2004). Changes in breast cancer detection and mammography recall rates after the introduction of a computer-aided detection system. *Journal of the National Cancer Institute*, Vol. 96, No. 3, (February 2004), pp.185-190, ISSN 0027-8874

Haralick, R.M.; Shanmugam, K. & Dinstein, I. (1973). Textural features for image classification. *IEEE Transactions on Systems Man and Cybernetics*, Vol. SMC-3, No. 6, (November 1973), pp. 610-621, ISSN 0018-9472

Heath, M.; Bowyer, K.; Kopans, D.; Moore, R. & Kegelmeyer, P. (2000). The Digital Database for Screening Mammography. *Proceedings of the 5th International Workshop on Digital Mammography, IWDM*, ISBN, Toronto, Canada, June 11–14, 2000

Jiang, Y.; Nishikawa, R.M.; Wolverton, D.E.; Metz, C.E.; Giger, M.L.; Schmidt, R.A. et al. (1996). Malignant and benign clustered microcalcifications: automated feature analysis and classification. *Radiology*, Vol. 198, No. 3, (March 1996), pp. 671-678, ISSN 0033-8419

Karahaliou, A.; Boniatis, I.; Sakellaropoulos, P.; Skiadopoulos, S.; Panayiotakis, G. & Costaridou, L. (2007a). Can texture of tissue surrounding microcalcifications in mammography be used for breast cancer diagnosis. *Nuclear Instruments and Methods in Physics Research A*, Vol. 580, No. 2, (June 2007), pp. 1071-1074, ISSN 0168-9002

Karahaliou, A.; Skiadopoulos, S.; Boniatis, I.; Sakellaropoulos, P.; Likaki, E.; Panayiotakis, G. & Costaridou, L. (2007b). Texture analysis of tissue surrounding microcalcifications on mammograms for breast cancer diagnosis. *The British Journal of Radiology*, Vol. 80, No. 956, (August 2007), pp. 648-656, ISSN 0007-1285

Karahaliou, A.; Boniatis, I.; Skiadopoulos, S.; Sakellaropoulos, P.; Arikidis, N.; Likaki, E.; Panayiotakis, G. & Costaridou, L. (2008). Breast cancer diagnosis: Analyzing texture of tissue surrounding microcalcifications. *IEEE Transactions on Information Techonology in Biomedicine,* Vol. 12, No. 6, (November 2008), pp. 731-738, ISSN 1089-7771

Kocur, C.M.; Rogers, S.K.; Myers, L.R.; Burns, T.; Kabrisky, M.; Hoffmeister, J.W. et al. (1996). Using neural networks to select wavelet features for breast cancer diagnosis. *IEEE Engineering in Medicine and Biology,* Vol. 15, No. 3, pp. 95-102, ISSN 0739-5175

Kopans, DB. (Ed.). (2007). *Breast Imaging,* 3rd Edition, Lippincott Williams & Wilkins, ISBN/ISSN: 9780781747684, Baltimore, MD

Kramer, D. & Aghdasi, F. (1999). Texture analysis techniques for the classification of microcalcifications in digitizedmammograms. *Proceedings of the 5th IEEE AFRICON Conference Electrotechnical Service for Africa,* ISBN 0780355466, Cape Town, South Africa, September - October 1999

Laws, K.I. (1979). Texture energy measures. *Proceedings of DARPA Image Understanding Workshop,* Los Angeles, November 1979

Leichter, I.; Lederman, R.; Bamberger, P.; Novak, B.; Fields, S. & Buchbinder, S.S. (1999). The use of an interactive software program for quantitative characterization of microcalcifications on digitized film-screen mammograms. *Investigative Radiology,* Vol. 34, No. 6, pp. 394-400, ISSN 1536-0210

Mallat, S. & Zhong, S. (1992). Characterisation of signals from multiscale edges. *IEEE Transactions in Pattern Analysis and Machine Intelligence,* Vol. 14, No. 7, (July 1992), pp. 710–732, ISSN 0162-8828

Markey, M.K.; Lo, J.Y.; Floyd, C.E.; (2002). Differences between computer-aided diagnosis of breast masses and that of calcifications. *Radiology,* Vol. 223, No. 2, (May 2002), pp. 489-493, ISSN 0033-8419

Nakayama, R.; Uchiyama, Y.; Watanabe, R.; Katsuragawa, S.; Namba, K. & Doi, K. (2004). Computer-aided diagnosis scheme for histological classification of clustered microcalcifications on magnification mammograms. *Medical Physics,* Vol. 31, No. 4, (April 2004), pp. 789-799, ISSN 0094-2405

Nakayama, R.; Watanabe, R.; Namba, K.; Takeda, K.; Yamamoto, K.; Katsuragawa, S. & Doi, K. (2006). Computer-aided diagnosis scheme for identifying histological classification of clustered microcalcifications by use of follow-up magnification mammograms. *Academic Radiology,* Vol. 13, No. 10, (October 2006), pp. 1219–1228, ISSN 1076-6332

Nakayama, R.; Watanabe, R.; Namba, K.; Takeda, K.; Yamamoto, K.; Katsuragawa, S. & Doi, K. (2007). An improved computer-aided diagnosis scheme using the nearest neighbor criterion for determining histological classification of clustered microcalcifications. *Methods of Information in Medicine,* Vol. 46, No. 6, pp. 716–722, ISSN 0026-1270

Papadopoulos, A.; Fotiadis, D.I. & Likas, A. (2005). Characterization of clustered microcalcifications in digitized mammograms using neural networks and support vector machines. *Artificial Intelligence in Medicine,* Vol.34, No.2, (June 2005), pp. 141–150, ISSN 0933-3657

Papadopoulos, A.; Fotiadis, D.I & Costaridou, L. (2008). Improvement of microcalcification cluster detection in mammography utilizing image enhancement techniques. *Computers in Biology & Medicine,* Vol. 38, No. 10, (October 2008), pp. 1045–1055, ISSN 0010-4825

Paquerault, S.; Yarusso, L.M.; Papaioannou, J.; Jiang, Y.; Nishikawa, R.M. (2004). Radial gradient-based segmentation of mammographic microcalcifications: observer evaluation and effect on CAD performance. *Medical Physics,* Vol.31, No. 9, (September 2004), pp. 2648-2657, ISSN 0094-2405

Patrick, E.A.; Moskowitz, M.; Mansukhani, V.T.; Gruenstein, E.I. (1991). Expert learning system network for diagnosis of breast calcifications. *Investigative Radiology,* Vol. 26, No. 6, (June 1991), pp. 534-539, ISSN 1536-0210

Pisano, E.D. (2000). Current status of full-field digital mammography. *Radiology,* Vol. 214, No. 1, (January 214), pp. 26–28, ISSN 0033-8419

Sampat, P.M.; Markey, M.K. & Bovik, A.C. (2005). Computer-aided detection and diagnosis in mammography. In: *Handbook of image and video processing*. Bovik, A.C. (Ed.). pp. 1195–1217, Academic Press, ISBN 0121197921, New York

Shen, L.; Rangayyan, R.M. & Desautels, J.E.L. (1994). Application of shape analysis to mammographic calcifications. *IEEE Transactions on Medical Imaging,*Vol. 13, No. 2, (June 1994), 263-274, ISSN 0278-0062

Skaane, P.; Diekmann, F.; Balleyguier, C.; Diekmann, S.; Piguet, J.C.; Young, K.; Abdelnoor, M. & Niklason, L. (2008). Observer variability in screen-film mammography versus full-field digital mammography with soft-copy reading. *European Radiology,* Vol. 18, No. 6, (June 2008), pp. 1134-1143, ISSN 0938-7994

Sklansky, J.; Tao, E.Y.; Bazargan, M.; Ornes, C.J.; Murchinson, R.C. & Teklehaimanot, S. (2000). Computer-aided, case-based diagnosis of mammographic regions of interest containing microcalcifications. *Academic Radiology,* Vol. 7, No. 6, (June 2000), pp. 395-405, ISSN 1076-6332

Soltanian-Zadeh, H.; Rafee-Rad, F. & Pourabdollah-Nejad, D. (2004). Comparison of multiwavelet, wavelet, Haralick, and shape features for microcalcification classification in mammograms. *Pattern Recognition,* Vol. 37, pp. 1973-1986, ISSN 0031-3203

Theodoridis, S. & Koutroumbas, K. (Eds.). (1999). *Pattern recognition.* Academic Press, New York

Thiele, D.L.; Kimme-Smith, C.; Johnson, T.D.; McCombs, M. & Bassett, L.W. (1996). Using tissue texture surrounding calcification clusters to predict benign vs malignant outcomes. *Medical Physics,* Vol. 23, No. 4, (April 1996), pp. 549–555, ISSN 0094-2405

Tourassi, G.T. (1999). Journey toward computer-aided diagnosis: role of image texture analysis. *Radiology,* Vol. 213, No. 2, (November 1999), pp. 317-320, ISSN 0033-8419

Yuan, Y.; Giger, M..L.; Li, H.; Bhooshan, N. & Sennett, C.A. (2010). Multimodality Computer-Aided Breast Cancer Diagnosis with FFDM and DCE-MRI. *Academic Radiology,* Vol. 17, No. 9, (September 2010), pp. 1158-1167, ISSN 1076-6332

Van de Wouwer, G.; Scheunders, P. & Van Dyck, D. (1999). Statistical texture characterization from discrete wavelet representations. *IEEE Transactions on Image Processing*, Vol. 8, No. 4, pp. 592-598, ISSN 1057-7149

Veldkamp, W.J.H.; Karssemeijer, N.; Otten, J.D.M. & Hendriks, J.H.C.L. (2000). Automated classification of clustered microcalcifications into malignant and benign types. *Medical Physics*, Vol. 27, No. 11, (November 2000), pp. 2600–2608, ISSN 0094-2405

17

Photovoltaic GaAs Detectors for Digital X-Ray Imaging

V.F. Dvoryankin, G.G. Dvoryankina, Yu.M. Dikaev, M.G. Ermakov, A.A. Kudryashov, A.G. Petrov and A.A. Telegin
Institute for Radio Engineering and Electronics of Russian Academy of Sciences, Russia

1. Introduction

The short coming of the conventional film-screen systems arises from limited dynamic range due to the film latitude and Swank noise from the screen and film granularity that limits the system rather than quantum fluctuations. A thin intensifying screen is used to achieve better spatial resolution; however thin screens also have limited detector quantum efficiency. Most currently available digital X-ray systems use scanned-slit geometries to minimize tehe required detector area and minimize system complexity. Scanned-slit systems achieve also efficient rejection of Compton scattered X-rays by suffering significant X-ray tube loading in comparison to conventional large-field imaging geometries. There remains a significant clinical need in production of detection systems with sufficiently high spatial resolution and detection quantum efficiency. An improvement of digital radiography compared to conventional systems is the high dynamic range. Futhermore real-time data acquisition is possible and digital image processing can be performed. A digital image representation has become feasible because of the availability of digital mass storage media.

In the past years , considerable attention was paid to the fabrication of X-ray detectors based on LEC SI GaAs (Amendolia et al., 1999; Bates, 1998; Bencivelly, 1994), LPE GaAs (Alexiev & Butcher, 1992), LP VPE GaAs (Adams et al., 1997; Bates et al., 1998) and GaAs pin structures fabricated by combining LPE and VPE (Bates et al., 1999). Early bulk devices suffered from poor charge collection efficiency and intermittent burst noise and, while later devices fabricated by LPE, LP VPE and the combination of LPE and VPE epitaxial deposition techniques proved to be good detectors, they suffered from poor detector efficiency due to the difficulties in producing thick low-doped epitaxial layers. Two types of semiconductor devices are used usually: pin diodes (McGregor&Hermon, 1997) and Schottky diodes (Buttar, 1993) operating at reverse bias voltages. A rather high (1 - 2 V/μm) operating bias voltage leads to an increase of detector noise arising from the leakage currents.

In order to reduce that noise it is necessary to operate at low temperatures. We have developed a new photovoltaic X-ray detector based on an epitaxial p^+-n-n′-n^+ GaAs structure (Achmadullin, 2002) which ensures high performance without bias voltage at room temperature. The photovoltaic effect (i.e. the emergence of a photoelectromotive force) is observed in a semiconducting structure absorbing photons, which generate current carriers (electron-hole pairs). These current carriers must be separated by the intrinsic electric field emerging in a heterogeneous semiconducting structure consisting of regions with different types of conductivity. There is some similarity between the X-ray detector and a solar cell based on GaAs (Jenny et al., 1956;Moizhes, 1960). But there is a difference too. The difference arises from higher operating energies of X-ray detector, that leads to the cecessity to solve more challenges. In the X-ray detector developed in our laboratory the photovoltaic effect is obtained in the p^+-n-n′-n^+ GaAs structure.

2. Fabrication and characteristics of the photovoltaic GaAs detector

The epitaxial p^+-n-n'-n^+ GaAs structures were grown by vapor-phase epitaxy (VPE), on Si-doped n^+ -GaAs(100) substrates ($n = 10^{18}cm^3$), 2" diameter and 500 (μm thick. There were two basic problems solved by the fabrication of those structures: (i) growth of high-resistant n-GaAs epitaxial layers of maximum thickness and (ii) creation of the depletion region all over this thickness. The growth of thick gallium arsenide epitaxial layers by VPE is complicated by low growth rates and by the imperfections on the surface of the growing layer, such as piramides of growth. For the epitaxial layer growth we have used the technology permitting to obtain n-GaAs epitaxial layer with low concentration of EL-2 defects.

The epitaxial structure consists of three epitaxial layers: p^+ -GaAs top layer with a thickness of 1-2 μm and $p \approx 10^{18}cm^{-3}$, n-GaAs epitaxial layer with a thickness of 60-100 (μm and 10^{11}-$10^{13}cm^{-3}$ and n'-GaAs buffer layer with a thickness of 2-3 μm and $n' \approx 5 \times 10^{17}cm^{-3}$. The ohmic contacts were prepared by vacuum deposition of Al/Cr and Ni/Ga/Au thin films on the front and rear surface of the structure, respectively.

Investigations of the I-V characteristics of the photovoltaic X-ray detector have shown that those characteristics are similar to that of the conventional solar cells. The behavior of the reverse branch of I- V characteristic i0 (reverse saturation current) is of special importance, because it determines the detector dark current. Under illumination of the photovoltaic X-ray detector by X-rays its I-V characteristics are shifted along the current axis. The typical I-V characteristic of the photovoltaic X-ray detector without illumination is shown in Fig. 1. The small disturbance at approximately -3 V is caused by the fail of measuring system.

The photovoltaic X-ray detector can be used in two operation modes: short circuit mode and open circuit mode. It is preferable to use the detector in short circuit operation mode because, then the response of the detector varies linearly with the X-ray intensity, while the response of the detector in the open circuit mode varies logarithmically.

When the photovoltaic X-ray detector is illuminated, a short circuit current, isc, is generated in the n-GaAs epitaxial layer and the I- V characteristics are shifted along the current axis. The current generated in an ideal photovoltaic detector can be written as

$$i_{sc} = N_g q,$$

where q is electron charge, Ng is the incident flux of all X-ray photons with the energy greater than the bandgap E_g upon the device. For GaAs $E_g = 1.424$ eV. Fig. 2 shows the short circuit current as a function of incident X-ray doze. One can see that the short circuit current varies linearly with the X-ray doze.

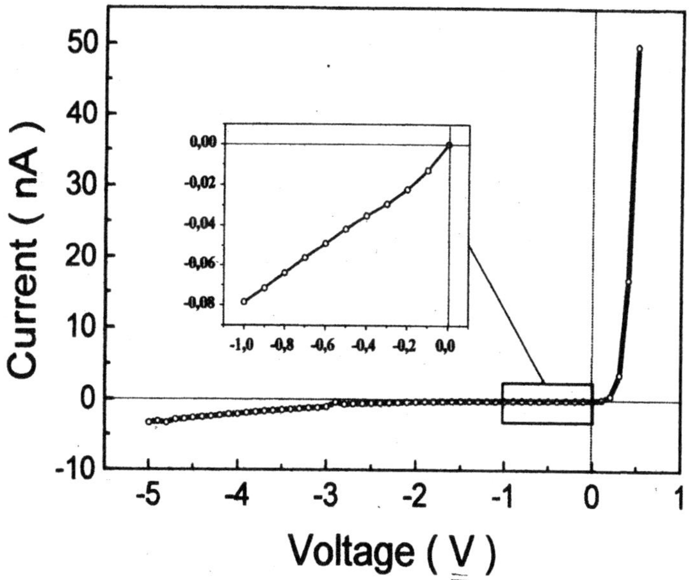

Fig. 1. Typical I-V characteristic of photovoltaic X-ray detector.

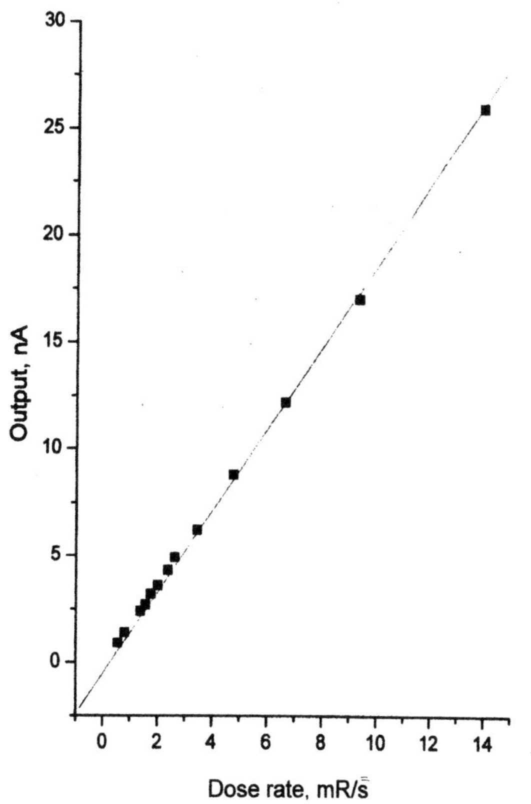

Fig. 2. Short-circuit current of X-ray detector as a function of X-ray dose rate.

The investigation of C-V characteristics has allowed us to control the depletion region in the epitaxial n-GaAs layer, to evaluate the carrier concentration $n = N_d - N_a$ (N_d is a donor concentration, N_a is a acceptor concentration), to spot the profile of the built-in electric field in the depletion region and, at last, to spot the energetic diagram for GaAs(p^+-n-n'-n^+) photovoltaic detector.

Fig. 3 shows the typical C-V characteristic of the photovoltaic X-ray detector. It can be seen that the capacitance is almost constant for reverse and forward biases up to 0.4 V. It is reasonable, therefore, to suppose that the depletion region extends over all the metallurgical thickness of the high resistant n-GaAs epitaxial layer. The presence of the depletion region over the entire thickness of a high-resistant n-GaAs is very important because it gives a opportunity to reduce the the long "tales" of the detector signal due to the carrier generation in the regions where the built-in electric field is neat zero.

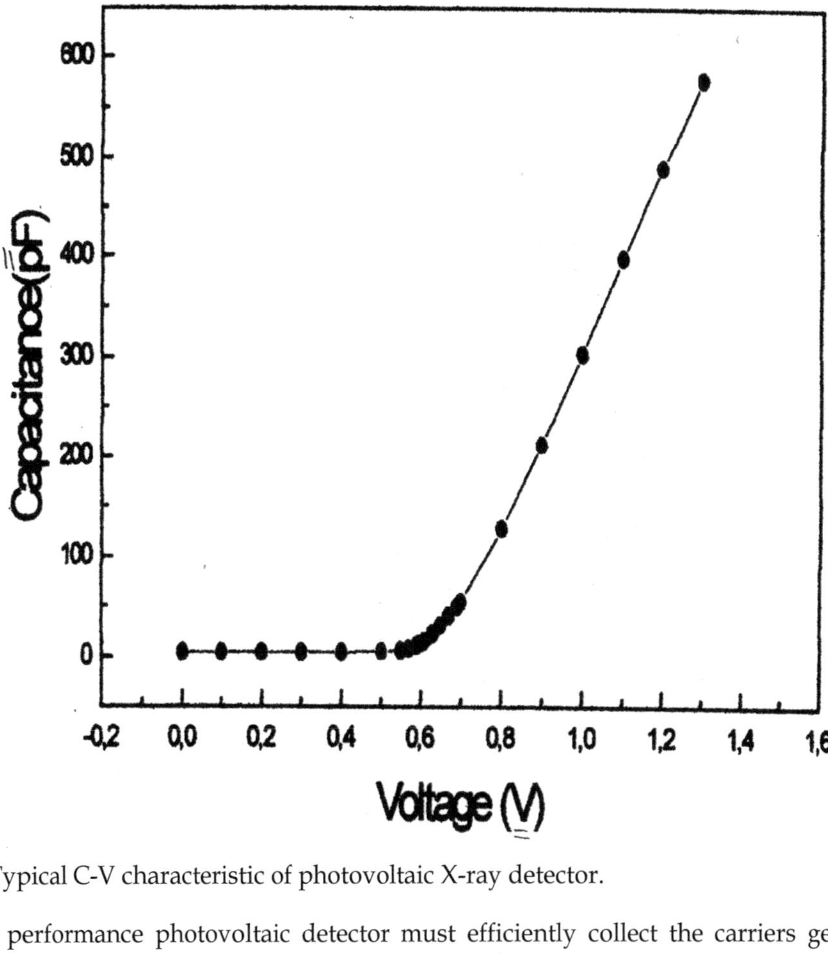

Fig. 3. Typical C-V characteristic of photovoltaic X-ray detector.

A high performance photovoltaic detector must efficiently collect the carriers generated. Maximum detector signal is obtained only when both electrons and holes created by x-ray irradiation in the depletion region are fully collected.

The charge collection efficiency is determined by the thickness of the depletion region and the collection length

$$L_c=(\mu_n\tau_n+\mu_p\tau_p)\cdot E\ ,$$

where μ_n and μ_p are electron and hole mobilities, τ_n and τ_p are electron and hole lifetimes, $\boldsymbol{E}$ is built-in electric field in the depletion region. The lifetime of excess free charge carriers produced by x-ray irradiation in the depletion region is an important parameter for the high charge collection efficiency. Poor collection efficiency is caused by deep level traps which reduce the mobility-lifetime product in GaAs layer. Generally large mobility-lifetime product and high resistivity are required for good transport characteristics resulting in high charge collection efficiency. The long lifetimes (of order of 200 ns) in epitaxial GaAs were obtained by decreasing of EL-2 center concentration to less as 10^{13} cm^{-3} in the *n*-GaAs epitaxial layer.

It should be noted that the carrier collection length decreases if forward bias voltage is applied to photovoltaic detector and transport of carriers via diffusion dominates as detector approaches the open-circuit mode. Let us now consider briefly the role of the depletion region. The concentrations of impurities and charge carriers out of the depletion region are balanced also charge density it is equal to zero. The depletion region almost doesn't contain mobile charges therefore there is here the large gradient of electric field due to the charges of ionized impurities. The thickness of a depletion region is given by

$$W=\left[\frac{\varepsilon}{2\pi e}\left(\frac{1}{N_A}+\frac{1}{N_B}\right)\left(V+\Phi_B\right)\right]^{1/2},$$

where ε is the dielectric constant, e is the charge of an electron, N_A and N_B are concentrations of acceptors and donors in the p^+ and n layers of the structure, V is the applied voltage and Φ_B is the built-in voltage of the junction. The width of the depletion region can be controlled by the epitaxial technique used to prepare GaAs p^+-n-n'-n^+ structure or by the application of reverse bias to the junction. Electron-hole pairs generated in the depletion region are separated and accelerated by the built-in electric field and enter the region where they are the majority carriers. Charge carriers generated out of the depletion region but on distance of the mean diffusion length from it will diffuse into the depletion region and drift there. The charge collection efficiency is the most important factor in detector operation. It is defined by three factors, namely by the charge carriers mobility's, by the charge carriers lifetimes and by the electric field in the p-n junction.

The built-in electric field is the origin of photocurrent in the photovoltaic X-ray detector. In order to obtain a reasonable built-in electric field in the depletion region it is important to control accurately the total number of impurities. Direct measurements of the built-in electric field by the EBIC method were made to determine its profile in the epitaxial GaAs (p^+-n-n′-n^+) structure. The junction structure was investigated by the use of Philips SEM 515 scanning electron microscope. In the built-in electric field profile studies the electron beam is incident normal to the edge of epitaxial structure. The profile of built-in electric field in epitaxial GaAs (p^+-n-n′-n^+) structure with depletion region of 80 μm thickness is shown in Fig. 4. One can see here that the built-in electric field exists over the entire epitaxial n-GaAs layer.

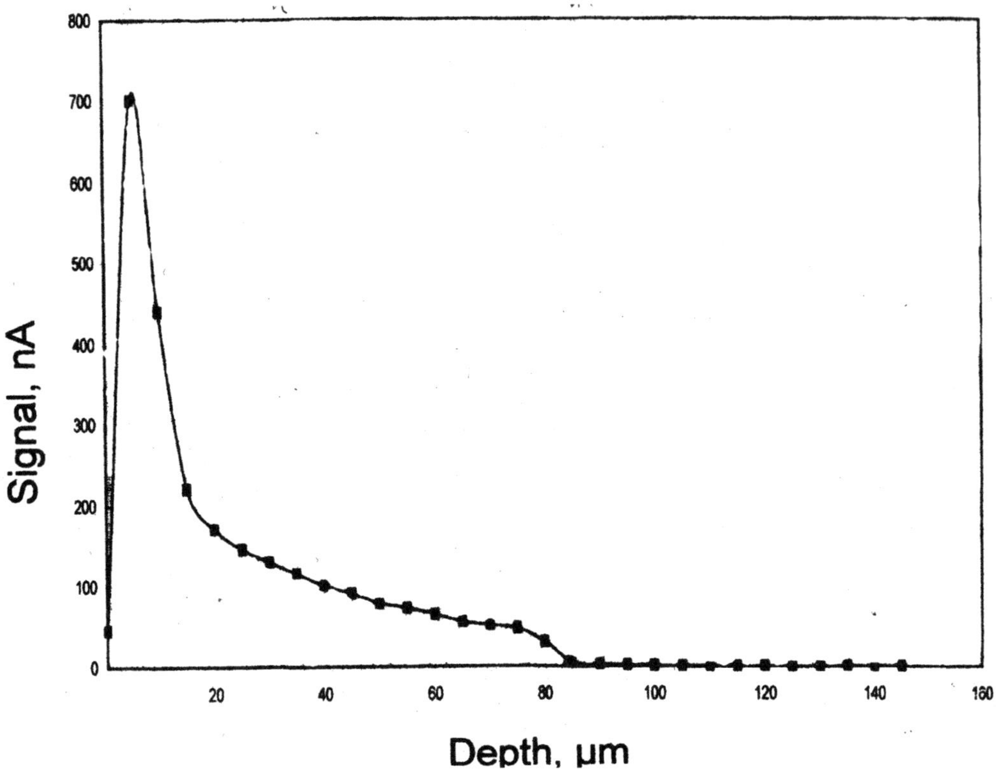

Fig. 4. Profile of the built-in electric field.

The response of the epitaxial GaAs (p^+-n-n′-n^+) detector to charged particles was investigated by the use of α-particles from radioisotope source. We have measured the charge collection efficiency and energy resolution.All measurements were made at room temperature. Registration of α-particles was performed at atmospheric pressure and in vacuum ($p \approx 10^{-4}$Torr) at 0 and 17 V bias voltages. Epitaxial GaAs (p^+-n-n′-n^+) detectors were tested by α-particles from a three-component source U^{233}[4824 keV]-Pu^{238}[5499 keV]-Pu^{239}[5156 keV]. The summary of the results is shown in table 1.

Here Vbias is the bias voltage, Eα(keV) is the energy of the α-particles, Qtheor(e) is the theoretical charge in the detector (in thousands of electron-hole pairs), N(Ch) is the position of peak in ADC counts, σ of the peak is also in ADC counts, Qcol is the measured charge collected in detector and CCE is the charge collection efficiency. The energy resolution better than 1% is obtained at air pressure. One can see on the Table that the charge collection efficiency at zero bias voltage is lower than at 17 V bias. Since the high concentration of electron-hole pairs created by α-particles disturbs significantly the built-in electric field, the electron-hole pairs are not fully collected without a bias voltage.

A photovoltaic X-ray detector was irradiated with ^{241}Am(60 keV) photons. Measurements of the charge collection efficiency obtained with bias voltages of 0 and 17 V show charge collection efficiency of 93.4% and 93.6%, respectively. In this case, the charge collection efficiencies without bias voltage and with the bias of 17 V are the same.

	E_α(keV)	Q_{theor}	N (Ch)	σ (Ch)	Q_{col}	CCE (%)	σ(e)
E_{bias}=0 V P = 740 mmHg	4824	1148.571	317	9.92	873.165	76.0	17.3
	5156	1227.619	375	9.08	974.375	79.4 ,	15.8
	5499	1309.286	431	7.72	1072.095	81.9	13.5
E_{bias}= 17 V P = 740 mmHg	4824	1148.571	378	9.4	979.61	85.3	16.4
	5156	1227.619	448	7.98	1101.76	89.7	13.9
	5499	1309.286	515	7.9	1218.675	93.1	13.8
E_{bias}=0 V P = 0 mmHg	4824	1148.571	519	9.22	905.655	78.9	16.1
	5156	1227.619	561	8.69	978.945	79.7	15.2
	5499	1309.286	599	7.1	1045.255	79.8	12.4
E_{bias} = 17 V P = 0 mmHg	4824	1148.571	622	5.1	1085.39	94.5	8.9
	5156	1227.619	675	4.71	1177.875	95.9	8.2
	5499	1309.286	729	5.2	1272.105	97.2	9.1

Table 1. The summary of α-particle measurements.

The quantum efficiency of the photovoltaic X-ray GaAs detector is limited by the thickness of the n-GaAs layer in the epitaxial structure. The use of a grazing incident angle geometry, which provides a larger absorption length for X-ray photons without increasing the actual thickness of the epitaxial layer, is the only way to increase the quantum efficiency of the photovoltaic GaAs X- ray detector. We have measured the sensitivity of the photovoltaic GaAs detector as a function of effective energy in the range 7-120 keV. The sesitibity S was calculated as

$$S = \frac{I_{ph}}{DA},$$

where I_{ph} is the photocurrent, D is the X-ray dose and A is the sensitive surface area of the detector. The results are shown in Fig. 5. The function has a maximum at 35 keV. The mean sensitivityat this energy was about 30 μA·min/Gy·cm2. Above 35 keV, the detector sensitivity decreases but at a lower rate compared to the decrease in X-ray linear absorption coefficient in GaAs. It can probably be explained by the cascade processes in the epitaxial structure.

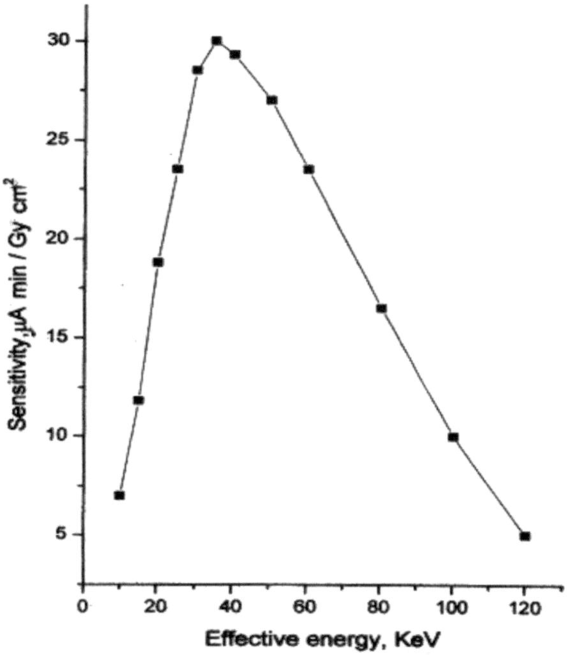

Fig. 5. Sensitivity of the photovoltaic GaAs detector as a function of effective energy.

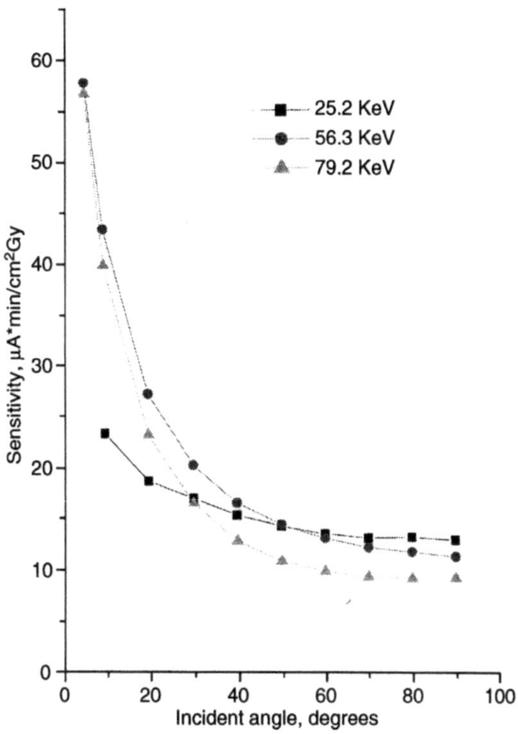

Fig. 6. Sensitivity of the photovoltaic GaAs X-ray detector as a function of the angle.

The quantum efficiency for the photovoltaic GaAs (p^+-n-n′-n^+) detector is limited by the thickness of the n′-GaAs epitaxial layer. To increase the sensitivity of the detector one can use the grazing-incident X-ray photons angle geometry which provides a larger absorption length in the depletion region without increasing the actual thickness. The measured sensitivity as a function of the angle is shown in Fig.6.

3. Multielement X-ray detector made by the use of photolitography

The scribing the channels on the depth greater than 100 µm to separate the pixels in active layer one from another made the linear detector very fragile if we want to decrease pixel size and pitch less than ~ 200 µm. So one cane make the pixel's row by the lithography and separate the pixel's photocurrent with the use of "guard" rings as it is shown in Fig. 7. In our case the pitch was 108 µm.

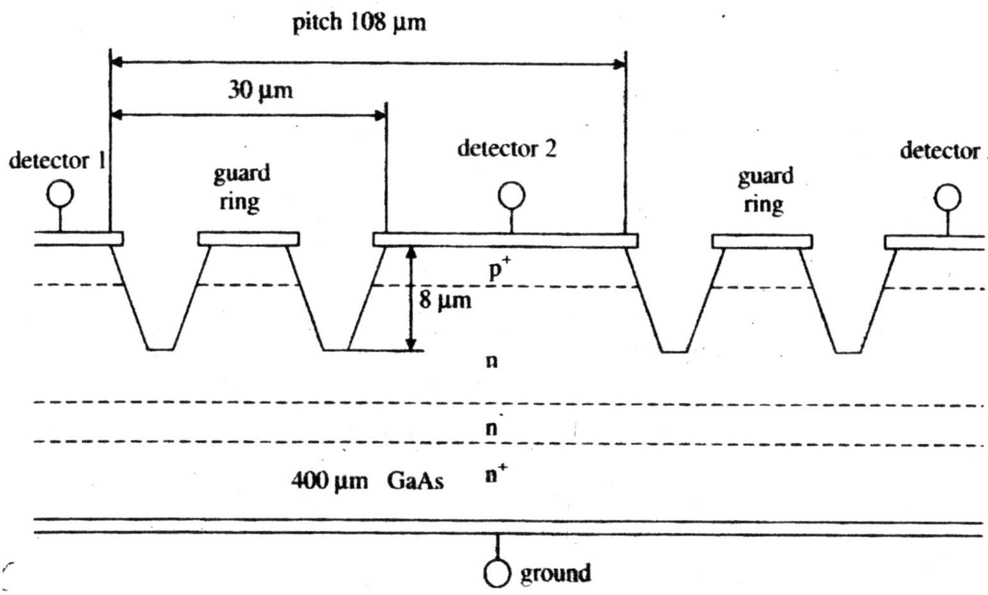

Fig. 7. Intrinsic structure of GaAs (p^+-n-n′-n^+) X-ray detector with guard rings.

In distance of 30 µm between pixels the aluminium conductor of a "guard" ring is located. The "guard" ring is connected to the full- wafer ohmic contact on n^+ side for all detectors (cathode). In p^+ layer and partially in n layer the grooves on depth of 8-10 µm are etched, which separate a conductive p^+ layer between contacts of anodes of detectors and "guard" ring. The anisotropic etch of a solution HCI-$KBr0_3$-H_20 was used with the purpose of decrease of lateral chemical etching of a GaAs material under aluminum contacts. That controlled process carries out the etching on determinate directions of crystallographic planes. The resistance between the nearby contacts is more than $10^6\Omega$. The potential of the full-wafer cathode is formed to suppress interchannel leakages of a photocurrent between anodes of detectors. Signal profiles on the three near-by contacts are shown in Fig. 8.

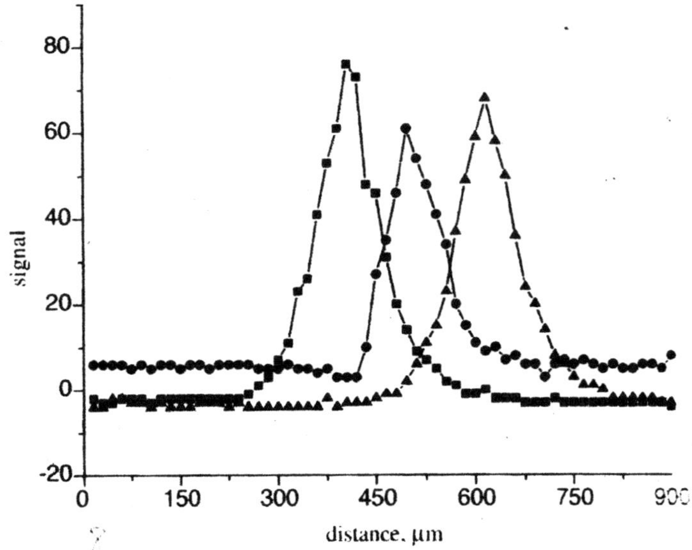

Fig. 8. Signal profiles on the three near-by contacts.

4. Bilinear X-ray detector

In order to increase the spatial resolution of the linear detector one can decrease the pitch and therefore the pixel size. But it leads to decreasing of the signal of the detector. To avoid this one can use a bilinear design of the detector. Let us see the difference between that two types of a detector.

The single or linear multielement detector is a row of pixels (Fig. 9) located along an axis 0X with periodic distance between their geometrical centres: d. The recording of the image is carried out by its scanning in an axis 0Y. The double or bilinear staggered photosensors (Fig. 9b,c) (Bosiers et al, 1995) consist of two rows of linear pixels shifted by one of them in relation to another along an axis OX on the half of pixel's period: d/2, and with distance centre to centre of axes of two rows in d/2. The step of scanning of bilinear row along an axis 0Y is equal d/2. For bilinear row, submitted in Fig. 9 b, the photosensitivity of sensors is lower, as the surface area of the aperture is twice as low as that for viewed here by us (Fig. 9c).

For harmonic intensity modulation in image the appropriate photosensor response, as it is easy to deduce from modulation transfer function (MTF), will correspond to

$$r(f_x, f_y, x, y) = SabMTF(f_x,f_y) \cos[2\pi(f_x x + f_y y)]$$

where S is the detector sensitivity, depending on absorbed photon energy and on detector matter; f_x, f_y are spatial frequencies of the image and a, b are geometrical sizes (apertures) of a rectangle on axes 0X and 0Y (Fig. 9). In a Fig. 10 the dependencies of response difference on value f for rectangular bilinear row with a step $\Delta x = d/2$ and $\Delta y = fy = 0$ for the photosensor moving in space with a step of scanning Δx, Δy, are shown: curve–1 (2a = d), curve–2 (2a/3 = d) and curve–3 (a= d;\ with $\Delta y = b$ and $\Delta x = fy = 0$: curve–1; and linear row: curve –4 ($\Delta x = a = d$, $\Delta y = 0$, $fy = 0$) and ($\Delta y = b = d$, $\Delta x = 0$, $f_x = 0$). For linear row

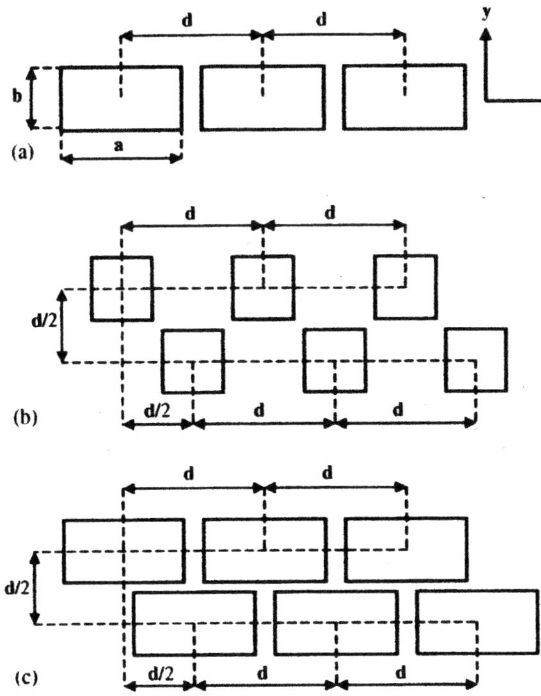

Fig. 9. Kinds of pixel rows.

response difference is higher at low spatial frequencies and lower (worse) at high spatial frequencies, than that for bilinear row. Minimum detectable contrast is evaluated from measurement of the smallest response difference (Munier et al., 1992).

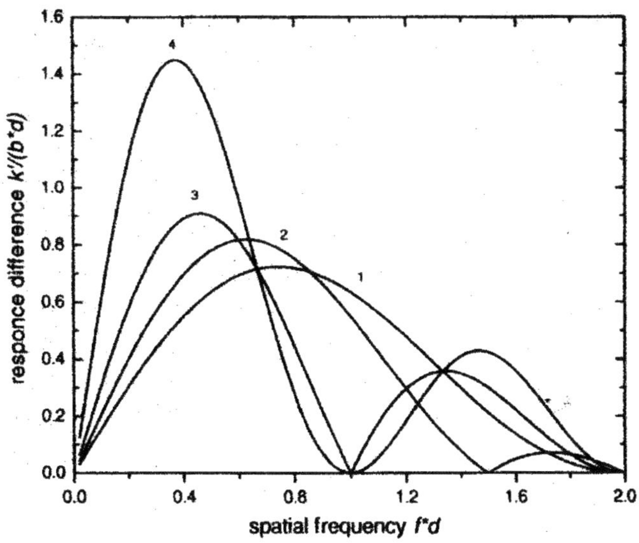

Fig. 10. Dependencies of detector response difference on spatial frequency for bilinear row (1,2,3) and linear row (4).

The multielement detector was made of 2 x 512=1024 pixels with pitch of 0.8 mm in our case. The spatial resolution of double staggered sensor row is twice as high as the resolution of that of single sensor row with the same pitch. Measured spatial resolution is 1.2 line-pairs/mm, contrast sensitivity not worse 1% and dynamic range defined as the ratio of maximum detectable X-ray signal to electronic noise level more than 2000 are received. Read-out operation of detector's signal was realized on near-to-short-circuit mode (Achmadullin et al., 2002). By combining the signal information from two linear rows of detectors a X-ray imaging with improved spatial resolution is received. One can see the X-ray image of fishes as an example of the use of bilinear detector in Fig 11. For comparison in the same figure is placed the image of fish received by the pin-diode detector with a pitch of 200 μm. The image is taken from the paper of G.I. Ayzenshtat et al.,2004. One can see that the noise in the pin-diode image makes the quality of the image much worse.

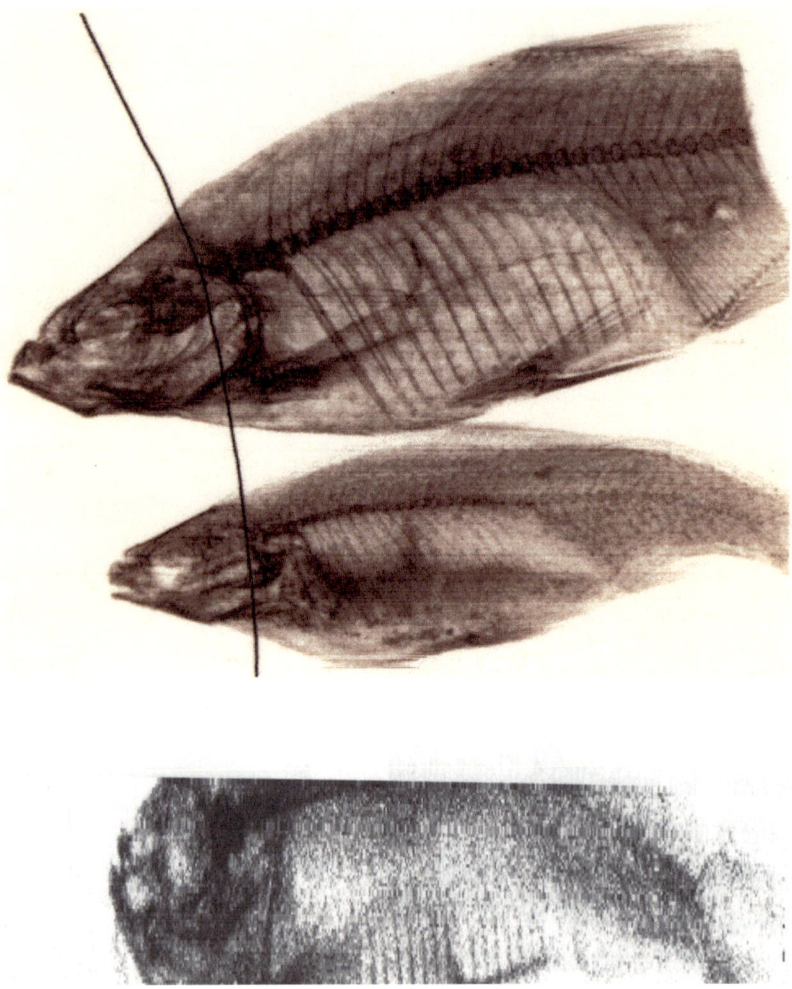

Fig. 11. The X-ray images of fishes. Left image is received by the bilinear detector with 800 μm pitch, right image is received by the pin-diode detector with the 200 μm pitch.

5. Conclusion

We have consicered here the basic features of the GaAs photovoltaic X-ray detector. The detector based on epitaxial p^+-n-n′-n^+ GaAs structures immediately converts X-ray photons to a photocurrent without bias. It has fast response and low noise level. All the measurements described above were made in short-circuit operation mode for the simplicity. To decrease a dose (it is very important in medicine) the detector can operate in pulse-count mode. Photovoltaic GaAs X-ray detectors can find their application in medicine, non-destructive testing, custom houses and other branches.

6. References

Adams R., Bates R., Da Via C., Johnson N.P., O'Shea V., Pickford A., Raine C. and Smith K.. Preliminary results for LP VPE X-ray detectors. *Nuclear Instruments and Methods in Physics Research Section A,* vol.395, Issue 1 (1997), pp. 129-131

Achmadullin R.A., Dvoryankin V.F., Dvoryankina G.G., Dikaev Yu.M., Ermakov M.G., Krikunov A.I., Kudryashov A.A., Petrov A.G., Telegin A.A. Photovoltaic X-ray Detectors Based on Epitaxial GaAs Structures. *Technical Physics Letters,* vol.28, № 1 (2002), pp.15-16

Р.А. Ахмадуллин, В.Ф. Дворянкин, Г.Г. Дворянкина, Ю.М. Дикаев, М.Г. Ермаков, О.Н. Ермакова, А.И. Крикунов, А.А. Кудряшов, А.Г. Петров, А.А. Телегин. Фотовольтаические детекторы рентгеновского излучения на основе эпитаксиальных структур GaAs. *Письма в ЖТФ* (2002), т.28, вып.1, стр. 34-38

Alexiev D., Butcher K.S.A. High purity liquid phase epitaxial gallium arsenide nuclear radiation detector. *Nuclear Instruments and Methods in Physics Research Section A,* vol.317, Issues 1-2 (1992), pp. 111-115

Amendolia C.R., Bertolucci E., Bisogni H.G. Bottigli U., Ciocci M.A., Conti M., Delogu P., Fantacci M.E., Maestro P., Marzulli V., Pernigotti E., Romeo N., Rosso V., Russo P., Stefanini A., Stumbo S. GaAs detector optimization for different medical imaging applications. *Nuclear Instruments and Methods in Physics Research Section A,* vol.434, Issue 1 (1999), pp. 14-17

Ayzenshtat G.I., Germogenov V.P., Guschin S.M., Okaevich L.S., Shmakov O.G., Tolbanov O.P., Vorobiev A.P. X-ray and γ-ray detectors based on GaAs epitaxial strictures. *Nuclear Instruments and Methods in Physics Research Section A,* vol.531, Issue 1 (2004), pp. 97-102

Bates R.L., Manopoulos S., Mathieson K., Meikle A., O'Shea V., Raine C., Smith K.M., Watt J., Whitehill C., Pospsil S., Wilhelm I., Dolezal Z., Juergensen H., Heuken M. Development of low-pressure vapour-phase epitaxial GaAs for medical imaging. *Nuclear Instruments and Methods in Physics Research Section A,* vol.434, Issue 1 (1999), pp. 1-13

Bates R., Campbell M., Cantatore E., D'Auria S., DaVià C., del Papa C., Heijne E.M., Middelkamp P., O'Shea V., Raine C., Ropotar I., Scharfetter L., Smith K. and Snoeys W. Gallium arsenide pixel detectors. *Nuclear Instruments and Methods in Physics Research Section A,* vol.410, Issue 1 (1998), pp. 6-11

Buttar C.M. GaAs detectors - a review. *Nuclear Instruments and Methods in Physics Research Section A,* vol.395, Issue 1 (1997), pp. 1-8

Bencivelli W., Bertolucci E, Bottigli U., Cola A., Fantacci M.E., Rizzo P., Rosso V. and Stefanini A. Electrical characterization and detector performances of a LPE GaAs detector for X-ray digital radiography. *Nuclear Instruments and Methods in Physics Research Section A,* vol.410, Issues 1-2 (1998), pp. 372-376

Bosiers J., Vermeiren J., Sevenhans J. High resolution linear arrays. *Proc. SPIE,* vol. 591 (1995), pp. 67-70

Jenny D.A., Loferski J.J., Rappoport P. Photovoltaic Effect in GaAs Junctions and Solar Energy Conversion. *Phys. Rev.,* vol.101, p.1208, 1956

McGregor D.S., Hermon H., Room-temperature compound semiconductor radiation detectors. *Nuclear Instruments and Methods in Physics Research Section A,* vol.395, Issue 1 (1997), pp. 101-124

Moizhes B.Ya. On the Theory of Photocells with a p-n Junction. *Soviet Physics- Solid State,* vol.2, №2, p.202, 1960

Munier B., Prieur-Drevon P., Roziere G., Ghabbal J. High resolution digital x-ray imaging with solid state linear detectors. *Proc. SPIE,* vol. 1651 (1992), pp. 106-115

18

Optimization of Digital Breast Tomosynthesis (DBT) for Breast Cancer Diagnosis

Nachiko Uchiyama[1], Takayuki Kinoshita[2], Takashi Hojo[2], Sota Asaga[2], Junko Suzuki[2], Yoko Kawawa[3] and Kyoichi Otsuka[4]
[1]*Research Center for Cancer Prevention and Screening, National Cancer Center, Tokyo*
[2]*Department of Breast Surgery, National Cancer Center, Tokyo,*
[3]*Department of Radiology, National Cancer Center, Tokyo,*
[4]*Siemens Japan K.K., Tokyo,*
Japan

1. Introduction

Recent papers have reported the usefulness of DBT as the latest diagnostic modality for breast cancer [1]-[6]. In this chapter, the author describes clinical evaluation of the usefulness regarding DBT with reference to other diagnostic modalities such as Full Field Digital Mammography (FFDM), contrast-enhanced (CE) MRI, contrast-enhanced (CE) CT, and ultrasound (US) in accordance with preliminary experiences in breast cancer diagnosis.

2. Diagnostic impact of adjunction of Digital Breast Tomosynthesis (DBT) to Full Field Digital Mammography (FFDM) and in comparison with Full Field Digital Mammography (FFDM)

Purpose: To evaluate the diagnostic impact of adjunction of DBT to FFDM and in comparison with FFDM only, in accordance with pathological findings and breast density.

Materials and Methods: This study was approved by the IRB at our institute. 303 women, having 333 lesions, (age 29-84, mean age 54.0 years old) that were recruited for this study gave informed consent. The images were taken as diagnostic mammograms from October in 2009 to October in 2011. 45 cases were referred from other institutions by US and 258 cases were referred by MMG or palpation. Clinical image data were acquired by an a-Se FFDM system with a spatial resolution of 85μm (MAMMOMAT Inspiration, Siemens, Germany).Two-view DBT was performed with the same rotation angle (±25°) and compression pressure as the FFDM. With one-view DBT, the radiation dose was 1.5 times compared to one-view FFDM. The radiation dose, utilizing ACR 156 phantom by FFDM, was 1.20mGy. Images were reconstructed by the shift and add method and the filtered back projection (FBP) method. FFDM and reconstructed slice images of DBT were reviewed at a dedicated workstation (MAMMO Report, Siemens, Germany). Two radiologists and four breast surgeons evaluated the findings by FFDM only and the adjunction of DBT to FFDM before surgery in accordance with BIRADS categories; BIRADS1-2 (no findings or benign),

BIRADS 3 (probably benign, but short-term follow-up or additional diagnostic procedure necessary), and BIRADS 4-5(highly suspicious or definitely malignant and a biopsy necessary). All cases were operated on and confirmed as malignant or borderline lesions pathologically.

Results: 181 cases were diagnosed as fatty or scattered (BIRADS density 1-2) and 122 cases were diagnosed as inhomogeneous dense or dense (BIRADS density 3-4). Of the pathological findings, 186 lesions were diagnosed as Invasive Ductal Carcinoma(IDC), 60 lesions were diagnosed as Ductal Carcinoma in Situ(DCIS), 33 lesions were IDC predominantly Ductal Carcinoma in Situ(DCIS),16 lesions were diagnosed as Invasive Lobular Carcinoma(ILC), 7 lesions were diagnosed as Lobular Carcinoma in Situ (LCIS), 5 lesions each were diagnosed as Mucinous Carcinoma (Muc Ca) and Intraductal Papilloma (IDP), 4 lesions were diagnosed as Apocrine Carcinoma, 3 lesions each were diagnosed as Mixed IDC+ILC and Intracystic Papillary Tumor(ICPT), two lesions each were diagnosed as Invasive Micropapillary Carcinoma(IMPC), DCIS with LCIS, and Phyllodes Tumor, and one lesion each was diagnosed as SCC, ILC with DCIS, ILC predominantly DCIS, ILC predominantly LCIS, and Muc Ca predominantly DCIS (Table1.). With FFDM only, the detection rate was 88.9% (176/198) for breasts with BIRADS density 1-2 and 83.7% (113/135) for breasts with BIRADS density 3-4. The findings by FFDM only were mass (n=142; 42.6%), Focal Asymmetry(FA) (n=31; 9.3%), distortion (n=15; 4.5%), microcalcifications (n=40; 12.0%), microcalcifications with FA (n=8; 2.4%), microcalcifications with distortion (n=7; 2.1%), microcalcifications with mass (n=46; 13.8%), and none (n=44; 13.2%).

With adjunction of DBT to FFDM, the detection rate (BIRADS 3-5) was 97.4% (193/198) for breasts with BIRADS density 1-2 and 94.8% (128/135) for breasts with BIRADS density 3-4. The average detection rate was 86.8% by FFDM only and 96.4% by adjunction of DBT to FFDM. There was a statistically significant difference between the FFDM only and adjunction of DBT to FFDM among BIRADS density 1-2 and BIRADS density 3-4 ($P<0.05$). On the other hand, there was no statistically significant difference according to breast density (FFDM only: $P=0.221$, 3-4; adjunction of DBT to FFDM: $P=0.202$).By BIRADS category with FFDM only, 44 lesions (13.2%) were diagnosed as BIRADS 1 or 2, 75 lesions (22.5%) were diagnosed as BIRADS 3, 214 lesions (64.3%) were diagnosed as BIRADS 4 or 5; on the other hand, 12 lesions (3.6%) were diagnosed as BIRADS 1 or 2, 21 lesions (6.3%) were diagnosed as BIRADS 3, 300 lesions (90.1%) were diagnosed as BIRADS 4 or 5 (Table 2.,Fig1).

In addition, regarding radiological findings, diagnostic accuracy was improved in 96 lesions (BIRADS 1-2 to BIRADS 3-5 or BIRADS 3 to BIRADS 4-5). These included 93 mass-related lesions (mass, FA, or distortion) and 3 microcalcifications-related lesions (microcalcifications, microcalcifications and FA, or microcalcifications and distortion). However, diagnostic confidence was improved in cases of microcalcifications-related lesions owing to the presence of masses or focal dense areas with microcalcifications. In addition, by adjunction of DBT to FFDM, 32 more lesions were detected in comparison with FFDM only (Table 3.)

Discussion. According to recent reports, DBT is a useful diagnostic procedure compared to 2D mammography because breast structures are superimposed onto a two-dimensional (2D) image [6]. The outline of the lesion can be potentially obscured. Our preliminary results also indicated that adjunction of DBT to FFDM contributed not only to detecting the lesion, but also to clarifying the diagnostic accuracy, especially with regard to mass-related lesions. On the other hand, regarding microcalcifications-related lesions, only using DBT slice image, it is difficult to recognize the overview of the clustered microcalcifications and analyze the morphology of each microcalcification's outline at current settings for image acquisition and reconstruction. As a result, adjunction of DBT to FFDM is the best current option. 32 more lesions were detected by adjunction of DBT to FFDM. Not only 14 invasive cancers (IDC n=11, ILC n=2, ILC pred LCIS n=1), but also 18 non-invasive cancerous or borderline lesions (DCIS n=15, LCIS n=1, IDP n=2).

Adjunction of DBT to FFDM was useful to detect early stage breast cancer and it is not affected by breast density.

Conclusion. In this study, the results indicated that adjunction of DBT to FFDM was superior to FFDM only, regarding diagnostic performance.

333 Lesions	**303 cases with**
IDC	n=186
DCIS	n=60
IDC Pred DCIS	n=33
ILC	n=16
LCIS	n=7
Muc Ca	n=5
IDP	n=5
Apocrine Ca	n=4
IDC with ILC	n=3
ICPT	n=3
IMPC	n=2
DCIS with LCIS	n=2
Phyllodes Tumor	n=2
SCC	n=1
ILC with DCIS	n=1
ILC Pred DCIS	n=1
ILC Pred LCIS	n=1
Muc Ca Pred DCIS	n=1
Total	**n=333**

Table 1. Subtypes of Pathological Findings of the Lesions.

FFDM only		**Adjunction of DBT to FFDM**	
BIRADS 1 or 2	n=44	BIRADS 1 or 2	n=12
		BIRADS 3	n=10
		BIRADS 4 or 5	n=22
BIRADS 3	n=75	BIRADS 3	n=11
		BIRADS 4 or 5	n=64
BIRADS 4 or 5	n=214	BIRADS 4 or 5	n=214
Total		**n=333**	

Table 2. Categorical Changes of FFDM Only Vs. Adjunction of DBT to FFDM.

FFDM Only	Adjunction of DBT to FFDM	
DCIS	n=22	n=7
IDC	n=13	n=2
LCIS	n=3	n=2
ILC	n=2	n=0
IDP	n=2	n=0
ILC Pred LCIS	n=1	n=0
ICPC	n=1	n=1
Total	**n=44**	**n=12**

Table 3. Missed Lesions in Pathological Findings by FFDM Only Vs. Adjunction of DBT to FFDM.

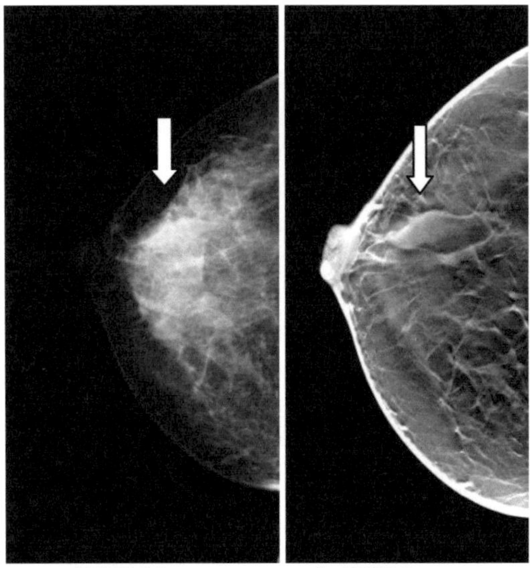

a. FFDM image b. DBT image

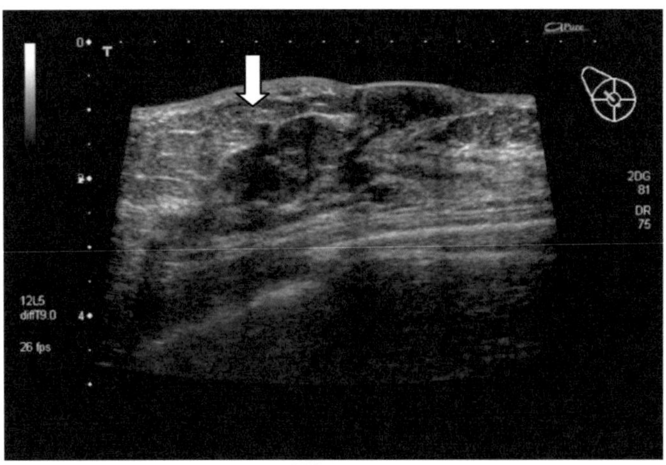

c. US image

Fig. 1. Radiological Findings of Adjunction of DBT and US images.

FFDM (Fig.1a) showed distortion only in the right breast by CC view (white arrow).DBT (Fig.1b) showed an irregularly shaped mass corresponding to the distortion shown by FFDM (white arrow). US (Fig.1c) showed hypo-echoic masses corresponding to the lesion shown by DBT (white arrow). The pathological diagnosis was IDC (Sci Ca).

3. Evaluation of correlation between pathological size and diagnostic size

Purpose

To compare the diagnostic performance between combined Full Field Digital Mammography (FFDM) and Digital Breast Tomosynthesis (DBT) in comparison with US and contrast enhanced MRI with regard to the extent of the lesion.

Materials and methods

This study was approved by the IRB at our institute. 196 women having 217 lesions (age 29-77, mean age 53.0 years old) that were recruited for this study, gave informed consent. The images of FFDM, DBT, US, and contrast enhanced MRI were taken for diagnosis before surgery from October, 2009 to October, 2011. Regarding FFDM and DBT, clinical image data were acquired by an a-Se FFDM system with a spatial resolution of 85μm (MAMMOMAT Inspiration, Siemens, Germany). Two-view DBT was performed with the same compression angle and compression pressure as the FFDM. With one-view DBT, the radiation dose was 1.5 times that of one-view FFDM. The radiation dose, utilizing ACR 156 phantom by FFDM, was 1.20mGy. FFDM and reconstructed slice images of DBT were reviewed at a dedicated workstation. Regarding contrast enhanced MRI, MIP images and MPR images (coronal, axial, sagittal) of 3mm thickness reconstructed from dynamic MRI (four phases) at 3.0 tesla were evaluated. Two radiologists and three breast surgeons evaluated the findings regarding extent of the lesion by FFDM only, FFDM plus DBT, US, and contrast enhanced MRI in a non-blind consensus study before surgery, and compared the total size of the lesion with the actual pathological size of the lesion. The coefficient of correlation was analyzed by Pearson's Product Moment Correlation Coefficient (SPSS Statistics 17.0, IBM, USA).

Results

Of the pathological findings, 125 lesions (57.6%) were diagnosed as IDC, 39 lesions (18.0%) were diagnosed as DCIS, 21 lesions (9.7%) were diagnosed as IDC predominantly DCIS, 11 lesions (5.1%) were diagnosed as ILC, five lesions (2.3%) were diagnosed as LCIS, three lesions each (2.4%) were diagnosed as Muc ca and Apocrine Ca, two lesions each (0.9%) were diagnosed as Phyllodes Tumor and IMPC, one lesion (0.5%) each was diagnosed as ILC with DCIS, Mixed ILC and IDC, Muc Ca pred DCIS, and ICPC(Table1.).The sensitivity of the lesion was 0.908 (197/217) by MMG, 0.972(211/217) by adjunction of DBT to FFDM, 0.927(201/217) by US, and 0.977 (212/217) by MRI.MMG missed 20 lesions (DCIS n=14, IDC n=5, and ICPC n=1), adjunction of DBT to FFDM missed 6 lesions (DCIS n=5 and ICPC n=1), US missed 16 lesions (DCIS n=12, IDC n=2, IDC pred DCIS n=1, and LCIS n=1) , and MRI missed 5 lesions (DCIS n=5).

The coefficient of correlation between pathological diagnostic size and each modality was 0.352 with FFDM ($P<0.01$), 0.586 with adjunction of DBT to FFDM ($P<0.01$), 0.472 with US ($P<0.01$), and 0.628 with MRI ($P<0.01$) regarding IDC and ILC (n=136; pathological size; 3-

108mm, average 35.4mm), 0.516 with FFDM ($P<0.05$), 0.590 with adjunction of DBT to FFDM ($p<0.01$), 0.375 with US ($P>0.05$), and 0.688 with MRI($P<0.01$) regarding IDC predominantly DCIS (n=21; pathological size; 14-104mm, average 46.9mm), and 0.454 with FFDM ($P<0.01$), 0.589 with adjunction of DBT to FFDM ($P<0.01$), 0.130 with US ($P>0.05$), and 0.558 ($P<0.01$) with MRI regarding DCIS(n=39; pathological size; 4-100mm, average 32.6mm) (Fig.2).

Discussion

According to recent reports, CE-MRI is sensitive in evaluating the extent of cancerous lesions; on the other hand, it involves the risk of overestimation of the size of the lesion [7]. In this study, we evaluated the sensitivity and the tumor size determined by FFDM only, adjunction of DBT to FFDM, US, and MRI compared with that determined by pathological diagnosis. In this study, regarding the sensitivity of the lesion, MRI showed the highest sensitivity and adjunction of FFDM to DBT showed comparable performance as well. Regarding the tumor size, MRI showed the strongest correlation with that determined by pathological diagnosis in IDC and ILC ($r = 0.628$) and IDC pred DCIS ($r=0.688$). The tumor size determined by adjunction of DBT to FFDM showed the second strongest correlation with that determined by pathological diagnosis in IDC and ILC ($r = 0.586$) and IDC pred DCIS ($r=0.590$) and the strongest correlation with that determined by pathological diagnosis in DCIS ($r=0.589$). By MRI, the lesions of DCIS were over-estimated compared with adjunction of DBT to FFDM (Fig.2c). In addition, the coefficient of correlation between adjunction of DBT to FFDM and MRI showed strong correlation compared to other diagnostic modalities, FFDM only and US. According to the results, the adjunction of DBT to FFDM combined with MRI can contribute to more accurate diagnosis with regard to evaluation of the extent of the lesion.

Conclusion

In this study, the results indicated that the adjunction of FFDM to DBT was superior compared with US or FFDM only, with regard to sensitivity and in evaluating the extent of the lesion. In addition, the adjunction of FFDM to DBT showed a strong correlation with MRI.

	196 Cases 217 Lesions (29-77y.o.; Averag Age 53y.o)
IDC	n=125
ILC	n=11
IDC Pred DCIS	n=21
DCIS	n=39
LCIS	n=5
Muc Ca	n=3
Apocrine Ca	n=3
Phyllodes Tumor	n=2
IMPC	n=2
ILC with DCIS	n=1
Mixed ILC and IDC	n=1
Muc Pred DCIS	n=1
ICPC	n=1
Total	**n=217**

Table 4. Subtypes of Pathological Findings of the Lesions.

FFDM	Pathology			
Coefficient of Correlation	0.352**			
Significant Probability	P<0.001			
*** FFDMDBT	Pathology	FFDM		
Coefficient of Correlation	0.586**	0.632**		
Significant Probability	P<0.001	P<0.001		
US	Pathology	FFDM	FFDMDBT	
Coefficient of Correlation	0.472**	0.480**	0.583**	
Significant Probability	P<0.001	P<0.001	P<0.001	
MRI	Pathology	FFDM	FFDMDBT	US
Coefficient of Correlation	0.628**	0.424**	0.586**	0.660**
Significant Probability	P<0.001	P<0.001	P<0.001	P<0.001

***FFDMDBT: Adjunction of DBT to FFDM

a. IDC,ILC (n=136) (Pathological Size; 3-108mm, Average 35.4mm)

FFDM	Pathology			
Coefficient of Correlation	0.516*			
Significant Probability	0.017			
FFDMDBT	Pathology	FFDM		
Coefficient of Correlation	0.590**	0.932**		
Significant Probability	0.005	P<0.001		
US	Pathology	FFDM	FFDMDBT	
Coefficient of Correlation	0.375	0.587**	0.589**	
Significant Probability	0.094	0.005	0.005	
MRI	Pathology	FFDM	FFDMDBT	US
Coefficient of Correlation	0.688**	0.869**	0.909**	0.542*
Significant Probability	0.001	P<0.001	P<0.001	0.011

b. IDC Predominantly DCIS (n=21) (Pathological Size; 14-104mm, Average 46.9mm)

FFDM	Pathology			
Coefficient of Correlation	0.454**			
Significant Probability	0.004			
FFDMDBT	Pathology	FFDM		
Coefficient of Correlation	0.589**	0.883**		
Significant Probability	P<0.001	P<0.001		
US	Pathology	FFDM	FFDMDBT	
Coefficient of Correlation	0.130	0.202	0.272	
Significant Probability	0.431	0.217	0.094	
MRI	Pathology	FFDM	FFDMDBT	US
Coefficient of Correlation	0.558**	0.535**	0.699**	0.266
Significant Probability	P<0.001	P<0.001	P<0.001	0.101

* Coefficient of correlation is significant at a 5% standard
** Coefficient of correlation is significant at a 1% standard

c. DCIS (n=39) (Pathological Size; 4-100m, Average 32.6mm)

Table 5. Coefficients of Correlation among Pathological Sizes and Diagnostic Sizes.

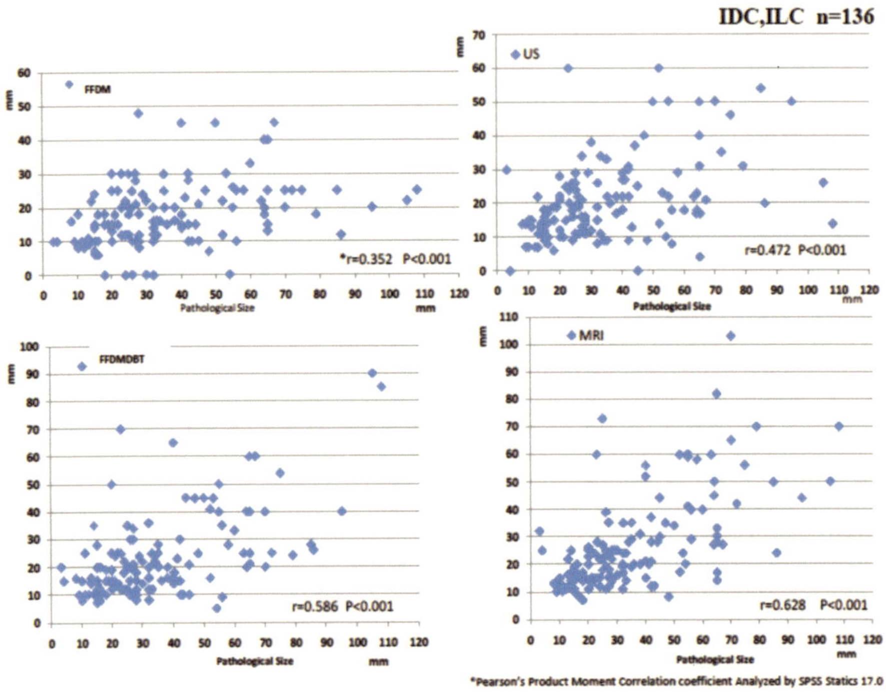

a. Coefficients of Correlation regarding IDC and ILC

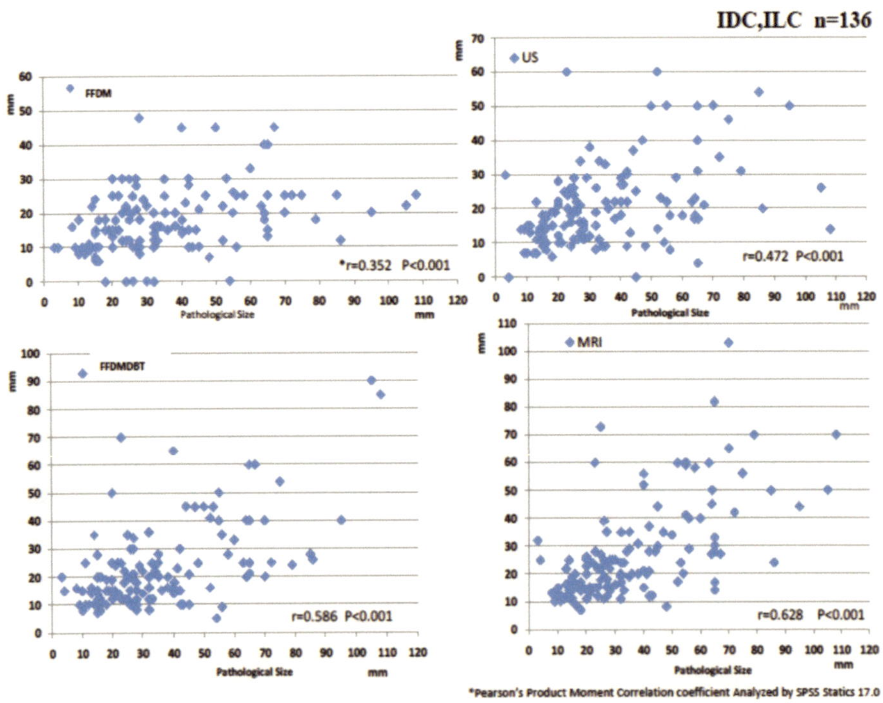

b. Coefficients of Correlation regarding IDC pred DCIS

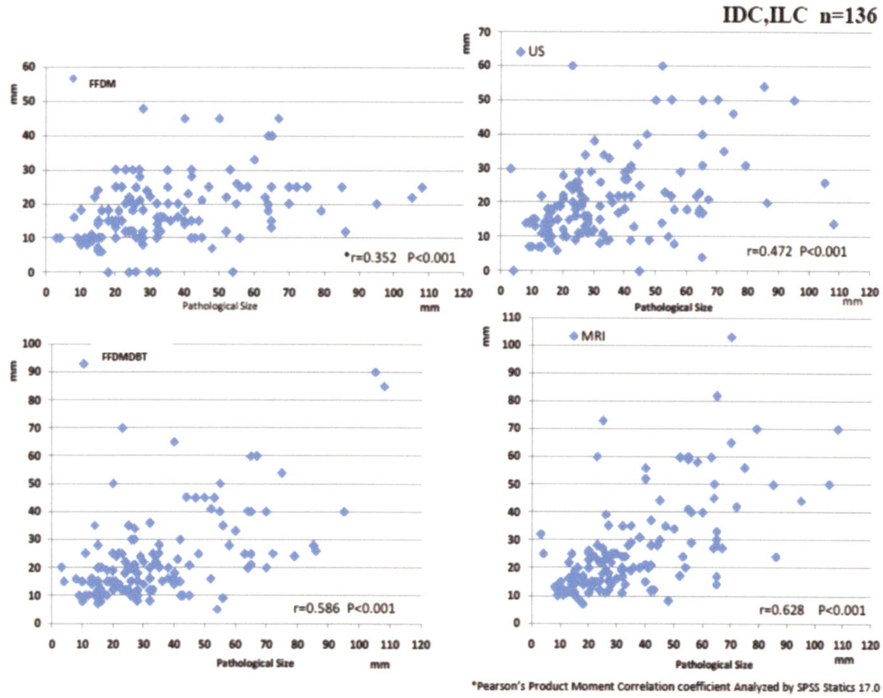

c. Coefficients of Correlation regarding DCIS

Fig. 2. Scatter diagrams of coefficients of correlation among pathological sizes and diagnostic sizes.

4. Usefulness of adjunction of Digital Breast Tomosynthesis (DBT) to Full-Field Digital Mammography (FFDM) in evaluation of pathological response after Neoadjuvant Chemotherapy (NAC) for breast cancer

Purpose

Neoadjuvant chemotherapy (NAC) is performed to reduce tumor size prior to surgery in women with breast cancer. The imaging methods that have been used until now to assess tumor response to neoadjuvant chemotherapy have serious limitations; for example, mammography alone cannot identify mass lesions in very dense breasts or distinguish viable residual lesions from the surrounding fibrous reaction after NAC [8]-[10]. Digital breast tomosynthesis has been only recently applied clinically and the diagnostic advantages in comparison to mammography have been reported on, including the fact that the slice images can be evaluated because tomosynthesis decreases the overlap in breast tissue [1]-[6]. In this study, we assessed the radiological findings and capability of DBT in adjunction to FFDM to predict response to chemotherapy in comparison with other diagnostic modalities.

Materials and methods

This study was approved by the IRB at our institute. 25 women (ages 29-73, mean age, 53.0 years old) having 26 lesions were recruited for this study and gave informed consent. The images were taken for diagnosis from December, 2009 to October, 2011. Pathological diagnosis was confirmed by Core Needle Biopsy (CNB) and the pathological subtypes were Invasive Ductal Carcinoma (n=20), Invasive Lobular Carcinoma (n=3), Invasive Micropapillary Carcinoma (n=2), and Mucinous Carcinoma (n=1).The clinical stages of the patients before NAC were II or III. All patients underwent surgery based on their response to NAC and residual tumor size estimated by diagnostic imaging was compared with the residual tumor size determined by surgical pathology. The diagnostic procedures were performed within one month prior to surgery. MMG and US were performed on each of the patients before and after NAC. Contrast-enhanced MRI was performed on 15 patients, and contrast-enhanced CT was performed on 10 patients both before NAC and after NAC. Adjunction of DBT to FFDM was performed before and after NAC in 10 out of 25 cases. In 15 out of 25 cases, adjunction of DBT to FFDM was performed only after NAC. Whole-breast US was performed with an 8 MHz wide-band high-resolution transducer (aplio™ XV, Toshiba Medical Systems, Japan). Transverse and longitudinal scans were acquired. Breast MRI was performed with a 3-Tesla system (Magnetom Trio, Siemens, Germany).Patients were studied in the prone position with a dedicated breast surface coil. The entire breast was imaged once before and four times after intravenous injection of 0.1mmol of Gd-DTPA/Kg of body weight (Magnevist; Schering, Germany). The post-processing procedures included digital image subtraction, Maximum Intensity Projection (MIP) and Multiplanar Reconstruction (MPR) by slices of 3mm thickness. Breast CT was performed with multi-detector raw CT (MDCT) (Aquilion64, Toshiba Medical Systems, Japan). The images were acquired before injection an iodine contrast medium, and 60 seconds after, and 3 minutes after injection of the total amount of 100ml, at the rate of 3ml/second (Iopamidol 300, Bayer AG, Germany). The images were reconstructed as slices of 2mm thickness and evaluated. With regard to DBT and FFDM, clinical image data were acquired by an a-Se FFDM system with a spatial resolution of 85μm (MAMMOMAT Inspiration, Siemens, Germany).Two-view DBT was performed with the same compression angle and compression pressure as the FFDM. With one-view DBT, the radiation dose was 1.5 times compared to one-view FFDM. The radiation dose with ACR 156 was 1.2mGy with FFDM. FFDM and reconstructed 1mm slice images from DBT were reviewed at a dedicated workstation. Two radiologists and four breast surgeons evaluated the findings of each diagnostic modality before surgery. The clinical response to chemotherapy was classified into the following categories, based on the "response evaluation criteria in solid tumors" (RECIST), using the measurements obtained with the different imaging methods: 1) Responders: a: Complete Response (CR): no clinical evidence of residual tumor or b: Partial Response, (PR), reduction in size of the tumor by more than 30%; 2) Non-Responders : a: Stable disease (SD): reduction in size of the tumor by less than 30% or b: Progressive disease (PD): increase in size of tumor or presence of new lesions. Pathological response to chemotherapy was classified into four categories: Grade 0 (No Response), Grade 1(Slight Response), Grade 2 (Fair Response), and Grade 3 (Complete Response) [11].

Results

Pathological responses of the lesions to NAC were Grade 0 (n=1), Grade 1 or Grade 2 (n=21), and Grade 3 (n=4).MMG findings of pathological Grade 3 were microcalcifications only (n=1), scar only (n=1), and microcalcifications with reduced mass lesion (n=2). Two out of four (50.0%) lesions demonstrated CR, and two out of four lesions demonstrated PR (50.0%).

Regarding the Grades 1-2 cases, lesions were diagnosed as reduced mass with or without microcalcifications (n=19) demonstrated PR (19/21, 90.5%) and 2 lesions diagnosed as only distortion or scar demonstrated CR (2/21, 9.5%). Regarding the Grade 0 case, the lesion detected as an enlarged mass (n=1) was diagnosed as PD (1/1, 100.0%). Adjunction of DBT findings of pathological Grade 3 were microcalcifications only (n=1), Scar only (n=1), and microcalcifications with scar without any density (n=2) that suggest CR (Fig.1). Regarding pathological Grades 1-2, the lesions were detected as reduced masses with or without microcalcifications (n=20) that suggested 20 cases were PR (20/21, 95.2%), and 1 case of only distortion or scar (n=1) that suggested CR (1/21, 4.8%). Regarding the Grade 0 case, the lesion was detected as an enlarged mass (n=1) that suggested PD (1/1, 100.0%). US findings of pathological Grade 3 (n=4) were diagnosed as CR (n=2, 50.0%), SD (n=1, 25.0%) and PR (n=1, 25.0%). US findings of pathological Grades 1-2 (n=21) were diagnosed as PR (n=17, 81.0%), SD (n=3, 14.3%) and CR (n=1, 4.8%). In the case of US findings of pathological Grade 0 (n=1), the lesion was diagnosed as PD (n=1, 100.0%). MRI (n=15) findings of pathological Grade 3 (3 lesions) were diagnosed as CR (n=2, 66.7%) and PR (n=1, 33.3%). MRI (n=15) findings of pathological Grades 1-2 (11 lesions) were diagnosed as PR (n=10, 90.5%) and CR (n=1, 9.5%). In the case of MRI findings of Grade 0(n=1), the lesion was diagnosed as PD (n=1, 100.0%). CT (10 cases with 11 lesions) findings of pathological Grade 3 (n=1) were diagnosed as CR (n=1, 100.0%). CT findings of pathological Grades 1-2 (n=10) were diagnosed as PR (n=10, 100.0%). MMG only resulted in two under-diagnosed lesions (2/26, 7.7%) and two over-diagnosed lesions (2/26, 7.7%).US resulted in one under-diagnosed lesion (1/26, 3.8%) and five over-diagnosed lesions (5/26, 19.2%). MRI resulted in one under-diagnosed lesion (1/15, 6.7%) and one over-diagnosed lesion (1/15, 6.7%) (Table1).

Discussion

Accurate evaluation of tumor response to NAC is necessary for optimization of preoperative planning. MRI and CT have recently developed the potential to assist the other traditional imaging methods in the evaluation of response to NAC [12]-[20]. By mammography, it is difficult to identify a mass lesion in dense breasts or to distinguish a viable lesion from a fibrous reaction owing to NAC. Using US only can result in over-diagnosis of chemotherapy-induced fibrosis, because in the case of a hypo-echoic lesion, it is difficult to differentiate between a fibrotic change induced by neoplastic change and a reduction in the tumor by NAC. In addition, it is difficult to measure by hand-held probe the overview of a large mass lesion or multi-centric lesions, such as locally advanced tumors that could be treated by NAC (Fig.1). On the other hand, adjunction of DBT to FFDM has potential diagnostic advantages. In accordance with our study, compared to FFDM only, adjunction of DBT to FFDM can evaluate the inside of and the outline of the lesion. Compared to US, adjunction of DBT to FFDM can evaluate the overview of the lesion objectively. Accurate evaluation of tumor response to the pharmacological treatment is fundamental for optimal surgical planning. CE-MRI and CE-CT have recently developed the potential to assist the other traditional imaging methods in the evaluation of response to chemotherapy. These are able to discriminate between neoplastic and fibrotic tissue, based on the rate of contrast media enhancement [12]-[17]. In addition, the higher sensitivity of MRI can detect non-invasive lesions as enhanced lesions that can be over-diagnosed as residual invasive components (Fig.2). According to our study, compared to CE-CT or CE-MRI, with adjunction of DBT to FFDM, it is possible to correlate the macroscopic evaluation with the pathological diagnosis without utilizing a contrast medium. The combination of adjunction of DBT to FFDM with other diagnostic modalities will contribute to improved diagnostic accuracy with regard to NAC response to locally advanced breast cancer.

Conclusion

The adjunction of DBT to FFDM combined with other diagnostic modalities will contribute to more accurate assessment of pathological response to NAC.

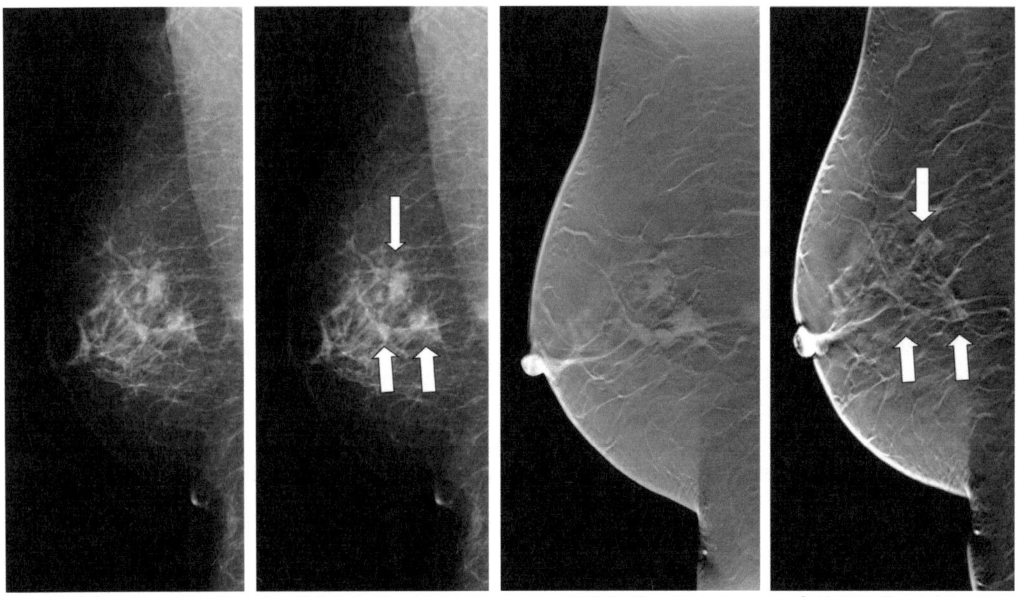

a. FFDM: Pre NAC b. FFDM: Post NAC c. DBT: Pre NAC d. DBT: Post NAC

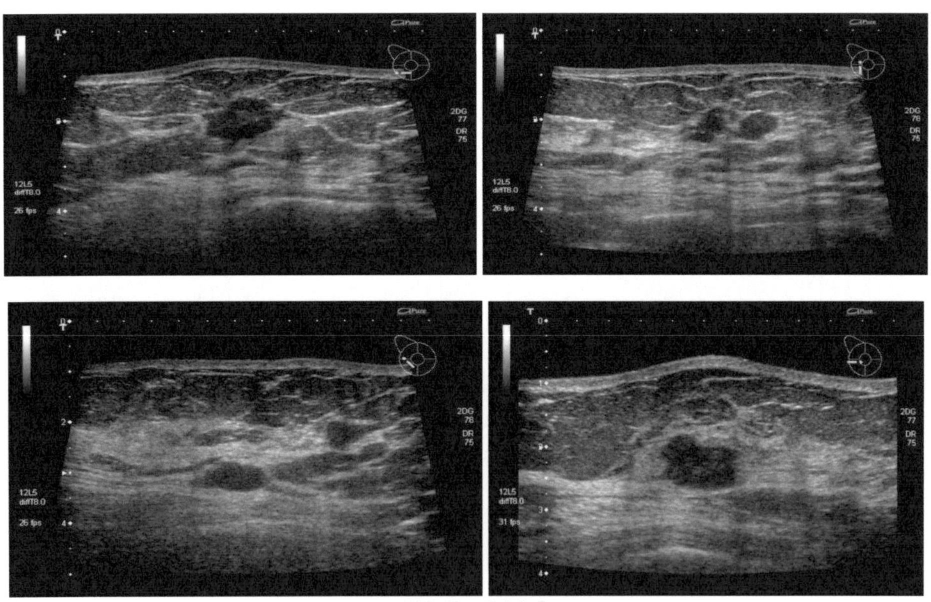

e. US: Pre NAC

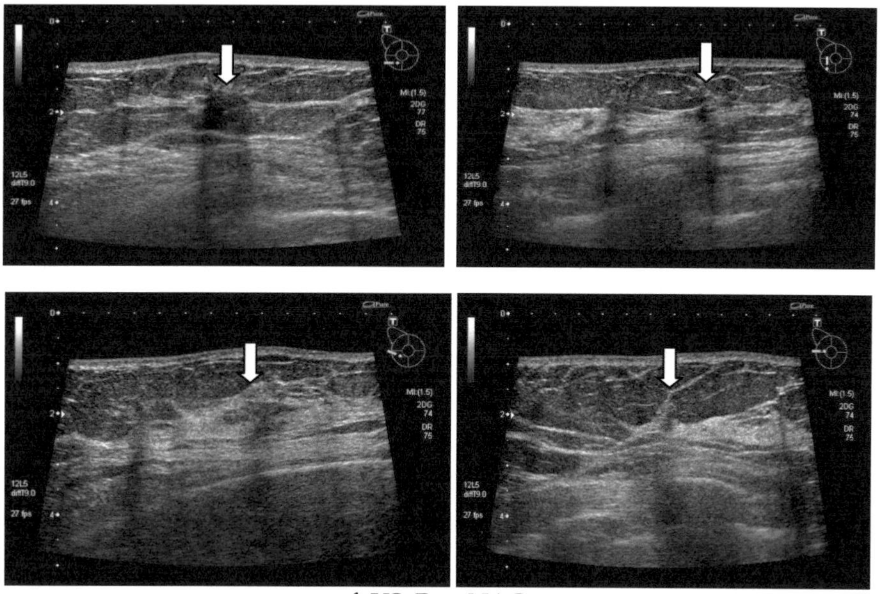

f. US: Post NAC

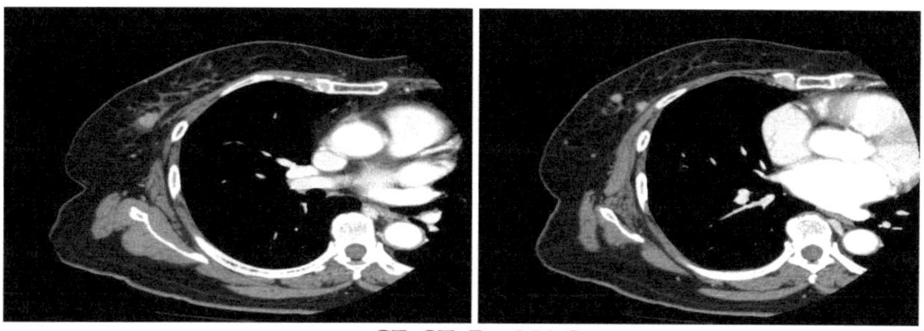

g. CE-CT: Pre NAC

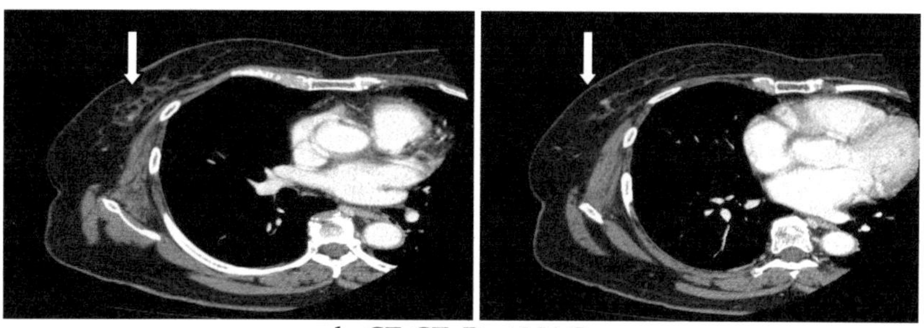

h. CE-CT: Post NAC

FFDM (Fig.1a-b) showed reduced masses after NAC (white arrow).
DBT (Fig.1c-d) showed reduced masses with scar with partial density inside of the corresponding lesion after NAC (white arrow).
US (Fig.1e-f) showed reduced hypo-echoic masses as suspicious residual lesions after NAC (white arrow).
The images of CE-CT (Fig.1g-h) showed reduced small enhanced nodules as suspicious residual lesions after NAC (white arrow).

Fig. 3. Pathological Grade 1 Case.

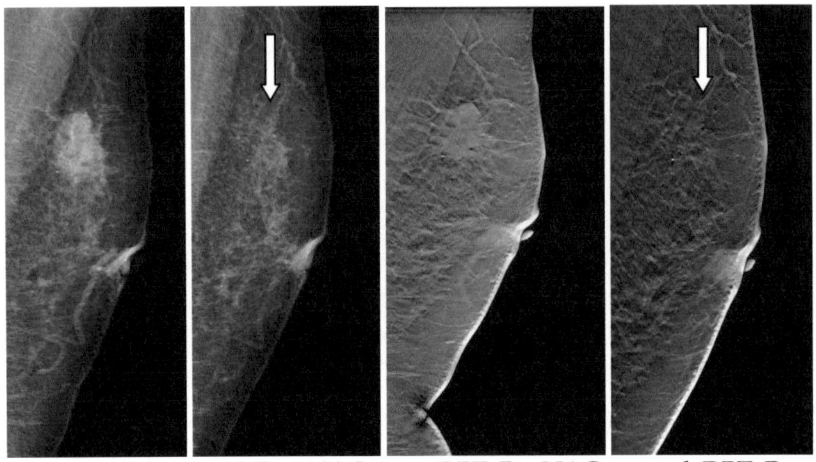

a. FFDM: Pre NAC b. FFDM: Post NAC c. DBT: Pre NAC d. DBT: Post NAC

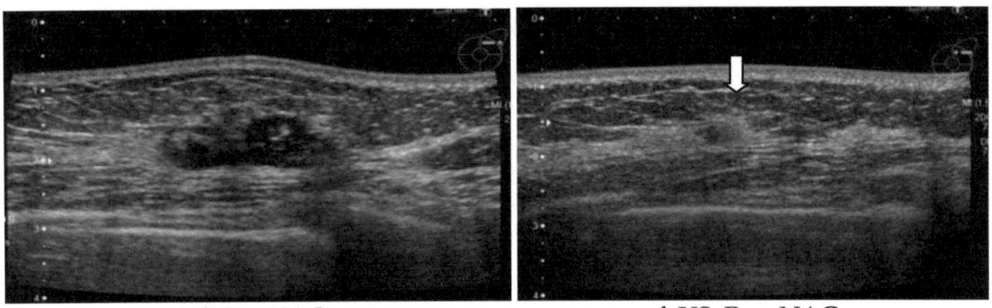

e. US: Pre NAC f. US: Post NAC

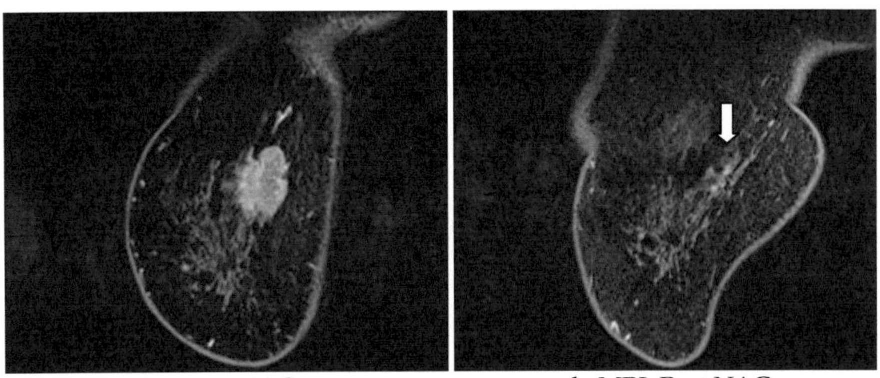

g. MRI: Pre NAC h. MRI: Post NAC

FFDM (Fig.2a-b) demonstrated a reduced mass with microcalcifications after NAC (white arrow).
DBT (Fig.2c-d) demonstrated microcalcifications with scar without core density inside of the corresponding lesion after NAC (white arrow).
US (Fig.2e-f) demonstrated a reduced hypo-echoic mass as a suspicious residual lesion after NAC (white arrow).
The coronal image of CE-MRI (Fig.2g-h) demonstrated small enhanced nodules as a suspicious residual lesion after NAC (white arrow). Pathological diagnosis demonstrated residual DCIS corresponding to the enhanced lesions by CE-MRI.

Fig. 4. Pathological Grade 3 Case.

Pathological Response	MMG	US (n=26)
Grade 0 (n=1)	*PD: n=1(100.0%)	PD: n=1(100.0%)
Grades 1-2 (n=21)	PR: n=19(90.5%), CR: n=2(9.5%)	PR: n=17(81.0%), SD: n=3(14.3%), CR: n=1(4.8%)
Grade3 (n=4)	CR: n=2(50.0%), PR: n=2(50.0%)	CR: n=2(50.0%), PR: n=1(25.0%), SD: n=1(25.0%)
Pathological Response		**CT (n=11)**
Grades 1-2 (n=10)		PR: n=10 (100.0%)
Grade 3 (n=1)		CR: n=1 (100.0%)
Pathological Response		**MRI (n=15)**
Grade 0 (n=1)		PD: n=1(100.0%)
Grades 1-2 (n=11)		PR: n=10(90.9%), CR: n=1(9.1%)
Grade 3 (n=3)		CR: n=2(66.7%), PR: n=1(33.3%)

* The clinical response to chemotherapy was classified in accordance with RECIST.

Table 6. Comparison of NAC Response by Diagnostic Evaluation and Pathological Evaluation.

5. Acknowledgment

This study was supported by Grant-in-Aid for Scientific Research (C) (No. 23591810) in Japan.

6. References

[1] Poplack SP, Tosteson TD, Kogel CA et al. (2007). Digital breast tomosynthesis: initial experience in 98 women with abnormal digital screening mammography. AJR 189(3): 616-23.

[2] Andersson I, Ikeda DM, Zackrisson S, et al. (2008). Breast tomosynthesis and digital mammography: a comparison of breast cancer visibility and BIRADS classification in a population of cancers with subtle mammographic findings. Eur Radiol 18(12): 2817-25.

[3] Good WF, Abrams GS, Catullo VJ, et al. (2008). Digital breast tomosynthesis: a pilot observer study. AJR 190(4): 865-9.

[4] Gennaro G, Toledano A, di Maggio C, et al. (2010) Digital breast tomosynthesis versus digital mammography: a clinical performance study. Eur Radiol. 20(7):1545-53.

[5] Uchiyama N, Kinoshita T, Akashi S, et al.(2011) Diagnostic Performance of Combined Full Field Digital Mammography (FFDM) and Digital Breast Tomosynthesis (DBT) in comparison with Full Field Digital Mammography (FFDM). CARS2011:32-33, Springer.

[6] Förnvik D, Zackrisson S, Ljungberg O, et al. (2010).Breast tomosynthesis: Accuracy of tumor measurement compared with digital mammography and ultrasonography. Acta Radiol. 51(3):240-7.

[7] Berg WA, Gutierrez L, NessAiver MS, et al.(2004).Diagnostic accuracy of mammography, clinical examination, US, and MR imaging in preoperative assessment of breast cancer. Radiology. 233(3):830-49.

[8] Helvie MA, Joynt LK, Cody RL, et al. (1996) Locally advanced breast carcinoma: accuracy of mammography versus clinical examination in the prediction of residual disease after chemotherapy. Radiology 198:327–332.

[9] Moskovic EC, Mansi JL, King DM, et al. (1993) Mammography in the assessment of response to medical treatment of large primary breast cancer. Clin Radiol 47:339–344.

[10] Keune JD, Jeffe DB, Schootman M, et al.(2010) Accuracy of Ultrasonography and Mammography in Predicting Pathologic Response after Neoadjuvant Chemotherapy for Breast Cancer. Am J Surg. 199(4): 477–484.

[11] Therasse P, Arbuck SG, Eisenhauer EA, et al. (2000) New Guidelines to evaluate the response to treatment in solid tumors. JNCI 92:205–216.

[12] Abraham DC, Jones RC, Jones SE, et al. (1996) Evaluation of neoadjuvant chemotherapeutic response of locally advanced breast cancer by Magnetic Resonance Imaging. Cancer 78:91-100.

[13] Londero V, Bazzocchi M, Del Frate C, et al. (2004)Locally advanced breast cancer: comparison of mammography, sonography and MR imaging in evaluation of residual disease in women receiving neoadjuvant chemotherapy. Eur Radiol. 14:1371–1379.

[14] Rosen EL, Blackwell KL, Baker JA, et al.(2003).Accuracy of MRI in the detection of residual breast cancer after neoadjuvant chemotherapy.AJR. 181:1275–1282.

[15] Yeh E, Slanetz P, Kopans D. (2005) Prospective Comparison of Mammography, Sonography, and MRI in Patients Undergoing Neoadjuvant Chemotherapy for Palpable Breast Cancer. A J R. 184:868–877.

[16] Balu-Maestro C, Chapellier C, Bleuse A, et al. (2002) Imaging in evaluation of response to neoadjuvant breast cancer treatment benefits of MRI. Breast Cancer Res Treat. 72:145–152.

[17] Partridge SC, Gibbs JS, Lu Y, et al.(2002) Accuracy of MR imaging for revealing residual breast cancer in patients who have undergone neoadjuvant chemotherapy. A J R. 179:1193–1199.

[18] Akashi T S, Fukutomi T, Sato N, et al.(2004) The use of contrast-enhanced computed tomography before neoadjuvant chemotherapy to identify patients likely to be treated safely with breast-conserving surgery. Ann Surg. 239(2):238-43.

[19] Vinnicombe SJ, MacVicar AD, Guy RL et al. (1996) Primary breast cancer: mammographic changes after neoadjuvant chemotherapy, with pathologic correlation. Radiology 198:333–340.

[20] Tozaki M, Kobayashi T, Uno S, et al. (2006) Breast-conserving surgery after chemotherapy: value of MDCT for determining tumor distribution and shrinkage pattern. AJR. 186(2):431-9.

Part 5

Clinical Case Reports

19

Fat Necrosis

Sergi Ganau, Lidia Tortajada, Fernanda Escribano,
F. Javier Andreu and Melcior Sentís
Women´s Imaging Department, UDIAT-CD,
Corporació Sanitària i Universitària Parc Taulí, Sabadell, Barcelona,
Spain

1. Introduction

Fat necrosis is a benign inflammatory process that arises from damage to breast adipose tissue. Knowledge about the pathophysiology of fat necrosis is fundamental to enable the correct diagnosis of this entity whose appearance on different imaging modalities ranges from typically benign findings to findings normally associated with malignant lesions.

In this chapter, we aim to provide a detailed description of the mechanisms involved in the development of fat necrosis as well as of the findings at mammography, sonography, magnetic resonance imaging, and other modalities. We also include a diagnostic algorithm that can be useful in the management of patients in whom fat necrosis is suspected.

2. Etiology

Breast fat necrosis is a benign inflammatory process. Although it is often considered idiopathic, breast fat necrosis is usually caused by trauma, and many idiopathic cases are probably due to microtrauma. Trauma leading to breast fat necrosis can result from accidents or clinical treatment. Among accidental agents, injury from safety belts in traffic accidents is common. Iatrogenic agents include breast surgery (including incisional biopsy; lumpectomy; breast reduction; breast augmentation by implants or injection of silicone, paraffin, or other exogenous substances; and flap breast construction techniques like TRAM, DIEP, etc.) and, less frequently, percutaneous procedures (including core biopsy, vacuum-assisted core biopsy, or fine-needle aspiration cytology), radiotherapy, and chemical irritation caused by anticoagulants or rupture of cysts or ductal ectasia. Some systemic diseases like panniculitis (Weber-Christian syndrome) have a pathogenesis and imaging manifestations similar to those of fat necrosis.

3. Clinical findings

Breast fat necrosis is often a clinically silent process. It most commonly debuts as a palpable mass, which may be accompanied by ecchymosis and erythema, or less frequently by skin thickening or retraction.

As Lee and Adair stated in the first report of breast fat necrosis (Lee&Adair, 1920), these clinical manifestations are so similar to those of breast cancer that we are obliged to use all the available means to differentiate between these two entities. Conventional imaging techniques like mammography or sonography can help in this differentiation, but they can also lead to confusion due to myriad appearances of fat necrosis on these modalities.

To better understand the wide spectrum of possible manifestations (ranging from perfectly differentiated benign findings to findings characteristic of malignant lesions), it is essential to know the pathogenesis of breast fat necrosis.

4. Pathophysiology

Fat necrosis occurs more often in breasts predominantly composed of adipose tissue; likewise, in breasts in which adipose tissue does not predominate, fat necrosis tends to occur close to the skin, where adipose tissue is most abundant.

In breast trauma, damage occurs mainly to adipocytes and to the microvascularization, which is abundant in adipose tissue.

Vascular damage results in an immediate inflammatory reaction consisting of arteriolar contraction to check bleeding. This contraction leads to increased arteriolar and capillary pressure, which cause transudation of fluid to the interstitial space and increased pressure in the venules, which in turn increases the permeability of the venous walls, thus resulting in the loss of proteins and consequently of fluid. All these factors that contribute to the increase in the amount of fluid in the interstitial space lead to the **edema** that is characteristic of the hyperacute inflammatory phase.

On the other hand, the release of cytoplasmic triglycerides into the interstitial space after adipocyte rupture also leads to a series of chemical and inflammatory reactions.

Shortly afterward, the damaged vessels release fibrinogen into the interstitial space, where the enzyme thrombin will convert it to active fibrin. Fibrin, which is elastic and insoluble, combines with the platelets to form a mesh to control bleeding. Furthermore, the "free" fat from the adipocytes will be encompassed by a sort of defense conglomerate, **granulation tissue**, which is mainly composed of macrophages, leukocytes (mainly neutrophils), fibrin, fibroblasts, and angioblasts. This fat-containing granulation tissue is called an **oil cyst**.

With time, the oil cyst can either calcify or it can be reabsorbed and replaced with connective tissue. It is important to understand each of these processes.

The fatty acids that make up the triglycerides can react with the calcium ions in the interstitial space to form calcium stearate, which will accumulate around the granulation tissue, resulting in a sphere of varying size contained within a shell of calcium, referred to as a **calcified oil cyst**.

On the other hand, the nonencapsulated fatty acids or even the granulation tissue itself can be attacked by the immune system and reabsorbed, leaving a **fibrous scar** that can also calcify with time.

These are the stages that can take place after trauma to breast adipose tissue. Although these stages tend to occur in the same order, the duration of each phase can differ widely, even within the same area of adipose tissue, so that different phenomena can be present at the same time (Ganau et al, 2009).

The wide variability of phenomena associated with fat necrosis and the wide time window in which they can appear can make the diagnosis challenging. For this reason, one of the main aims of this chapter is to provide the tools to ensure an accurate imaging diagnosis. It is essential to obtain a thorough clinical history including possible trauma or surgery.

5. Imaging&pathological findings

5.1 Mammographic findings

5.1.1 Edema

In many cases, edema does not manifest on the mammogram. When it does, the findings are very subtle, usually consisting of focal skin thickening, which may or may not be associated with an increase in the density of subcutaneous fat and trabecular thickening (1). These findings have low specificity, being similar to those of mastitis (although the clinical presentation tends to be different). In inflammatory carcinoma, these same findings tend to be more evident and to involve the entire breast.

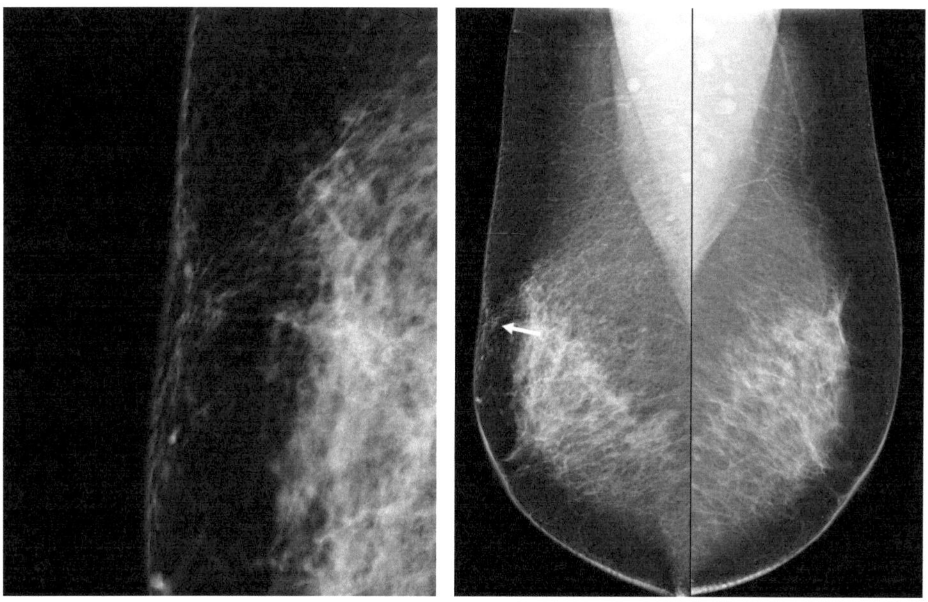

Fig. 1. Increased density and trabeculation of subcutaneous fat associated with slight skin retraction (arrow).

5.1.2 Granulation tissue

The density of granulation tissue is indistinguishable from fibroglandular breast tissue from a mass or from an asymmetry (2). However, granulation tissue is easy to recognize if other findings of fat necrosis are present.

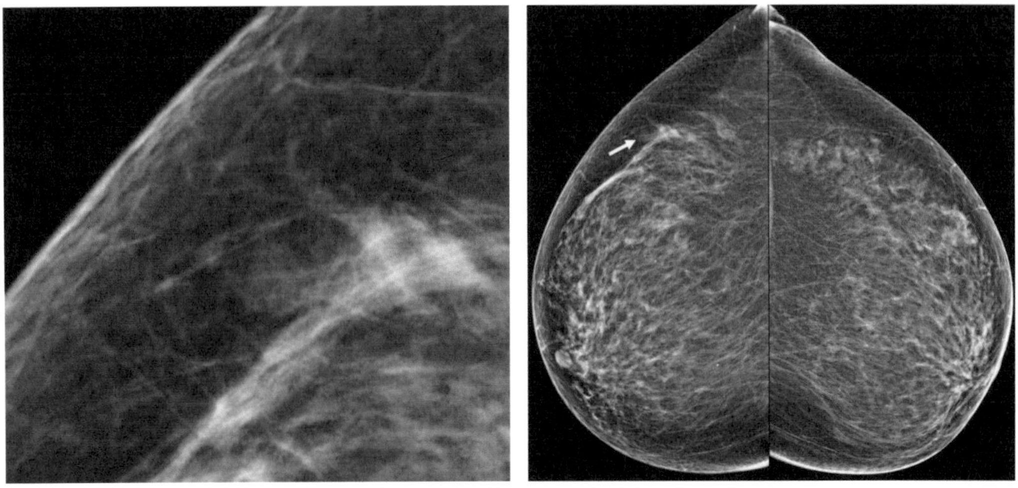

Fig. 2. Nodular image not present on previous mammograms (arrow), with a slightly lower density than the fibroglandular tissue in the same area, corresponding to a focus of fat necrosis.

5.1.3 Oil cyst

Oil cysts are easy to recognize. They are round or oval, with well-defined margins that may be partially or completely calcified or not at all, and their fatty content makes them radiolucent (3). The calcifications tend to be smooth and curvilinear and distributed from the periphery to the center (like an eggshell), although they may also adopt a more irregular shape (4). Oil cysts have been classified in function of their size as *liponecrosis microcystica calcificans* (< 3 mm in diameter) and *liponecrosis macrocystica calcificans* (> 3 mm in diameter) (Lanyi, 1986).

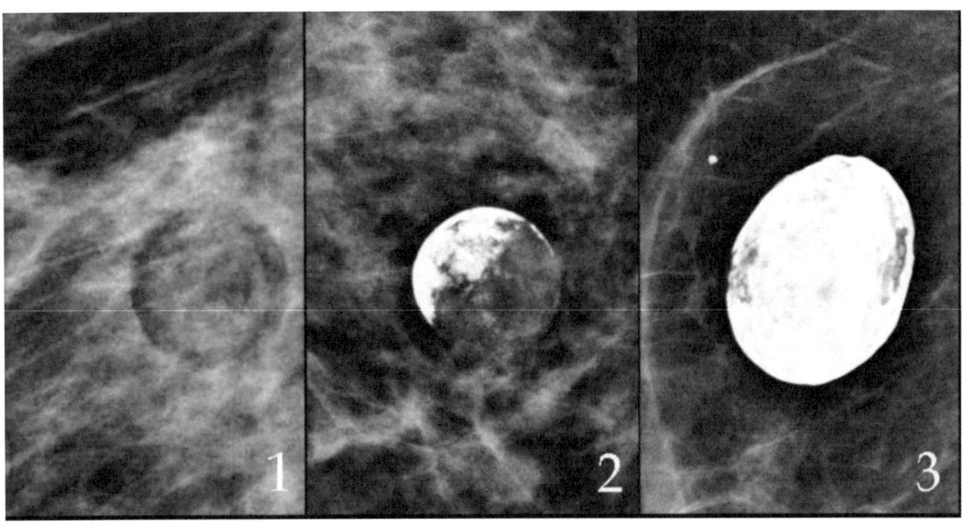

Fig. 3. Well-defined oil cysts: 1. Without calcified walls; 2. With partially calcified walls; 3. With nearly entirely calcified walls.

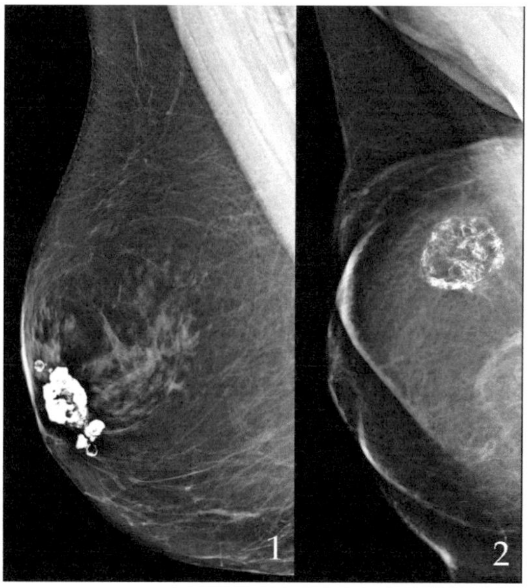

Fig. 4. Irregular oil cysts: 1. After breast reduction surgery; 2. After transverse rectus abdominus myocutaneous (TRAM) flap oncoplastic surgery.

If the salts have not precipitated completely in the peripheral granulation tissue they may remain "floating" on the cyst's fatty fluid, causing a level (5).

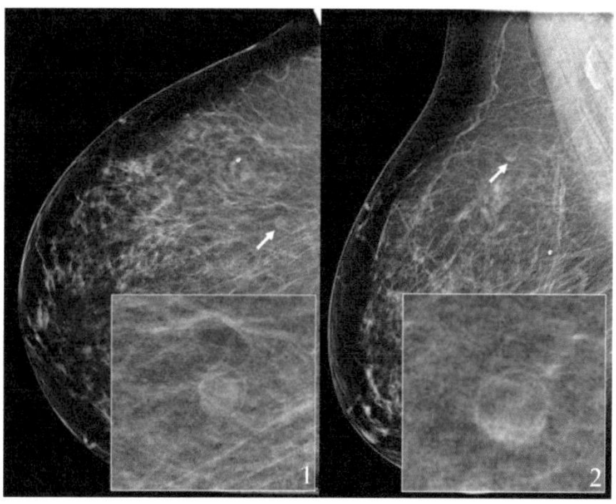

Fig. 5. Oil cyst with precipitated calcium salts (arrow) that separate from the oil in the mediolateral oblique projection to form a level (1. craniocaudal projection; 2. oblique mediolateral projection).

These findings are sometimes difficult to differentiate from a galactocele or from a bleeding oil cyst, although neither of these results are a reason for suspicion.

In some cases, the immune system can react when the cyst is still radiolucent due to its fatty content, and the walls of the cyst can thicken and adopt an irregular or ill-defined shape, simulating a malignant lesion (6).

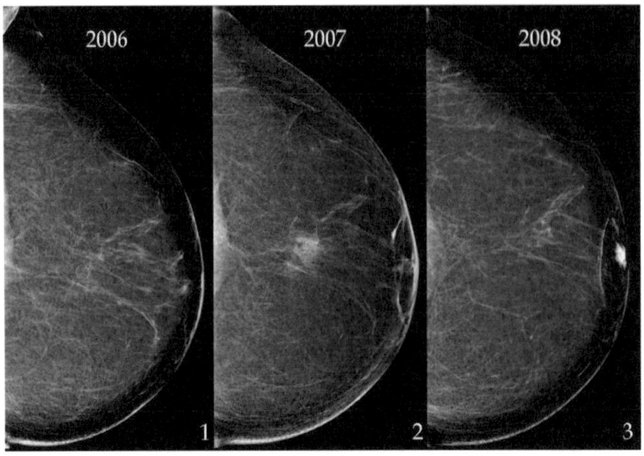

Fig. 6. Oil cyst (1). One year later, the patient had a reaction to a foreign body that simulated a malignant lesion (2). Core biopsy: fat necrosis. The disappearance of the lesion during follow-up (3) confirmed that this was a benign process.

Again, the clinical context and associated mammographic findings are important in distinguishing complicated oil cysts from other, less innocuous entities.

5.1.4 Fibrous scar

The fibrous scar that replaces the oil cyst can take on different shapes, and accordingly the mammographic findings can vary, ranging from asymmetry to an ill-defined or well-defined mass. These are the findings that make it most difficult to differentiate fat necrosis from a malignant mass, especially when the retraction of the scar tissue gives the mass a spiculated or irregular shape. When the scar also calcifies, the findings are completely different from those of a calcified oil cyst; the numerous amorphous and even pleomorphic calcifications that often occur with the scar (7) make histological study and the differential diagnosis with a neoplasm process essential.

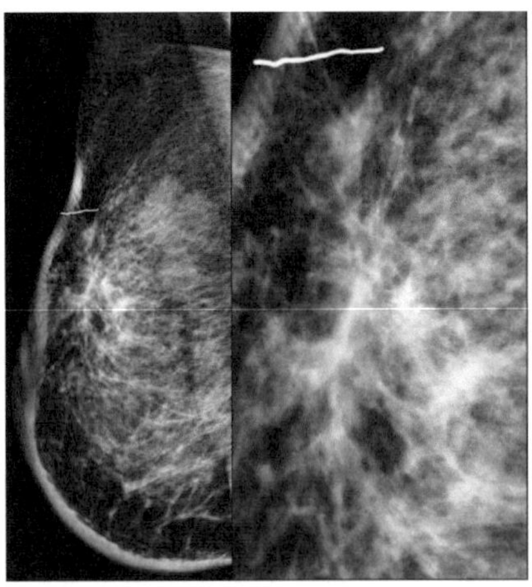

Fig. 7. Parenchymal distortion together with pleomorphic calcifications adjacent to the surgical scar. Vacuum-assisted biopsy: fat necrosis.

5.1.5 Summary of the most common findings over time

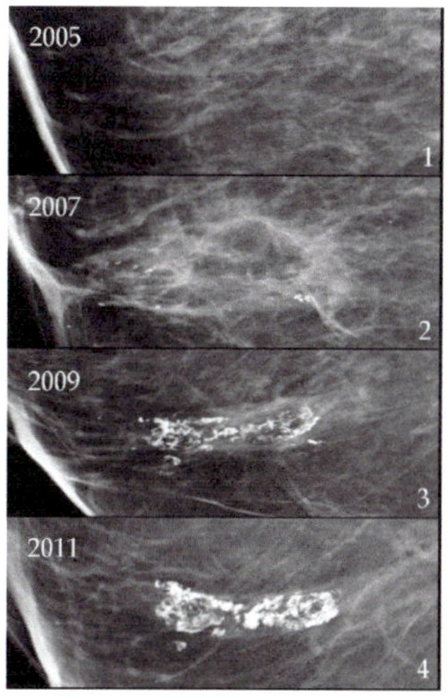

Fig. 8. Phases of fat necrosis: 1. Normal mammogram, with no history of trauma. 2. Retroareolar trauma in the left breast. Oil cyst and increased density around the cyst, together with calcifications, compatible with granulation tissue. 3. The oil cyst and granulation tissue are progressive replaced with coarse calcifications. 4. The calcifications replace the granulation tissue completely.

5.1.6 Other classic (and not so classic) examples

Mammograms in women with seat belt injuries of the breast show typical fat necrosis findings in a bandlike distribution corresponding to the path of the safety belt (DiPiro et al, 1995).

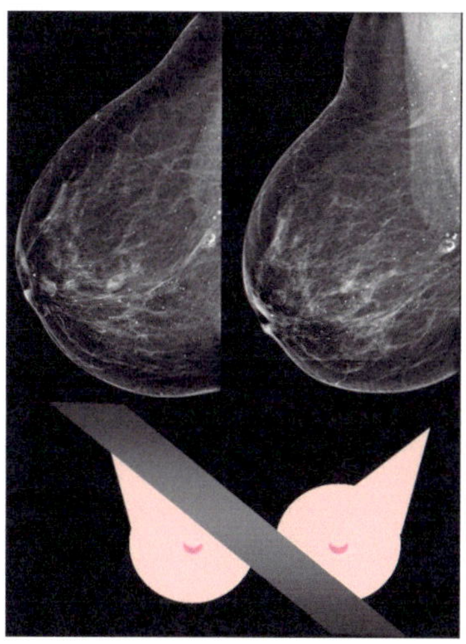

Fig. 9. Mammogram obtained a few months after a traffic accident shows calcifications compatible with fat necrosis; the calcifications are distributed throughout the anatomic region that comes in contact with the safety belt.

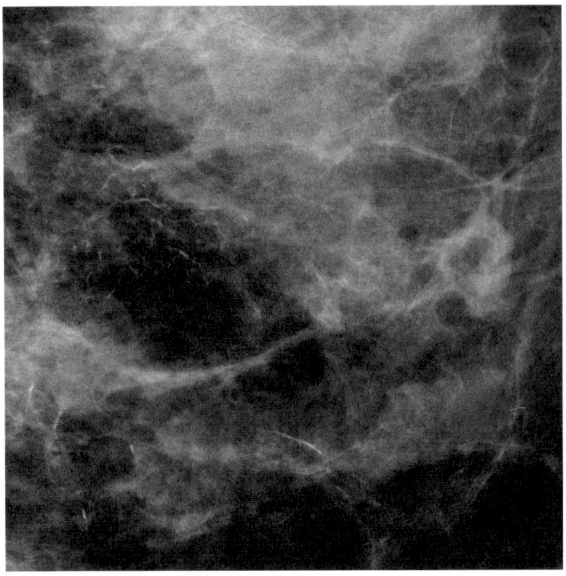

Fig. 10. Oil cysts in different phases. In this case, the lesions resulted from the injection of autologous fat for reconstructive-esthetic purposes (lipofilling).

5.2 Histologic findings.

Although fine-needle aspiration cytology can be sensitive and specific for the diagnosis of fat necrosis, core biopsy or vacuum-assisted biopsy are even more sensitive and specific. Nevertheless, in some cases diagnostic uncertainty may persist, requiring excisional surgical biopsy.

The histologic findings vary in function of the phase of the process of fat necrosis. Hemorrhagic changes in the adipocytes will give rise to a cavity filled with necrotized fat. The walls of this cavity will consist of a mesh of histiocytes, inflammatory cells, and giant multinucleated cells; with time, collagen-secreting fibroblasts responsible for scar formation will be progressively added. The calcifications mentioned in previous sections may also be identified.

5.3 Sonographic findings

5.3.1 Edema

Skin thickening (easily appreciable by comparison with the contralateral breast) and increased echogenicity of adipose tissue are characteristic of, although not specific to, fat necrosis (11). Other processes, most of them benign (e.g., lipomas) can cause the same findings. The clinical history is key. Malignant processes that can present as hyperechogenic areas must also be taken into account. Linda et al. found 0.4% of hyperechogenic lesions in a series of nearly two thousand malignant lesions (Linda et al., 2011).

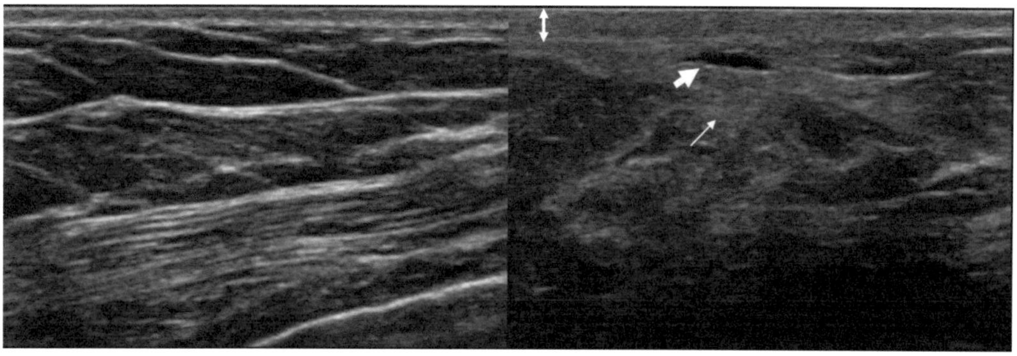

Fig. 11. 1. Normal breast adipose tissue. 2. Findings after trauma to the same breast: skin thickening (double-headed arrow), minimal free fluid (thick arrow), and increased echogenicity of the subcutaneous fat (thin arrow).

Sonoelastographic techniques can also be useful for evaluating the hardening of subcutaneous adipose tissue that occurs in these cases (12).

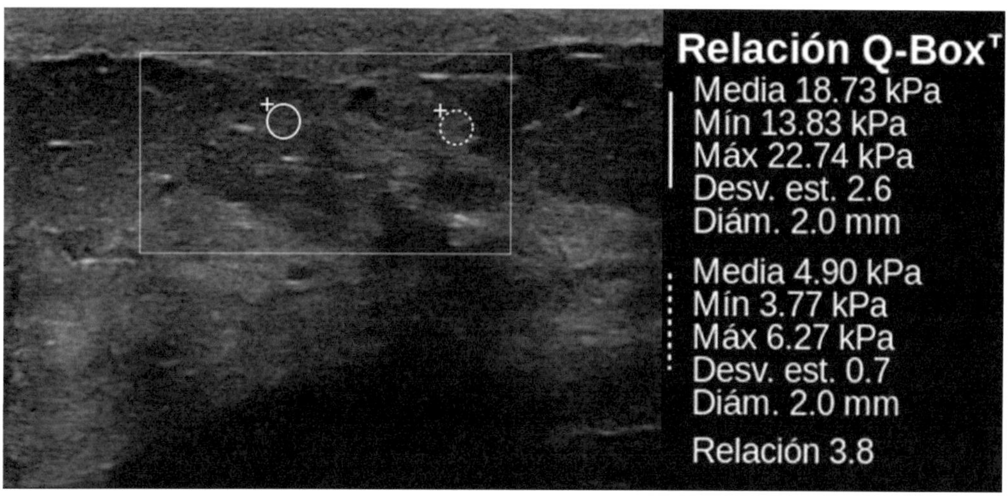

Fig. 12. Shear-wave quantitative sonoelastography. Variability in the maximum, mean, and minimum elasticity of the subcutaneous fat between two ROIs in the same area (continuous line: edematous fat; broken line: normal fat).

5.3.2 Granulation tissue

The only way to differentiate granulation tissue on sonography is by taking the absence of echogenicity of the oil cyst as a reference. The degree of calcification of the margins of these cystic cavities reflects their phase of development.

Color Doppler can also be useful for demonstrating the increased vascularization in the periphery of the cyst that occurs with the formation of the granulation tissue (13).

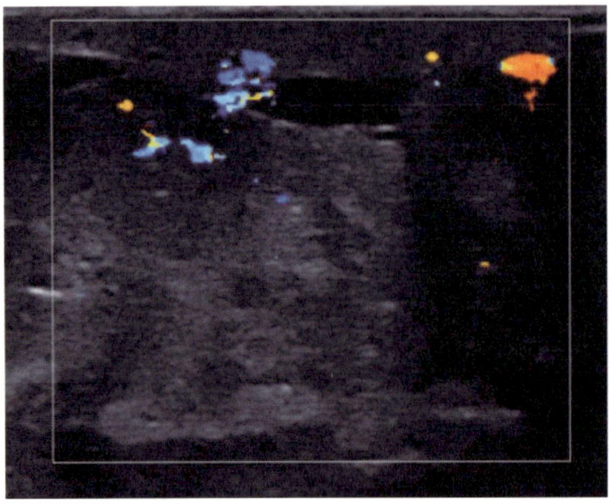

Fig. 13. Increased color Doppler signal reflects the increase in vascularization after trauma.

5.3.3 Oil cyst

Oil cysts are round or oval anechoic lesions with smooth, well-defined, generally hyperechoic margins. Therefore, they are very easy to recognize and practically impossible to differentiate from simple cysts, except for the adjacent structures (generally, areas of echogenic adipose tissue) or if we decide to puncture and drain them, thus obtaining an oily fluid.

Nevertheless, calcium stearate is often seen floating in oil cysts and accumulating in the base, forming a level that moves with patient's movement, simulating a galactocele.

Depending on the degree of calcification of the wall, we can identify a single or double echogenic ring as well as a posterior acoustic shadow which, if considerable, can cause an artifact that hinders the visualization of the cyst (14).

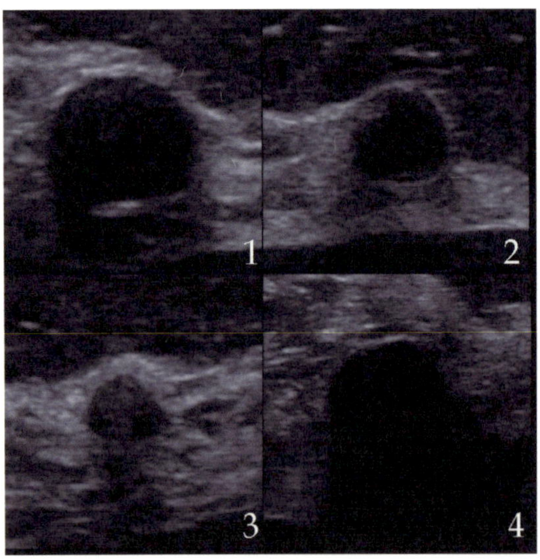

Fig. 14. Oil cysts with different degrees of calcification, In case 4, the posterior acoustic shadow hinders the visualization of the cyst.

5.3.4 Fibrous scar

As mentioned above, sonography can be very useful in the diagnosis during the initial phases of fat necrosis. However, in more advanced phases, the scars adopt the form of spiculated or irregular-shaped masses that can make it difficult to differentiate fat necrosis from malignant disease (15).

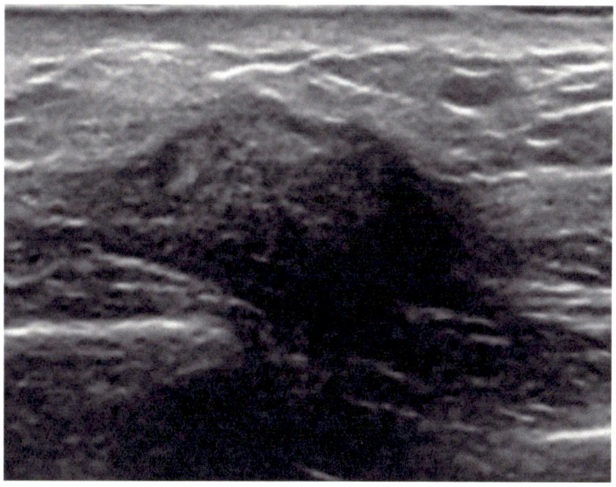

Fig. 15. A slightly heterogeneous mass with irregular margins. Core biopsy: fat necrosis.

Nevertheless, sonography is very useful for guiding interventional procedures that may be necessary when suspicious findings are present.

The role of color Doppler in these cases is uncertain, because like the formation of granulation tissue, which can persist for at least two years, some low grade tumors with a significant desmoplastic reaction can have scant vascularization.

Sonoelastography is also not useful for differentiating between a fibrous scar and a malignant lesion, because both are very stiff (16).

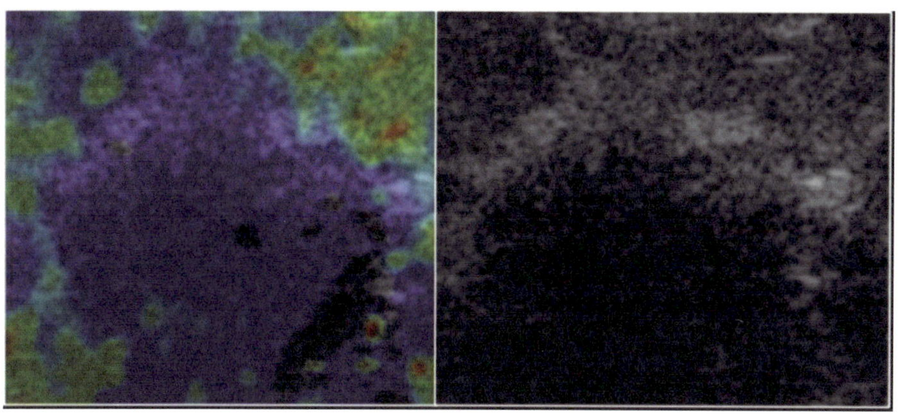

Fig. 16. A hypoechoic mass with an echogenic halo and irregular margins that has high stiffness on sonoelastography (score 5 in Ueno's classification) and is thus suggestive of malignancy. Core biopsy: fat necrosis.

5.4 MRI findings

5.4.1 Edema

Edema is hyperintense on T2-weighted sequences and hypointense on T1-weighted sequences (17). Edema does not enhance after the administration of intravenous contrast material.

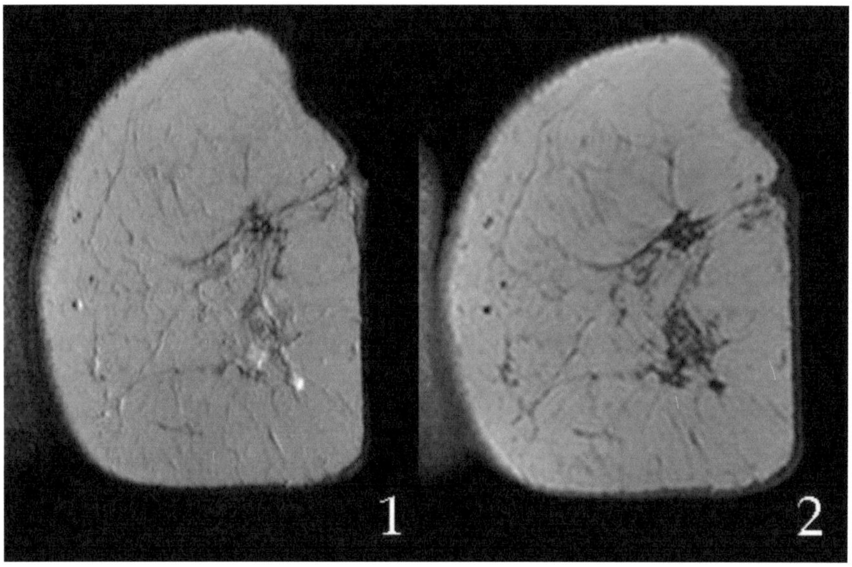

Fig. 17. Postsurgical changes in a breast treated for carcinoma. Some areas are hyperintense in T2-weighted sequences (1) and hypointense on T1-weighted sequences (2), corresponding to edema (fluid signal).

5.4.2 Granulation tissue

Granulation tissue is the main cause of contrast agent uptake in fat necrosis. Owing to the peripheral distribution of the granulation tissue around the oil cyst, ring enhancement, also characteristic of malignant lesions, is common. However, the nearly unequivocal MRI findings for oil cysts (see below) mean that the benign nature of this ring enhancement is rarely in doubt.

In some cases, however, the arrangement of the granulation tissue is less well defined, so it is important to consider the signal intensity in T1-weighted sequences. The presence of fat, which is typically hyperintense in T1-weighted sequences, together with the patient's clinical history, can help to rule out a neoplasm and diagnose fat necrosis (18). (Ganau et al., 2009; Taboada et al., 2009; Tan et al., 2005).

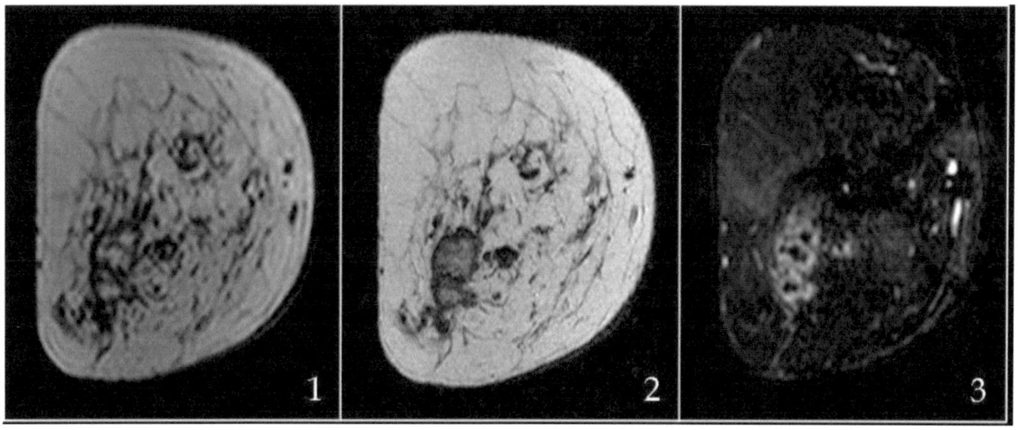

Fig. 18. Right breast three years after surgery for infiltrating ductal carcinoma. MRI shows an irregular mass with hyperintense foci in T1-weighted sequences (1) that are slightly hypointense in T2-weighted sequences (2); the mass has irregular peripheral enhancement after intravenous contrast administration (3). In this clinical context, it is imperative to rule out relapse of the tumor. Vacuum-assisted biopsy: fat necrosis.

5.4.3 Oil cyst

Oil cysts are shown as rounded or oval masses with well-defined margins; they are hyperintense in T1-weighted sequences and can be either hypo- or hyper-intense on T2-weighted sequences. Depending on whether granulation tissue surrounds the cyst, the typical ring enhancement may or may not be observed. Depending on the degree of calcification of the cyst, a signal void may be present in T1-weighted sequences.

The contents of oil cysts never enhance (19).

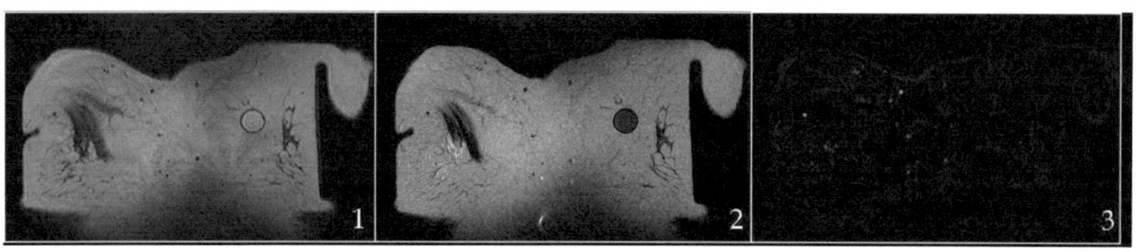

Fig. 19. Typical findings for an oil cyst: A nodular cystic lesion with well-defined margins; it is hyperintense on T1-weighted images (1), slightly hypointense on T2-weighted images (2), and does not enhance (3).

5.4.4 Fibrous scar

MRI is essential for imaging fibrous scars. The greater the fibrotic content of the scar, the less likely the scar can take up contrast material. However, the persistence of granulation tissue can cause enhancement of the scar. Hyperintense foci may also be seen within the scar in T1-weighterd sequences due to the persistence of fat (20).

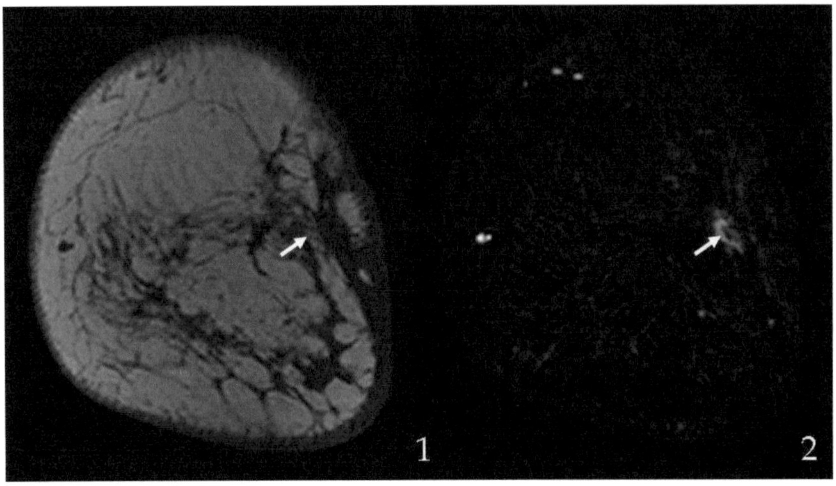

Fig. 20. A woman with a personal history of infiltrating ductal carcinoma of the left breast treated with surgery and radiotherapy. One and a half years later, hyperintense areas are seen adjacent to the surgical scar on T1-weighted images (1), with peripheral enhancement (2) (arrows). It is essential to rule out relapse. Vacuum-assisted biopsy: Fat necrosis.

The negative predictive value of screening with MRI approaches 100% in patients with a history of surgery for breast cancer. In these cases, it is important to evaluate the morphokinetic behavior of the contrast agent in scars. The absence of enhancement suggests the absence of malignancy. Nevertheless, uptake in the area of the scar requires relapse to be ruled out.

Echo-planar MRI techniques can be useful in these cases. Thus, for example, high apparent diffusion coefficients in diffusion-weighted sequences of these cicatricial lesions suggest the absence of tumor recurrence. On the other hand, on MR spectroscopy, choline peaks in a fibrous scar suggest tumor recurrence.

If any uncertainty persists about whether a lesion represents fat necrosis or a malignant process, histologic study is necessary.

In summary, fat necrosis is complex from both the clinical and diagnostic points of view. On the one hand, it can be extremely easy to diagnose in patients with a clear history of trauma and characteristic clinical and imaging findings. On the other hand, it can be very difficult to diagnose in patients with or without a known history of trauma in whom the imaging findings are identical to those of malignant breast disease.

For this reason, with the aim of preventing underdiagnosis (considering a malignant process to be an episode of fat necrosis) and avoiding unnecessary diagnostic procedures (considering an episode of fat necrosis to be a malignant process), we present a algorithm for the management of these patients that takes into account three fundamental factors: the clinical presentation, the personal risk of breast cancer, and the findings on different diagnostic imaging techniques.

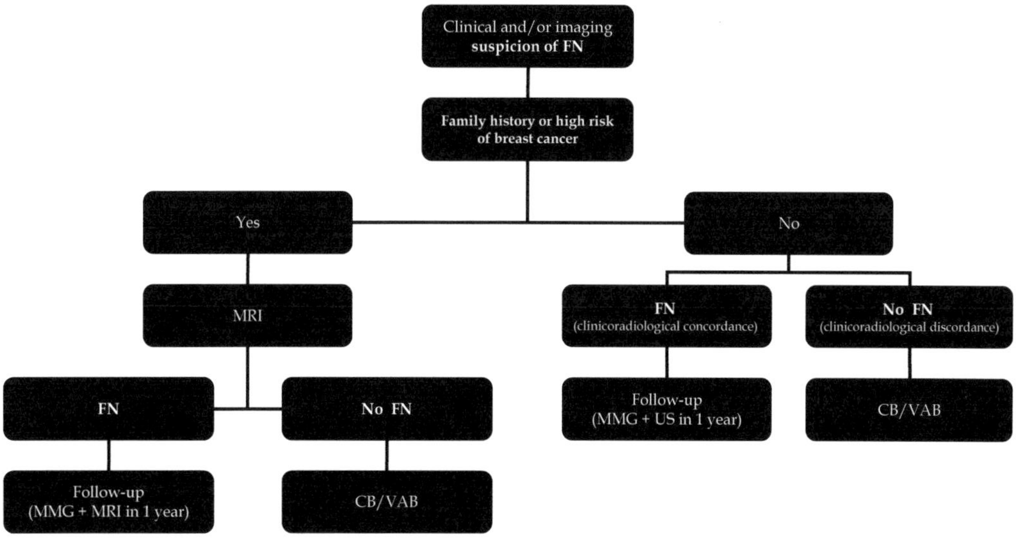

CB = core biopsy; FN = fat necrosis; MMG = mammography; MRI = magnetic resonance imaging; US = ultrasound; VAB = vacuum-assisted biopsy.

Table 1. Diagnostic algorithm for the management of patients with suspected fat necrosis.

6. Conclusions

Knowledge about the pathogenesis of fat necrosis is fundamental for recognizing the many different findings that can be seen on different imaging modalities. A multimodal approach, assessing the findings in the context of the patient's risk profile, can improve the accuracy of the diagnosis of fat necrosis.

7. Acknowledgement

The author thanks the patients, my colleagues in the Department of Women´s Imaging, and John Giba for assistance in manuscript preparation.

8. References

DiPiro, PJ.; Meyer, JE.; Frenna, TH. & Denison, CM. (1995). Seat belt injuries of the breast: findings on mammography and sonography. *American Journal of Roentgenology*, Vol.164, No.2, (February, 1995), pp.317-320, PMID 7839961

Ganau, S.; Tortajada, L.; Escribano, F.; Andreu, X. & Sentís, M. (2009). The great mimicker: Fat necrosis of the breast—Magnetic resonance mammography approach. *Current Problems in Diagnostic Radiology*, Vol.38, No.4, (July/August 2009), pp.189-197, ISSN 036300188

Lanyi M. (1988). Calcifications outside the lobular and ductal system of the breast, In: *Diagnosis and differential diagnosis of breast calcifications*, Springer-Verlag, pp.157-174, ISBN 3-540-16949-0, Berlin Heidelberg.

Lee, BJ.; Adair, F. (1920). Traumatic fat necrosis of the female breast and its differentiation from carcinoma. *Annals of Surgery*, Vol.72, No.2, (August 1920), pp. 188-195, PMID 1410519

Linda, A.; Zuiani, C.; Lorenzon, M.; Furlan, A.; Girometti, R.; Londero, V. & Bazzocchi, M. (2011). Hyperechoic lesions of the breast: Not always benign. *American Journal of Roentgeneology*, Vol.196, No.5, (May, 2011), pp. 1219-1224, PMID 21512095

Taboada, JL.; Stephens, TW.; Krishnamurthy, S.; Brandt, KR. & Whitman, GJ. (2009). The many faces of fat necrosis in the breast. *American Journal of Roentgenology*, Vol.192, No.3, (March 2009), pp. 815-825, PMID 19234281

Tan, PH.; Lai, LM.; Carrington, EV.; Opaluwa, AS.; Ravikumar, KH.; Chetty, N.; Kaplan, V.; Kelley, CJ. & Babu, ED. (2006). Fat necrosis of the breast—A review. *The Breast*, Vol.15, No.3, (June, 2006), pp. 313-218, PMID 16198567

20

A Case of a Secretory Carcinoma of the Breast: Radio-Pathological Correlation

Shinya Tajima[1], Ichiro Maeda[2], Yasuyuki Kurihara[1], Miyuki Fukushima[2], Yoshihide Kanemaki[1], Hiroshi Shimamoto[1], Keiko Kishimoto[1], Tomoko Uejima[3], Koichiro Tsugawa[3] and Yasuo Nakajima[1]

[1]*Department of Radiology,*
[2]*Department of Pathology,*
[3]*Department of Breast Surgery,*
St. Marianna University School of Medicine, Kanagawa,
Japan

1. Introduction

Secretory carcinoma of the breast is a rare variant (the frequency is below 0.15 %) of breast tumor[1, 2]. It was first described by McDivitt and Stewart in 1966, as a juvenile breast carcinoma as it was thought to occur only in childhood[3]. Subsequently, in 1970 Norris et al.[2] and in 1980 Tavassoli et al.[4] advocated "secretory carcinoma" based on histopathological feature. It is now well known to occur in all age groups. As review of available literature, about 100 cases of secretory carcinoma of the breast has been reported at histopathology[5]. However, its gene expression profiling and the imaging appearances of this carcinoma are not well described. We report the gene expression profiling and the imaging characteristics of the secretory carcinoma of the breast.

2. Case report

The patient had no palpable mass or nipple discharge or axillary lymph node swelling but she was pointed out abnormality in her left breast for the screening of mammography and ultrasonography. She visited our hospital for further examination and medical treatment. Mammography showed multiple iso-density masses with unclear and partly spiculated margin on the mid portion of left Mediolateral-oblique view and inner portion of left Cranio-caudal view (Figure1A, 1B). Ultrasonography revealed multiple nodular hypo-echoic masses measured 67 x 14 mm with high Depth/Width ratio, which suggested a malignant nature (Figure 2). Then HR-MRI on a 1.5-T system using a surface breast coil was performed. Diffusion weighted HR-MR image showed multiple mass-like high signal intensities. Contrast enhanced T1 weighted HR-MR image of early phase showed segmental distribution of multiple nodular mass-like enhancements measured by 60 x 40 mm (Figure 3A, 3B). Thus malignancy was suspected. Non-contrast enhanced T1 weighted image of HR-MRI revealed multiple dot-like high signal intensities in the mass (Figure 3C). Therefore this tumor was thought to contain rich protein or hemorrhage. Fat-saturated T2 weighted image of HR-MRI revealed nodular high signal intensities in the mass (Figure 3D).

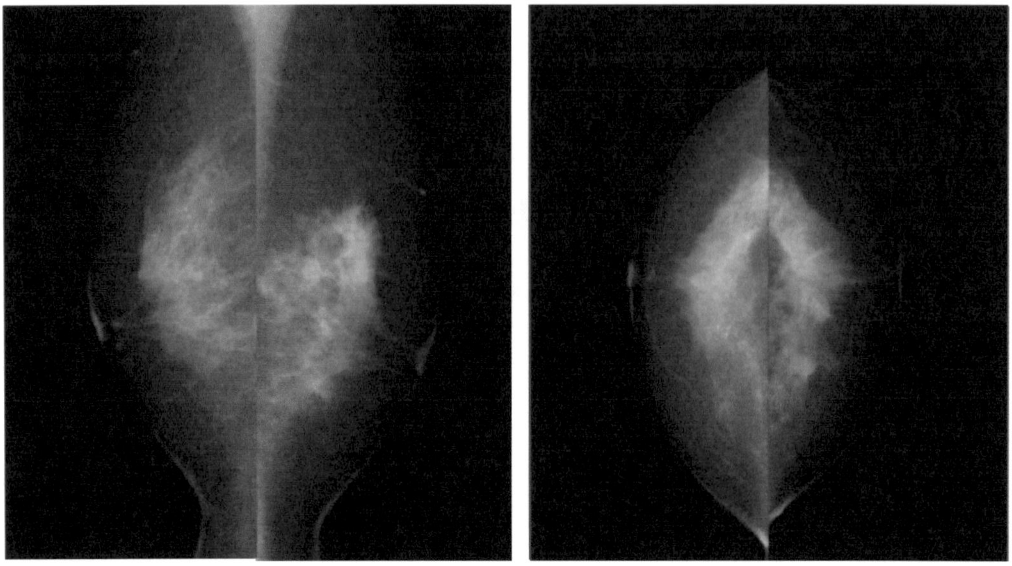

A B

Fig. 1. A. MLO view of mammography, B: CC view of mammography; Multiple iso-density masses with unclear and partly spiculated margin are seen on the mid portion of left MLO view (A) and inner portion of left CCview (B).

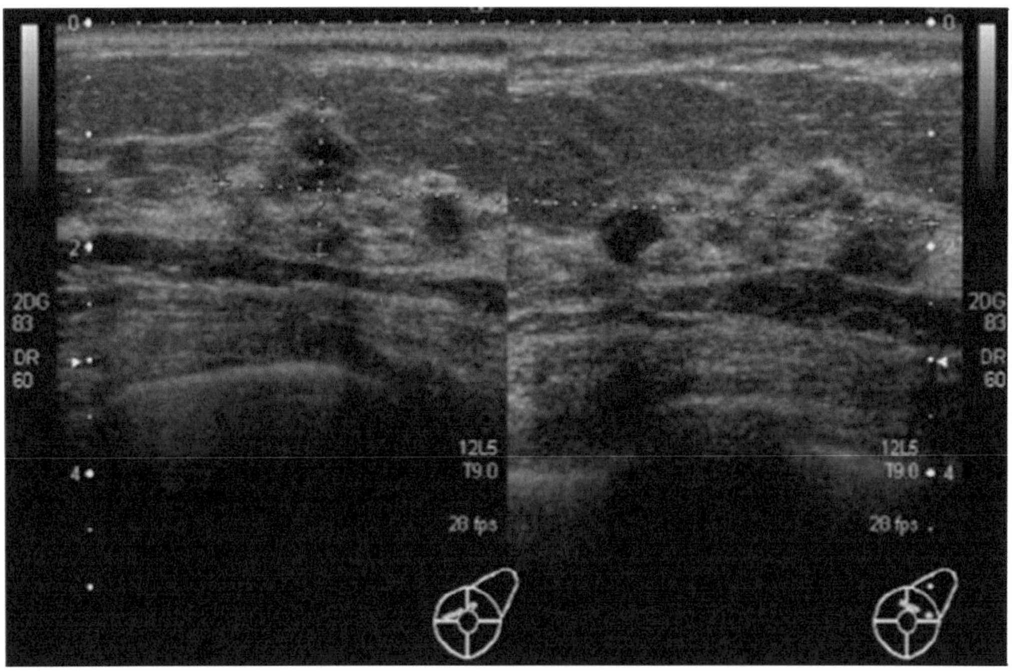

Fig. 2. Ultrasonography of the left breast; Multiple nodular hypo-echoic masses with high Depth/Width ratio are seen and which suggested a malignant nature.

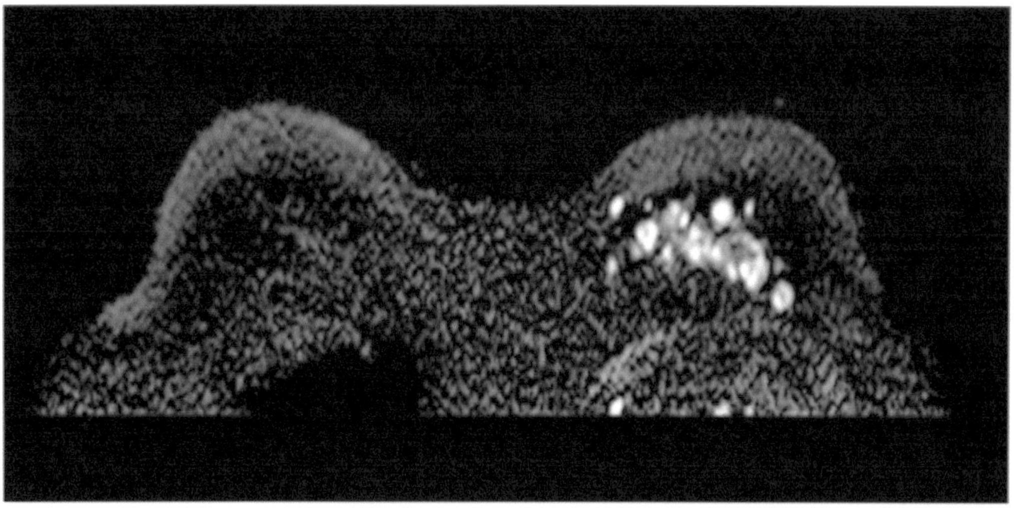

Fig. 3A. Diffusion weighted image of HR-MRI; Multiple mass-like high signal intensities are seen in the left breast.

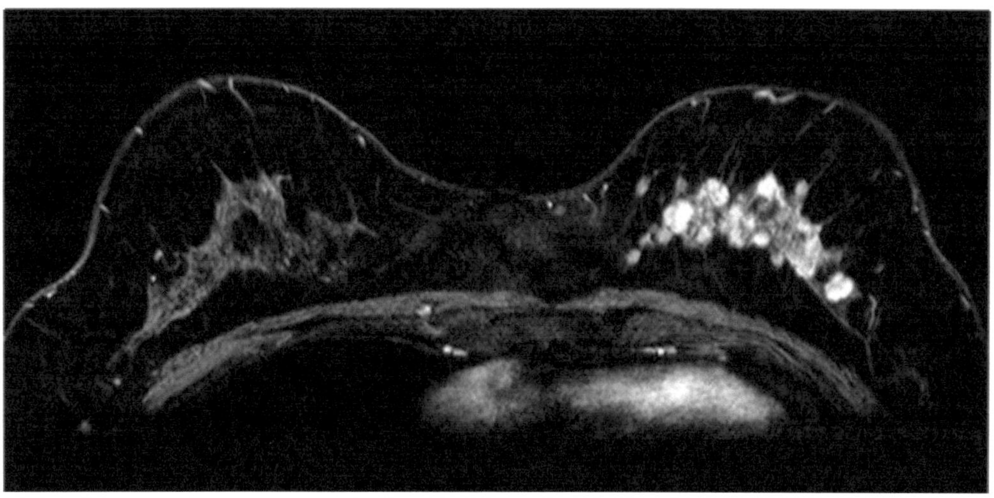

Fig. 3B. Contrast enhanced T1 weighted image on early phase of HR-MRI; Segmental distribution of multiple nodular mass-like enhancements are seen in the left breast. These mass-like enhancements might reflect the nodular growth of the secretory carcinoma.

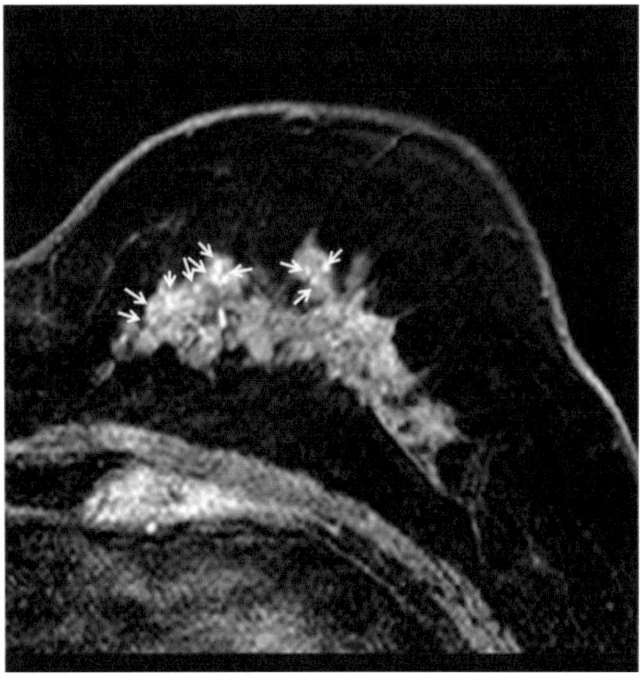

Fig. 3C. Non-contrast enhanced T1 weighted image of HR-MRI; Multiple dot-like high signal intensities are seen on the mass (arrows). These high signal intensities might reflect the secretory material of the secretory carcinoma.

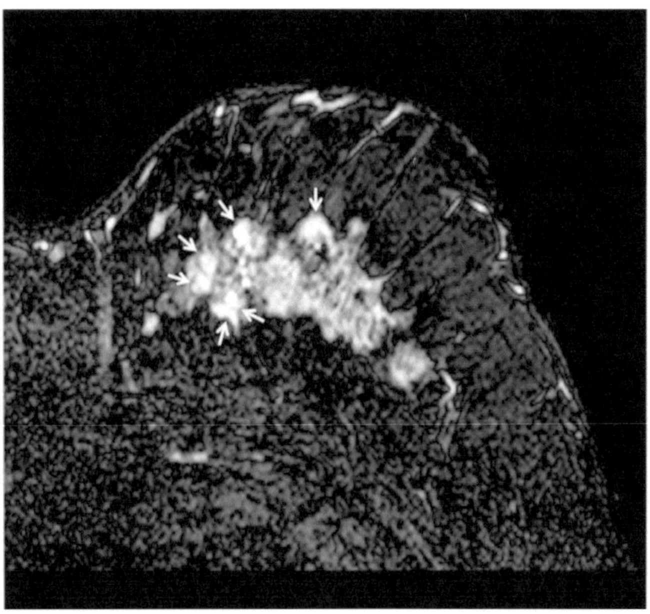

Fig. 3D. Fat-saturated T2 weighted image of HR-MRI; Multiple nodular high signal intensities are seen on the mass (arrows). These high signal intensities might reflect the secretory material of the secretory carcinoma.

Cytology showed typical aggregated forms of tumor cells like bunches of grapes and the cytologic smears revealed grapelike clusters of mucous globular structures (MGSs) and speculated as a secretory carcinoma (Figure 4). Then left mastectomy was performed as a curative operation. Grossly, the tumor measured 6.8 x 4.5 x 2.0 cm and was gray-whitish circumscribed multiple nodular firm mass. And the tumor size was concordant with HR-MR imaging findings. The resected specimen of histopathological feature was microcystic or glandular architecture and composed of cells that produce abundant intracellular and extracellular secretory material, and immunohistochemically the tumor was positive for periodic acid-Schiff (PAS) as well as S-100 protein. The tumor consisted cells of pale-to-clear or eosinophilic cytoplasm, and small, round, low-grade nuclei with inconspicuous nucleoli. The tumor cells showed nodular growth and invasion of the adipose tissue was seen part of the tumor. Hence that was diagnosed a secretory carcinoma (Figure 5A, 5B, 5C, 5D). Secretory carcinoma is associated with a genetic ETV-6-NTRK3 gene fusion leading to a chimeric protein tyrosinase kinase expression, however it was not experimented in the present case.

ER, PgR, and HER2 were all negative and triple negative cancer is suggested in our case. Immunohistochemically, the tumor cells are CK5/6, CK8/18, EGFR, vimentin, and c-kit all positive and our case of secretory carcinoma was considered to have the spectrum of basal-like type in gene expression profiling.

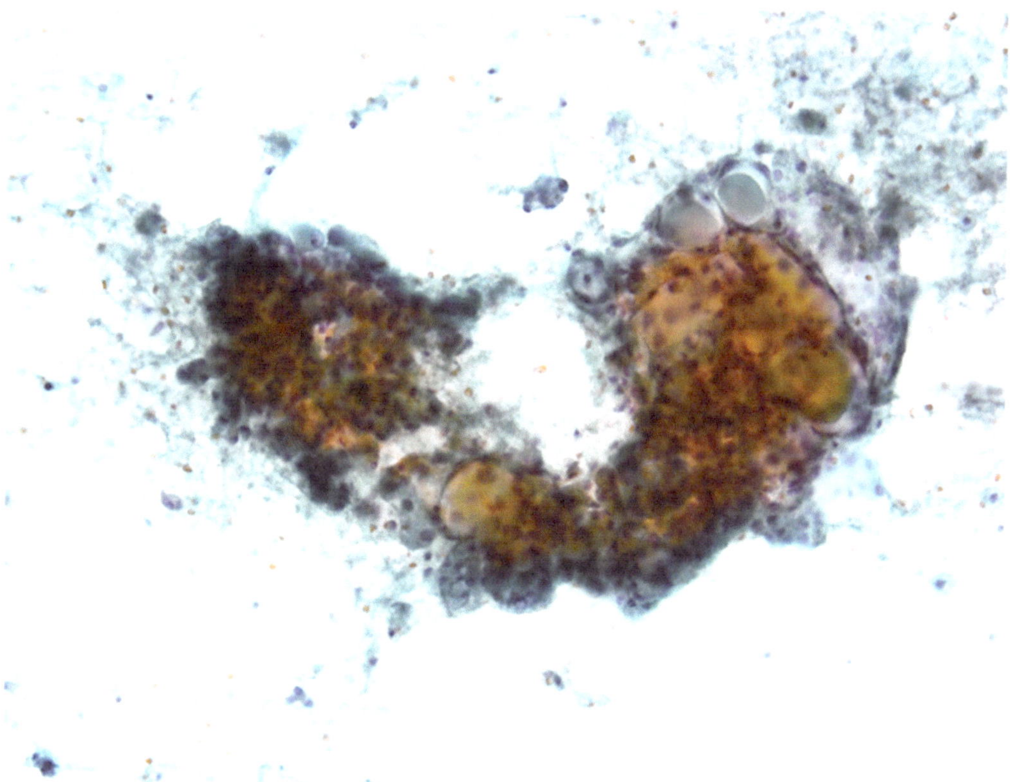

Fig. 4. Cytology of the secretory carcinoma (Papanicolaou stain, x400); Aggregated forms of tumor cells like "bunches of grapes" are seen.

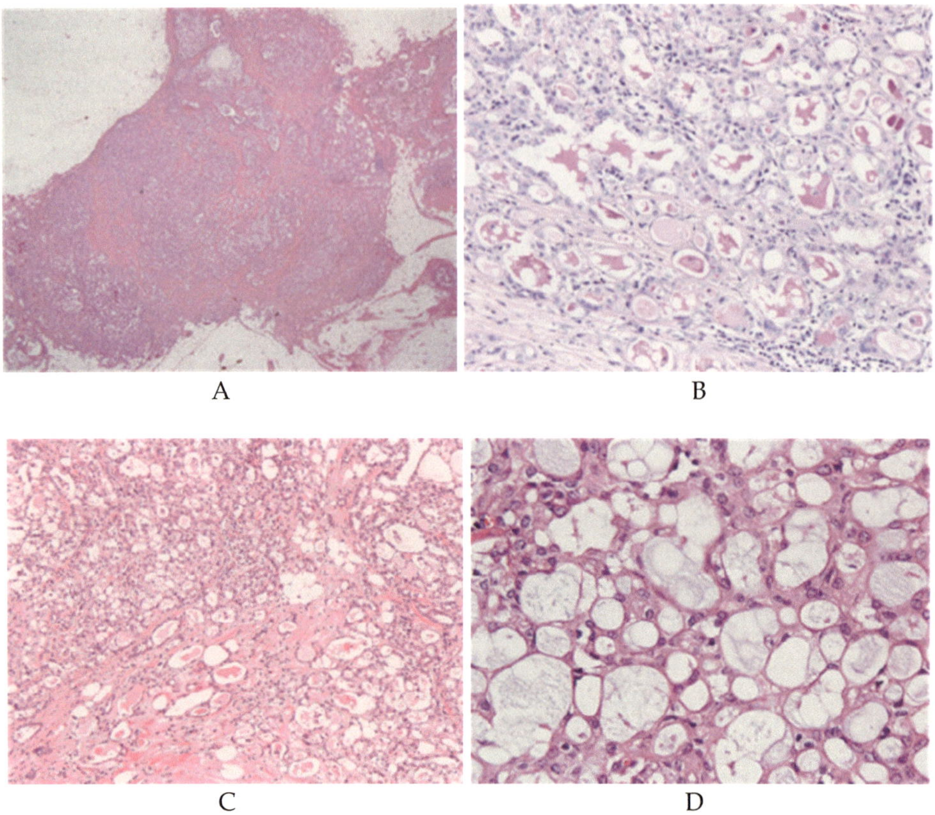

Fig. 5. A: Histology of the secretory carcinoma (Haematoxylin and Eosin stain, x2); Low magnification view of the secretory carcinoma. The secretory carcinoma of the nodular growth is seen. B: Histology of the secretory carcinoma (Periodic acid-Schiff stain, x200); Higher magnification view of the secretory carcinoma. The secretory material of the secretory carcinoma is positive for Periodic acid-Schiff stain. C, D: Histology of the secretory carcinoma (Figure 5C; Haematoxylin and Eosin stain x100, Figure 5D; Haematoxylin and Eosin stain, x400); Higher and high magnification view of the secretory carcinoma. The carcinoma cells arranged microcystic or glandular architecture and abundant intracellular and extracellular secretory material is seen.

3. Discussion

Secretory carcinoma of the breast is a rare but histopathologically distinct variant of invasive ductal carcinoma that thought to be indolent growth pattern and a more favorable prognosis than that of typical ductal carcinoma[6]. The frequency is thought to be below 0.15 % of all breast tumors[1, 2]. In our hospital, the frequency was 0.05 %.

By using DNA microarray techniques, it has been shown that breast cancers can be classified into biologically distinct groups based on their gene expression profiles. These groups comprise luminal A (ER positive and HER2 negative), luminal B (ER and HER2 positive), ERBB2 (ER negative and HER2 positive), and triple negative (ER and HER2 negative) subtypes[7]. Our case was ER, PgR and HER2 negative, hence the triple negative cancer is suggested. The triple negative cancer is a heterogeneous group and is further categorized into the basal-like and the normal breast subtypes, which are positive and negative, respectively, for myoepithelial/basal markers such as basal CKs. The consensus criteria for the basal-like subtype which has been reported is as follows. Nielsen et al. suggested four representative surrogate markers for the basal-like subtype: ER, HER2, EGFR, and CK5/6[8]. Other additional criteria used for the basal-like subtype comprise (1) ER negativity and HER2 negativity, and vimentin, EGFR, CK8/18, and/or CK5/6 positivity, and (2) triple negativity, and CK5/6 and/or EGFR positivity[7]. Other markers that have been included in the myoepithelial/basal biomarkers are laminin[9, 10], c-kit[11], p63[12], nestin[13], osteonectin[14], caveolin 1[15]. In the present case, the tumor cells were CK5/6, CK8/18, EGFR, vimentin, and c-kit all positive and our case of secretory carcinoma was considered to have the spectrum of basal-like type in gene expression profiling. Lae et al reported that secretory carcinomas in woman were ER negative, PgR negative and HER2 negative, so called triple negative[16]. The tumors were also reactive for S100 and E-cadherin and focally for CK8/18 and CK5/6[16]. Our case was compatible with the report of Lae et al.. Secretory carcinoma has been reported as low-grade carcinoma, however our case suggests that not always a secretory carcinoma is low-grade carcinoma. Triple negative cancer is considered to be a clinicopathological entity with aggressive behaviors and poor prognosis. Our case suggests that the secretory carcinoma of the breast should need careful therapeutic follow up.

Here we will discuss about the imaging features of the secretory carcinoma. Mammography of a secretory carcinoma usually reveals a discrete tumor with smooth or irregular borders[17]. Also, our case of mammography showed multiple iso-density masses with unclear and partly spiculated margin and this finding was not specific for the entity of a secretory carcinoma. On ultrasonography, secretory carcinoma of the breast is frequently shown as a small benign-looking nodule or group of nodules with low clinical stage[18]. And secretory carcinoma of ultrasonographic appearance is a solid, well-circumscribed mass and is not specific for this entity and mimics benign entities such as fibroadenoma, as well as other well-differentiated breast carcinomas[19]. Ultrasonography of the present case revealed multiple nodular hypo-echoic masses measured 67 x 14 mm with high Depth/Width ratio, which suggested a malignant nature, however was not specific for a secretory carcinoma. It is not well known that the HR-MR imaging feature of secretory carcinoma of the breast. However, in our case, dot-like high signal intensities within the mass were observed on T1 and high signal intensities on T2 weighted images on HR-MRI and additionally nodular multiple mass-like early enhancements were seen on contrast enhanced HR-MR imaging. Therefore this tumor was thought to contain rich protein or hemorrhage. The rich protein lesions reveal high signal intensity not only T1 weighted image but also T2 weighted image on HR-MR imaging by the concentration of protein[20, 21, 22]. Dot-like high signal intensities on T1 weighted image and nodular high signal intensities on fat-saturated T2 weighted image of HR-MRI might correspond to the groups of intracellular and extracellular secretory milk-like material of the secretory carcinoma (Figure 3C, 3D, 5C, 5D). And mass-like early enhancements on contrast enhanced T1 weighted HR-MR image might correspond to the nodular growth of the secretory carcinoma (Figure 3B, 5A). Moreover, these findings of dot-like high signal intensities on T1 weighted image with the distribution of scattered within the mass and high signal intensities on T2 weighted image of HR-MRI besides mass-like early enhancement on contrast enhanced T1 weighted HR-MR images are thought to be one of the imaging features of secretory carcinoma of the breast. Differential diagnoses of the secretory carcinoma on imaging characteristics including HR-MRI might theoretically be mucinous carcinoma of pure and mixed forms, sarcomas (angiosarcoma, myxofibrosarcoma and so on), and matrix-producing carcinoma as concerning about mucinous or rich protein lesion, and invasive ductal carcinoma with hemorrhage and angiosarcoma as concerning about hemorrhage on HR-MR images. Mucinous carcinoma of pure and mixed forms might typically reveal lobulated shape and very high signal intensity on T2 weighted images, and a pattern of gradual enhancement or heterogenous enhancement on dynamic HR-MR images[23]. And the most common appearance of mucinous carcinoma is a hypo-echoic lesion with heterogenous internal echo on ultrasonography[24]. Matrix-producing carcinoma might typically reveal hypo- or high-echoic zone in the tumor on ultrasonography and ring-shaped enhancement on contrast enhanced HR-MRI with high signal intensity in the central area of the tumor on T2 weighted imaging[25]. Angiosarcoma might typically reveal both a high- and hypo-echoic lesion without acoustic shadow on ultrasonography[26], and HR-MRI of angiosarcoma might reveal low intensity tumor on T1 weighted images, markedly high intensity on T2 weighted images and prolongation of enhancement on the dynamic study and the presence of multiple regions without enhancement in the tumor[27]. Sarcomas might contain mucinous lesion, however the distribution of mucin might not be typically dot-like and scattered in the mass on T1 weighted image of HR-MRI. Invasive ductal carcinoma with hemorrhage and angiosarcoma might have hemorrhagic lesion and sometimes reveal high signal intensity on T1 weighted image of HR-MRI, however their distribution might rarely be scattered in the mass on T1 weighted image of HR-MRI.

In conclusion, these findings of dot-like high signal intensities on T1 weighted image with their distribution of scattered within the mass and high signal intensities on T2 weighted image of HR-MRI besides mass-like early enhancement on the dynamic HR-MR image are thought to be one of the imaging features of secretory carcinoma of the breast. And our findings of HR-MR images might be helpful to diagnose the secretory carcinoma of the breast on HR-MR imaging.

4. References

[1] Tokunaga M, Wakimoto J, Muramoto Y, et al: Juvenile secretory carcinoma and juvenile papillomatosis. Jpn J Clin Oncol 1985;15:457-465

[2] Norris HJ, Taylor HB.: Carcinoma of the breast in woman less than thirty years old. Cancer 1970;26:963-969

[3] Mcdivitt RW, Stewart FW.: Breast carcinoma in children. JAMA 1966;195:388-390

[4] Tavassoli FA, Norris HJ.: Secretory carcinoma of the breast. Cancer 1980;45:2404-2413

[5] Madhusmita J, Shameem S.: Cytodiagnosis of secretory carcinoma of the breast: A report on two cases. Diagn Cytopathol 2009;38(12):921-924

[6] Paeng MH, Choi HY, Sung SH, et al.: Secretory carcinoma of the breast. J Clin Ultrasound 2003 Oct;31(8):425-429

[7] Yuka S, Hitoshi T.: Clinicopathological characteristics of triple-negative breast cancers. Breast Cancer 2009;16:254-259

[8] Nielsen TO, Hsu FD, Jensen K, et al.: Immunohistochemical and clinical characterization of the basal-like subtype of invasive breast carcinoma. Clin Cancer Res 2004;10:5367-5374

[9] Livasy CA, Karaca G, Nanda R, et al.: Phenotypic evaluation of the basal-like subtype of invasive breast carcinoma. Mod Pathol 2006;19:264-271

[10] Rodriguez-Pinilla SM, Sarrio D, Honrado E, et al.: Vimentin and laminin expression is associated with basal-like phenotype in both sporadic and BRCA1-associated breast carcinomas. J Clin Pathol 2007;60:1006-1012

[11] Kim MJ, Ro JY, Ahn SH, et al.: Clinicopathologic significance of the basal-like subtype of breast cancer: a comparison with hormone receptor and HER-2/neu-overexpressing phenotypes. Hum Pathol 2006;37:1217-1226

[12] Laakso M, Loman N, Borg A, et al.: Cytokeratin 5/14-positive breast cancer: true basal phenotype confined to BRCA1 tumors. Mod Pathol 2005;18:1321-1328

[13] Li H, Cherukuri P, Li N, et al.: Nestin is expressed in the basal/myoepithelial layer of the mammary gland and is a selective marker of basal epithelial breast tumors. Cancer Res 2007;67:501-510

[14] Lakhani SR, Reis-Filho JS, Fulford L, et al.: Prediction of BRCA1 status in patients with breast cancer using estrogen receptor and basal phenotype. Clin Cancer Res 2006;11:5175-5180

[15] Savage K, Lambros MB, Robertson D, et al.: Caveolin 1 is overexpressed and amplified in a subset of basal-like and metaplastic breast carcinomas: a morphologic, ultrastructural, immunohistochemical, and in situ hybridization analysis. Clin Cancer Res 2007;13:90-101

[16] Marick L, Paul F, Xavier S-G, et al.: Secretory breast carcinomas with ETV6-NTRK3 fusion gene belong to the basal-like carcinoma spectrum. Mod Pathol 2009;22:291-298

[17] Beatty SM, Orel SG, Kim P, et al.: Multicentric secretory carcinoma of the breast in a 35-year-old woman: Mammographic appearance and the use of core biopsy in preoperative management. Breast J 1998;4:200-203

[18] Mun SH, Ko EY, Han BK, et al.: Secretory carcinoma of the breast: sonographic features. J Ultrasound Med 2008 Jun;27(6):947-954

[19] Siegel JR, Karcnik TJ, Hertz MB, et al.: Secretory carcinoma of the breast. Breast J 1999 May;5(3):204-207

[20] Brown JJ, van Sonnenberg E, Gerber KH, et al.: Magnetic resonance relaxation times of percutaneously obtained normal and abnormal body fluids. Radiology 1985;154:727-731

[21] Mitchell DG, Burk DL Jr, Vinitski S, et al.: Review article. The biophysical basis of tissue contrast in extracranial MR imaging. AJR 1987;149:831-838

[22] Mitchell DG, Mintz MC, Spritzer CE, et al.: Adnexal masses: MR imaging observations at 1.5 T, with US and CT correlation. Radiology 1987;162:319-324

[23] Shuichi M, Masaki Y, Toshiko S, et al.: Mucinous carcinoma of the breast: MRI features of pure and mixed forms with histopathologic correlation. AJR 2009;192:W125-W131

[24] Liu H, Tan H, Cheng Y, et al.: Imaging findings in mucinous breast carcinoma and correlating factors. Eur J Radiol 2010 Jul 6.

[25] Yamaguchi R, Tanaka M, Yokoyama T, et al.: Clinicocytopathology of breast cancers with a ring-like appearance on ultrasonography and/or magnetic resonance imaging. Pathol Int 2010 Jan;60(1):22-26

[26] Grant EG, Holt RW, Chun B, et al.: Angiosarcoma of the breast: Sonographic, Xeromammographic, and Pathologic appearance. AJR 1983;141:691-692
[27] Yuichiro K, Yutaka K, Yoshihiko N, et al.: Angiosarcoma of the breast-Specific findings of MRI. Breast Cancer 2006 Oct;13:369-373

21

Radiologic Features of Triple Negative Breast Cancer

Yasuyuki Kojima, Reika In and Hiroko Tsunoda
Division of Breast and Endocrine Surgery, Department of Surgery, St.Marianna University School of Medicine
Department of Radiology, St. Luke's International Hospital
Japan

1. Introduction

Triple negative (TN) breast cancer is defined as cancer with negative expressions of hormone receptors and human epidermal growth factor receptor 2 (HER2). This subtype is characterized as a cancer with a high malignancy potential and a poor prognosis. Endocrine therapy and anti-HER2 therapy are ineffective in the treatment of TN breast cancer as they have less specific targets compared with other subtypes of breast cancer. At present, chemotherapy is the only option to treat this type of cancer. This subtype is found in approximately 15.5% of all breast cancer cases in Japan (Iwase et al., 2010). The percentage of other subtypes are as follows; Luminal A (hormone receptors positive and HER2 negative), 69.0%; Luminal B (hormone receptors positive and HER2 positive), 7.3% and HER2-enriched (hormone receptor negative and HER2 positive), 8.2%. Some reports described a subtype of DCIS that correlates to the progression to invasive carcinoma; comedo type DCIS progresses to invasive carcinoma, both more often and more rapidly than low-grade DCIS (Pinder SE & Ellis IO, 2003; Ketcham AS & Moffat FL, 1990). This may be a reason for the rarity of TN DCIS. The incidence of TN DCIS accounts for less than 5% of DCIS. If this is true, early detection of this particularly aggressive type of breast cancer is vital. (Moriya et al, 2010) There have been reports claiming that TN IDC occurs from ER negative, HER2 positive DCIS lesion and loses its HER2 expression when it progresses to an invasive cancer, which may indicate a precursor process is at work (Bradley BB et al., 2006; Livasy CA et al., 2007; Flora Z et al., 2007). To clarify these hypotheses, comparison between TN IDC and TN DCIS is also essential. There are no other reports that we were able to find that focus specifically on TN DCIS. We cannot predict the outcome of TN DCIS, if it is not diagnosed and treated, because this has not been researched nor documented (Page DL et al., 1995; Page DL et al., 1982; Betsill WLJ et al., 1978). We reviewed another report on a series of cases in which DCIS was not completely excised. The findings from those reports indicate that a more frequent and rapid progression from DCIS to invasive cancer is related to the comedo subtype of DCIS, which is comparable to low-grade DCIS (Pinder SE & Ellis IO, 2003; Simpson JF, 2009). We need to investigate the specific features of this subtype, and we need to determine the radiological and pathological features of TN breast cancer via retrospective evaluation in a large population, in order to make a more precise diagnosis.

2. Patients and methods

TN breast cancer cases were studied by conducting chart reviews between January 2007 and January 2011 to assess mammogram (MMG), ultrasound (US), magnetic resonance imaging (MRI), methods of detection, and pathology findings. Routine diagnostic breast mammography, ultrasound, and MRI were performed before surgeries in our hospital.

2.1 Mammography

For each patient, mammograms with mediolateral oblique and craniocaudal view were carried out. In all cases, mammograms were retrospectively reviewed by two breast radiologists, and classified as focal asymmetric density (FAD), masses, calcifications, or architectural distortion, according to the Japanese mammography guidelines (The Committee of Mammography Guideline, 2010). Margins of masses were reviewed for being circumscribed, microlobulated, indistinct, and speculated. Mammography was performed by using Senographe 800T and Senographe DMR units from GE (films, MIN-R EV; screen, EV150) till August 2008. In August 2008, digital mammography with the Selenia from Hitachi was introduced.

2.2 Ultrasound

Each patient underwent whole-breast US which was performed and diagnosed by one of two radiologists, specialized in breast imaging. The ultrasound findings were classified as masses, low echoic area, distortions, and calcifications. Noted features included shapes (oval, lobulated, polygonal, or irregular), patterns of the internal echoes (hypoechoic, isoechoic, or hyperechoic), the posterior echoes (accentuating, no change, or attenuating), vascularity (avascular, spotty signals, hypovascular, hypervascular) and elasticity scores (1–5; scores defined as previously reported (Itoh A et al., 2006)).

For patients, ultrasound was performed by using 10 MHz linear-array transducers (LOGIQ 7 system, GE) and 12 MHz linear-array transducers (HDI 5000, Philips) until September 2007, and from October 2007, 12 MHz linear-array transducers (SSA 790A, Toshiba Medical Systems) and 14 MHz linear-array transducers (EUB 7500, Hitachi Medical) were used. All elasticity images were obtained by using EUB 7500.

2.3 Magnetic resonance imaging

The equipment used for MRI was a Signa Excite HD ver. 12 (1.5 Tesla) from GE with 4- or 8-channel breast coil. The protocol was as follows: fat-suppressed T1WI, sagittal (pre-and post-enhancement) fast SPGR: TR/TE 6.5/1.5, FA 15°, FOV 16 cm, matrix 256 9 192, slice thickness 2 mm, scan time 2 min 10 s; fat-suppressed T2WI, sagittal FSE: TR/TE; 3,000/85, FOV 16 cm, matrix 256 9 224, slice thickness 5 mm, gap 1 mm, scan time 2 min 24 s; and delayed axial scan with VIBRANT: TR/TE 6.4/3.0, FOV 34 cm, matrix 350 9 350, slice thickness 1.2 mm, ASSET 2.0, scan time 2 min 40 s.

2.4 Pathological findings

All resected specimens were diagnosed by whole sectioning. Hematoxilin–eosin staining was performed in formalin-fixed, paraffin-embedded material for pathological diagnosis.

Immunohistochemistry of estrogen receptor (ER), progesterone receptor (PgR), and HER2 were evaluated. The assessments of ER and PgR were done using Allred score, and the HER2 status was graded as 0, 1+, 2+, and 3+. HER2 score 3+ was defined as positive, and 2+ was checked by fluorescence in situ hybridization for its positivity. Five cases were eliminated, because the postoperative hormonal status turned out to be positive. In this cohort, 61 patients underwent neoadjuvant chemotherapy.

3. Results

Our cohort included 2,868 operations performed for primary breast cancer diagnosed in our institute between January 2007 and January 2011. Table 1 shows the characteristics of all triple-negative cases. Women with triple-negative invasive breast cancer were likely to have histologically higher-grade tumors compared to ductal carcinoma in situ.

Age	56.3 (26-91)
Ductal carcinoma in situ	n=20
Size (cm)	2.9 (0.5-6.6)
Nuclear grade	
1	14
2	3
3	3
Invasive cancer	n=101
Size (cm)	2.6 (0.7-6.0)
Nuclear grade	
1	21
2	26
3	54

Table 1. Characteristics of TN breast cancer patients (n=121).

3.1 DCIS

Our cohort included 657 DCIS patients, who were diagnosed and treated in our institute between January 2007 and January 2011. Among all 657 DCIS cases, 20 cases (3.0%) were ER-negative, PgR-negative, and HER2-negative. Ages in this group ranged from 40 to 73 years old, with an average age of 55.8. In 12 cases, patients underwent partial resection, and in 8 cases, patients underwent total mastectomy. DCIS was confirmed in all patients by whole sectioning of the resected specimens.

The radiology and pathology findings are shown in Table 2. Mammographic findings of TN DCIS were as follows: there were no abnormal findings in six cases, masses were revealed in two cases, FAD was detected in three cases, and architectural distortion was noted in five cases. However, calcifications, which have been considered as typical radiologcal findings in DCIS, were observed in only four cases (20.0%) out of our TN DCIS (Tables 2, 3). US findings were as follows: low echoic masses were noted in 7 cases, low echoic areas were noted in 14 cases, architectural distortion was noted in four cases. MRI findings revealed typical DCIS findings, including 7 masses and 12 non-mass-like enhancements (one patient did not undergo MRI). The average lesion size measured 2.9 cm in diameter (with a range of

0.5–8.5 cm). Fourteen cases were classified as nuclear grade (NG) 1, three cases were classified as NG2, and three cases were classified as NG3. Histological findings confirmed non-comedo type in 9 cases; mixed types, including some comedo components, were found in 8 cases; comedo type in 3 cases. In seven cases, apocrine metaplasia was observed, and in seven cases we noted a remarkable sclerosing adenosis in the background breast tissue areas of DCIS.

case	MMG	US	MRI	NG	Type of DCIS
1	mass	low echoic mass	Non-mass like, segmental clumped enhancement	1	mixed
2	distortion	low echoic area, distortion	Non-mass like, ductal enhancement	1	non-comedo, SA
3	distortion	low echoic mass	Non-mass like, segmental homogenous enhancement	1	non-comedo, SA
4	no findings	low echoic mass	Mass	1	non-comedo, apocrine metaplasia
5	no findings	low echoic area	Mass	1	mixed
6	no findings	low echoic area	Non-mass like, segmental homogenous enhancement	3	mixed
7	mass	low echoic mass	Not performed	1	comedo
8	no findings	low echoic area	Non-mass like, segmental clumped enhancement	2	mixed, apocrine metaplasia
9	FAD	low echoic area, distortion	Non-mass like, segmental clumped enhancement	1	non-comedo, SA
10	calcifications	low echoic area	Mass, foci	3	mixed
11	distortion	low echoic mass	Non-mass like, segmental heterogenous enhancement	1	non-comedo, SA, apocrine metaplasia
12	distortion	low echoic area, distortion	Mass	1	non-comedo, SA, apocrine metaplasia
13	calcifications	low echoic area	Non-mass like, segmental heterogenous enhancement	2	mixed
14	FAD	low echoic area	Non-mass like, segmental heterogenous enhancement	1	mixed
15	FAD	low echoic mass	Mass	2	mixed
16	no findings	low echoic area	Non-mass like, segmental heterogenous enhancement	1	non-comedo, apocrine metaplasia
17	calcifications	low echoic area	Non-mass like, segmental clumped enhancement	3	comedo
18	calcifications	low echoic area	Mass	1	comedo
19	no findings	low echoic area	Non-mass like, segmental heterogenous enhancement	1	non-comedo, SA, apocrine metaplasia
20	distortion	low echoic mass	Mass	1	comedo, SA, apocrine metaplasia

Table 2. Radiology and pathology findings of TN DCIS cases.

Findings	Number (%)
Calcifications	4 (20)
Mass	2 (10)
Focal asymmetric density	3 (15)
Architectural destortion	5 (25)
No abnormal findings	6 (30)

Table 3. Mammogram findings of triple negative ductal carcinoma in situ.

Representative cases are shown in Figs. 1 and 2. In the first case, the MMG revealed an architectural distortion in the right breast. Spot view revealed no abnormal calcifications. US revealed an irregularly shaped low echoic area with architectural distortion. The MRI revealed a non-mass like, segmental heterogenous enhancement. The pathological findings confirmed non-comedo DCIS, with sclerosing adenosis and apocrine metaplasia.

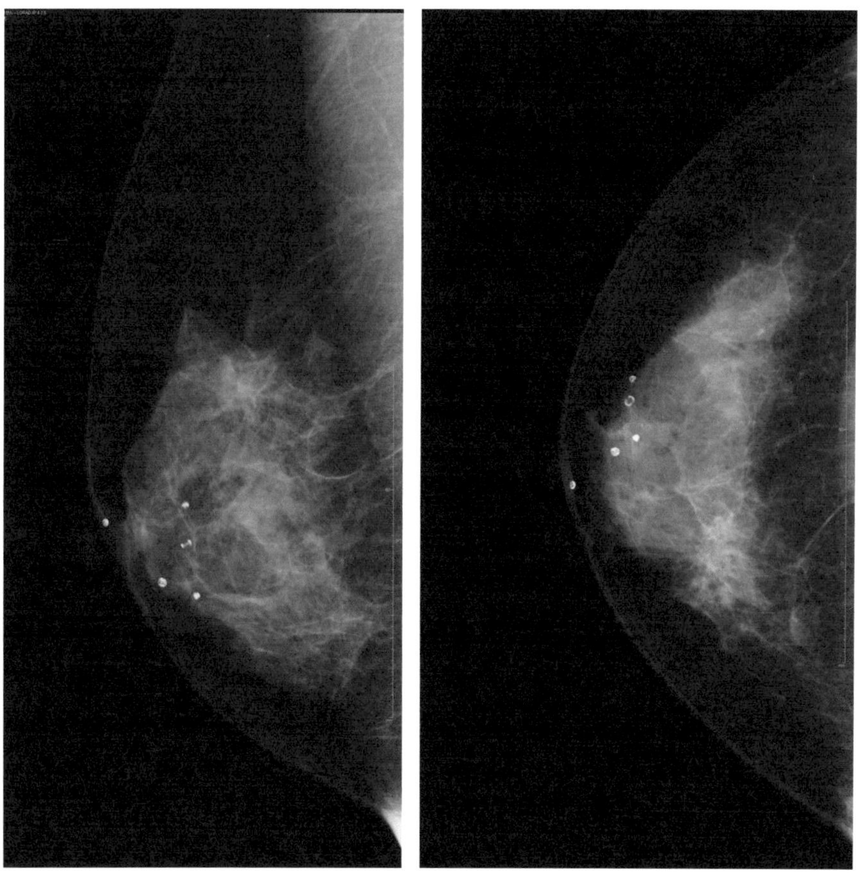

Fig. 1.1. A first representative case of DCIS, mammography of the right breast.

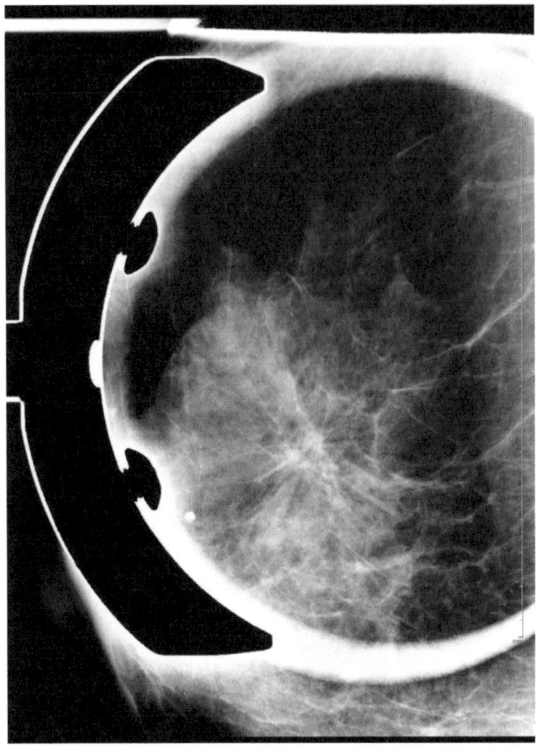

Fig. 1.2. A first representative case of DCIS, mammography with spot view.

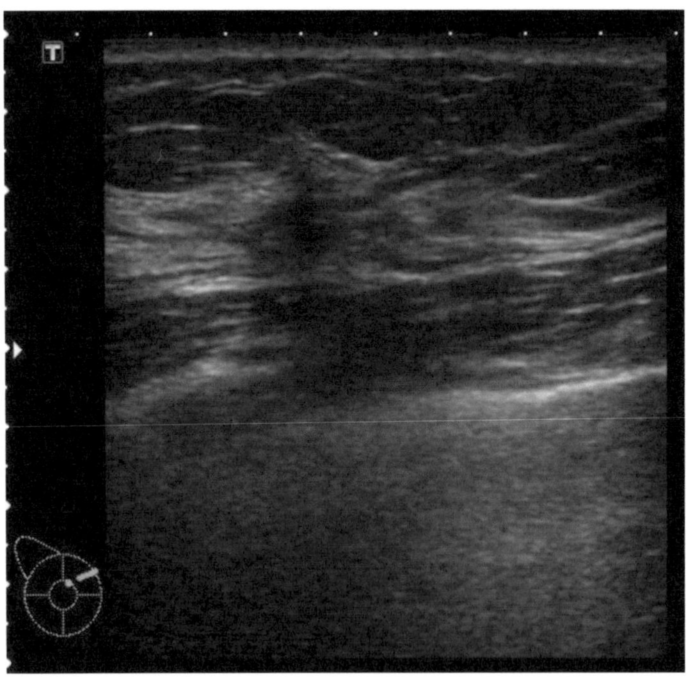

Fig. 1.3. A first representative case of DCIS, Ultrasound.

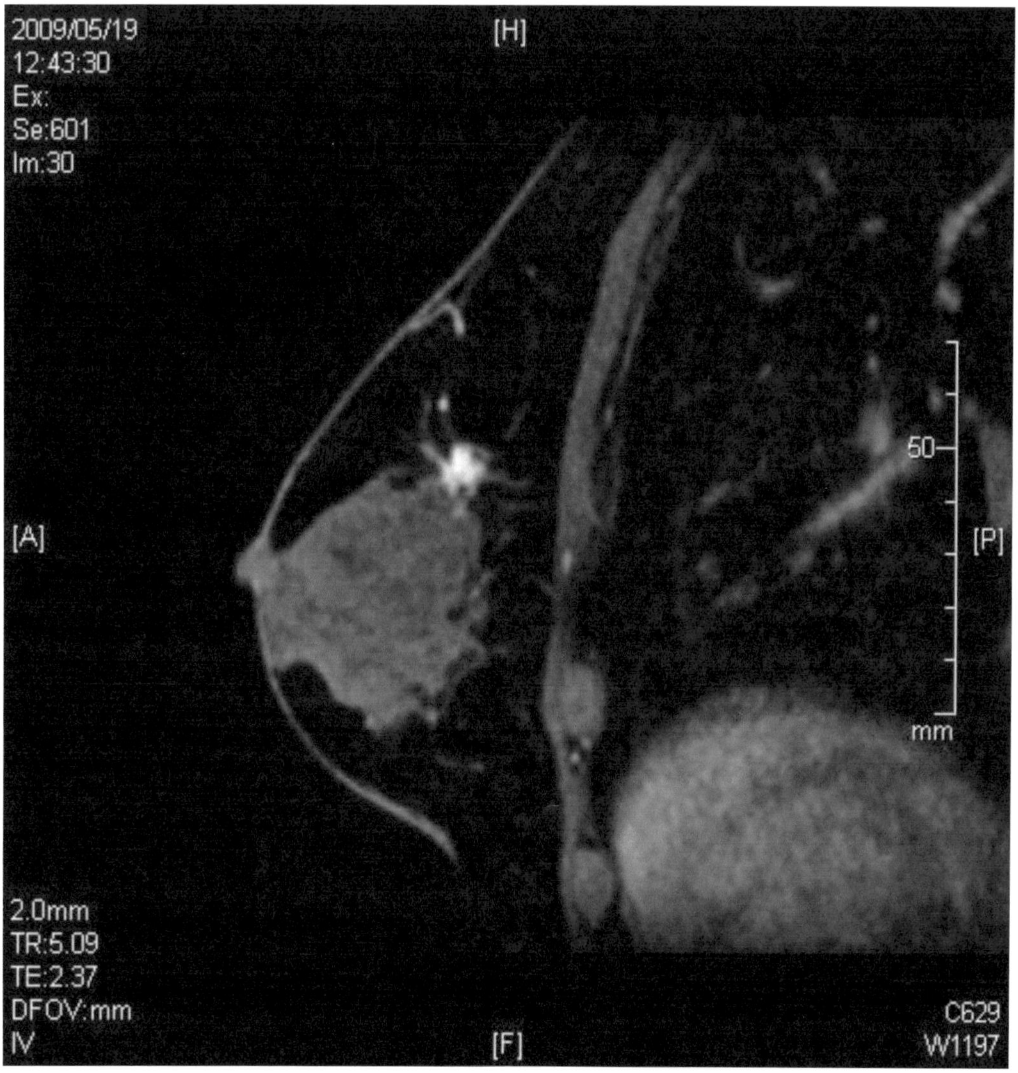

Fig. 1.4. A first representative caseof DCIS, MRI.

In the second case, MMG revealed a focal asymmetric density with architectural distortion in the right breast. US revealed an irregularly shaped low echoic mass. The MRI revealed a segmental enhancement with an architectural distortion. Pathological diagnosis confirmed DCIS with sclerosing adenosis.

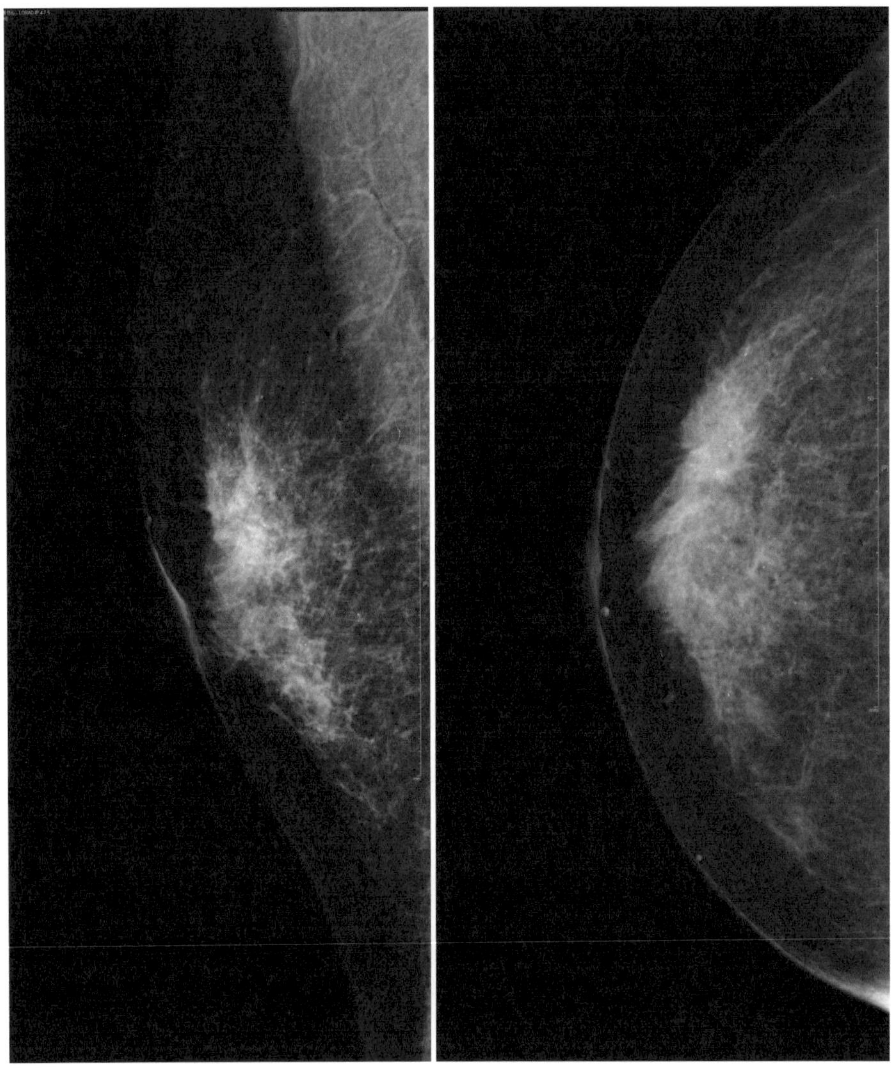

Fig. 2.1. A second representative case of DCIS, mammography of the right breast.

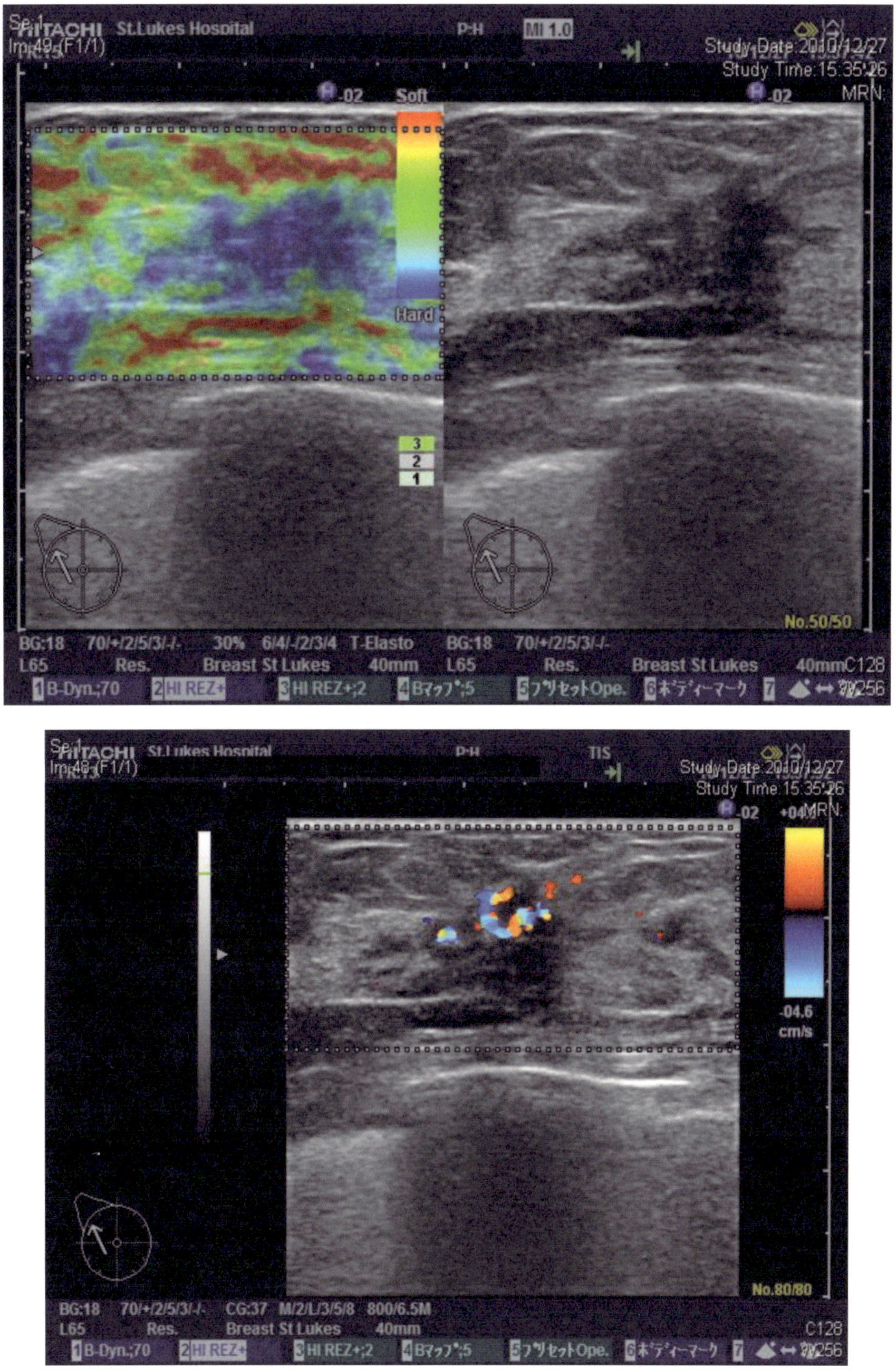

Fig. 2.2. A second representative case of DCIS, Ultrasound; elastography (above) and collar Doppler view (below).

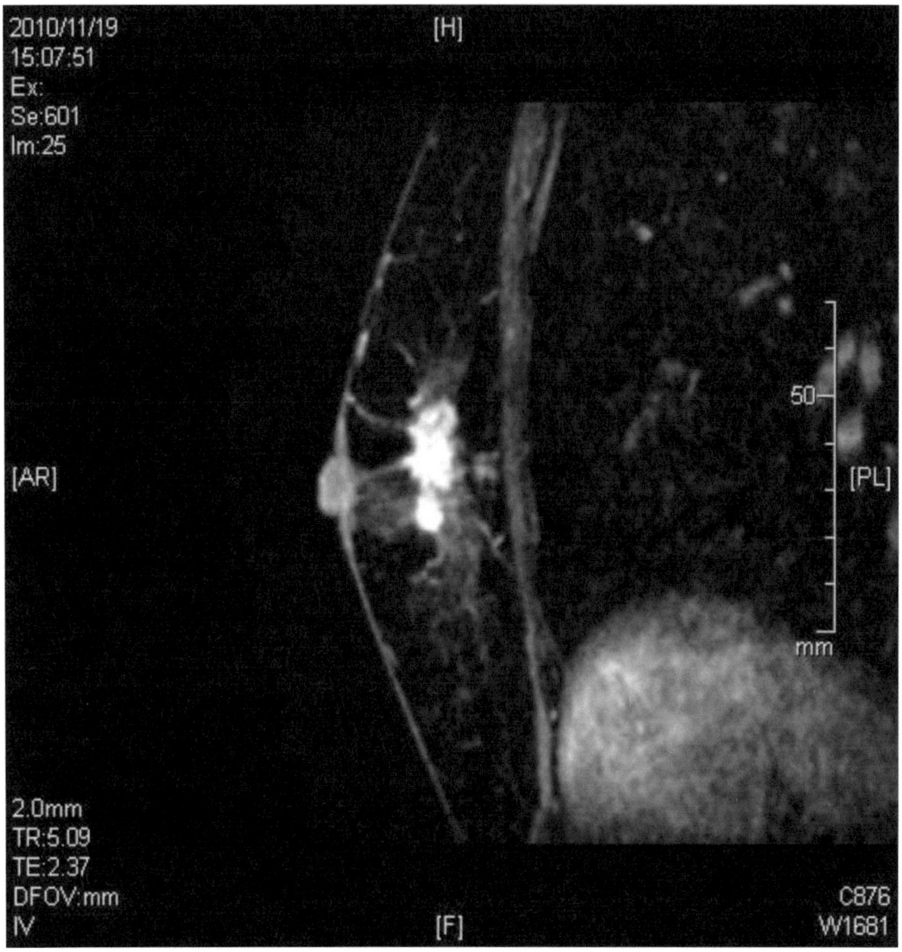

Fig. 2.3. A second representative case of DCIS, MRI.

3.2 IDC

Table 4 shows the radiological findings of TN invasive cancer in our study. On mammography, in almost all patients scattered fibrograndular (44/100, 44%) to heterogeneous (46/100, 46%) breast density was noted. Triple-negative breast cancers frequently presented with a mass (63/100, 63%) and were less associated with focal asymmetric density (13/100, 13%), calcifications (10/100, 10%), and distortion (5/100, 5%). Margins of masses were assessed. Masses with microlobulated margins were the most frequent (26/63, 41.3%), indistinct margins (19/63, 30.2%) and circumscribed margins (12/63, 19.0%) were commonly observed, but spiculated margins were rare (6/63, 9.5%).

On ultrasound, cancers were less frequently observed as non-mass lesions (7/97, 7.2%), and were more likely to present as a mass (90/97, 92.8%); these were lobulated (42/90, 46.7%), irregular (17/90, 18.9%), or oval (24/90, 26.7%) in shape, and less likely to show attenuating posterior echoes (8/97, 8.2%). Of the 42 cases obtained via elasticity imaging, 35 (83.3%) lesions were scored as 4 or 5.

Mammography	n=100	Ultrasound	n=97
Density		Findings	
Predominant fatty	6	Mass	90
Scattered fibrograndular	44	Non-mass like	7
Heterogeneously dense	46	Architectural distortion	0
Dense	4	Calcifications	0
Findings		Shape of mass	n=90
No abnormal findings	10	Oval	24
Focal asymmetric density	13	Lobulated	42
Mass	63	Irregular shape	17
Calcifications	10	Indistinct	7
Architectural distortion	5		
		Posterior echoes	
Border of mass	n=63	Accentuating	43
Circumscribed	12	No change	46
Microlobulated	26	Attenuating	8
Indistinct	19		
Spiculated	6	Vascularity	
		Avascular	7
		Spotty signals	32
		Hypovascular	38
		Hypervascular	14
		Elasticity score	n=42
		1~3	7
		4, 5	35

Table 4. Mammography and ultrasound findings for triple negative breast cancer patients

Representative cases are shown in Figs. 3 and 4. On the mammogram of the first case, there were scattered fibroglandular elements in both breasts. There was a 2.3 cm oval high density mass with circumscribed margin in the left breast in the posterior depth of the superior region seen on the mediolateral oblique view which likely represents expansively growing tumor. On the ultrasound, there was an oval mass with circumscribed margin in the inner upper quadrant of the left breast. The tumor size was approximately 2.0 cm, slight spotty vasculature was seen at the edge of the tumor, and poor elasticity via elastography (elasticity score 4). MRI also showed an oval enhanced mass with circumscribed margin. The pathological findings confirmed invasive ductal carcinoma, nuclear grade 3, with fat invasion and lymphovascular invasion.

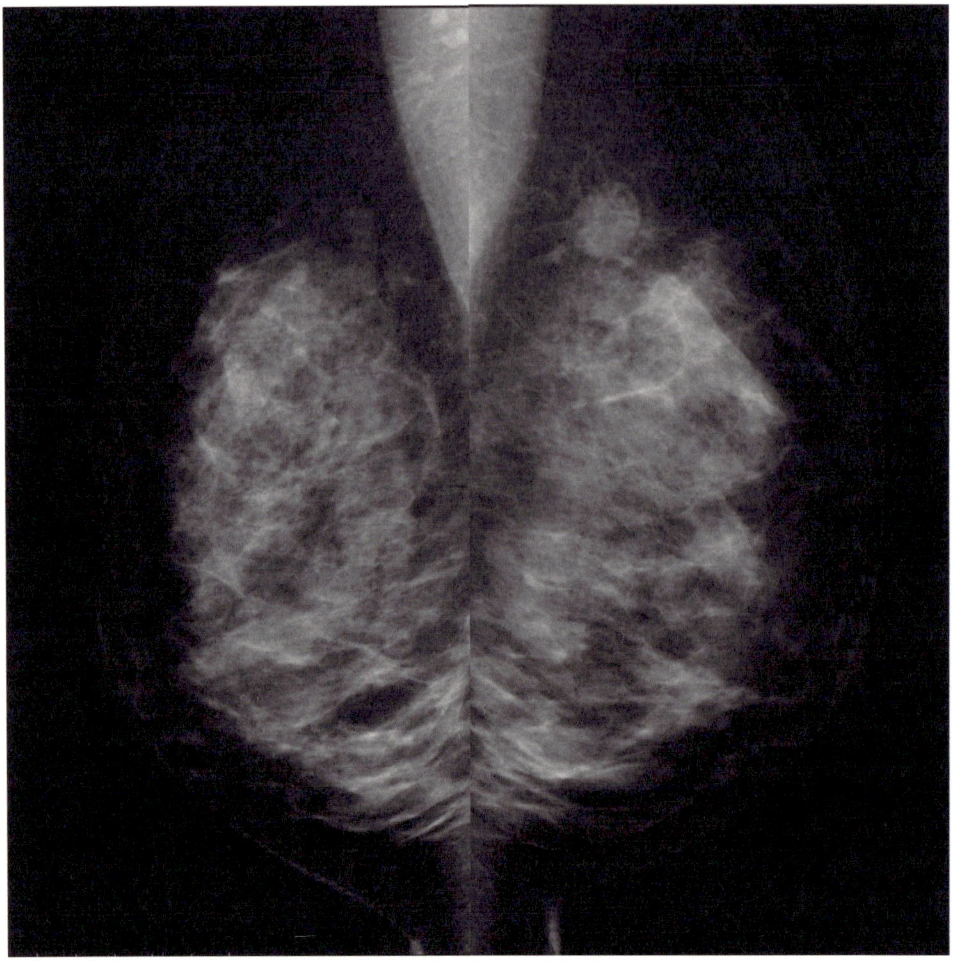

Fig. 3.1. A first representative case of IDC, mammography.

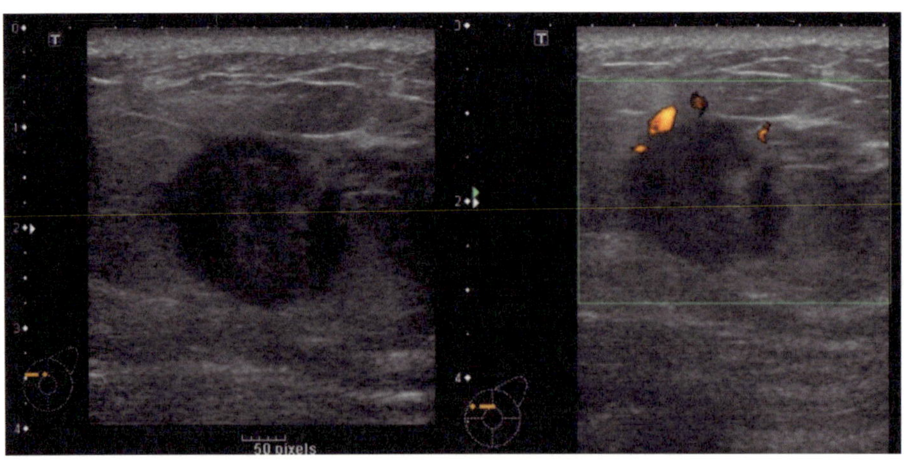

Fig. 3.2. A first representative case of IDC, Ultrasound; B-mode and power Doppler.

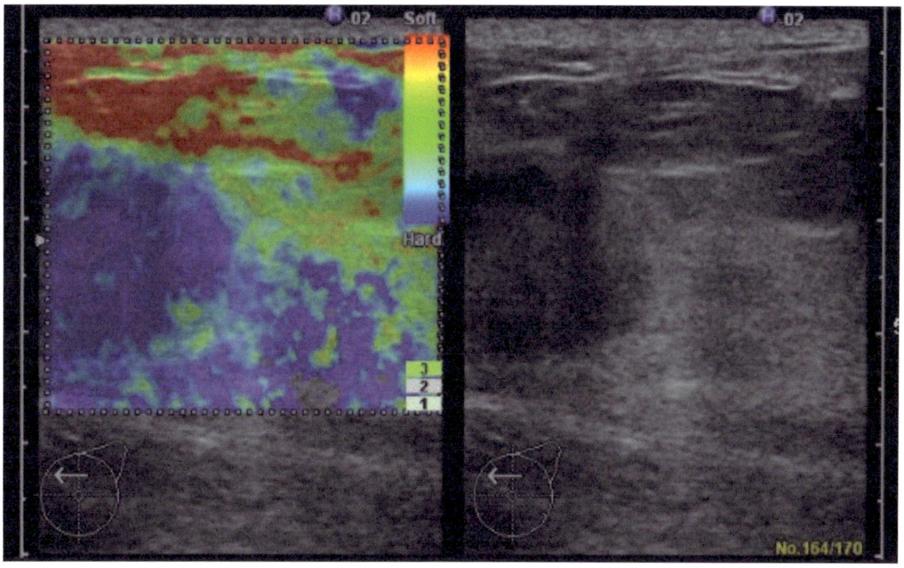

Fig. 3.3. A first representative case of IDC, Ultrasound; elastography.

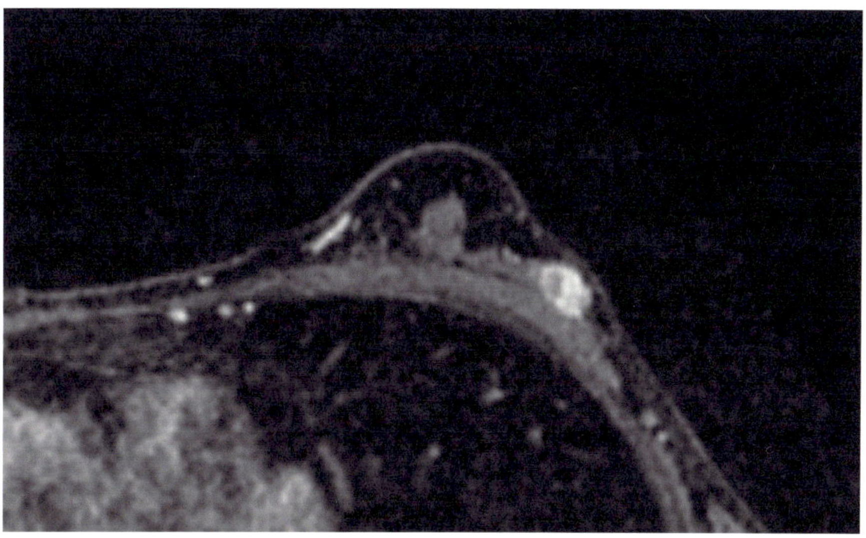

Fig. 3.4. A first representative case of IDC, MRI.

On the second case, mammogram revealed scattered fibroglandular elements in both breasts. There was an oval high density mass with microlobulated margins in the posterior depth of the superior region seen on the mediolateral oblique view of the right breast. The tumor sizes was 1.8 cm in diameter. On the ultrasound, there was a lobulated mass with circumscribed margin in the outer upper quadrant of the right breast. The mass showed mosaic pattern vasculature indicating hypervascularity of the tumor, and poor elasticity via elastography (elasticity score 4). MRI showed a circumscribed enhanced mass in the upper portion of the right breast. Pathological findings revealed invasive ductal cancer, nuclear grade 2.

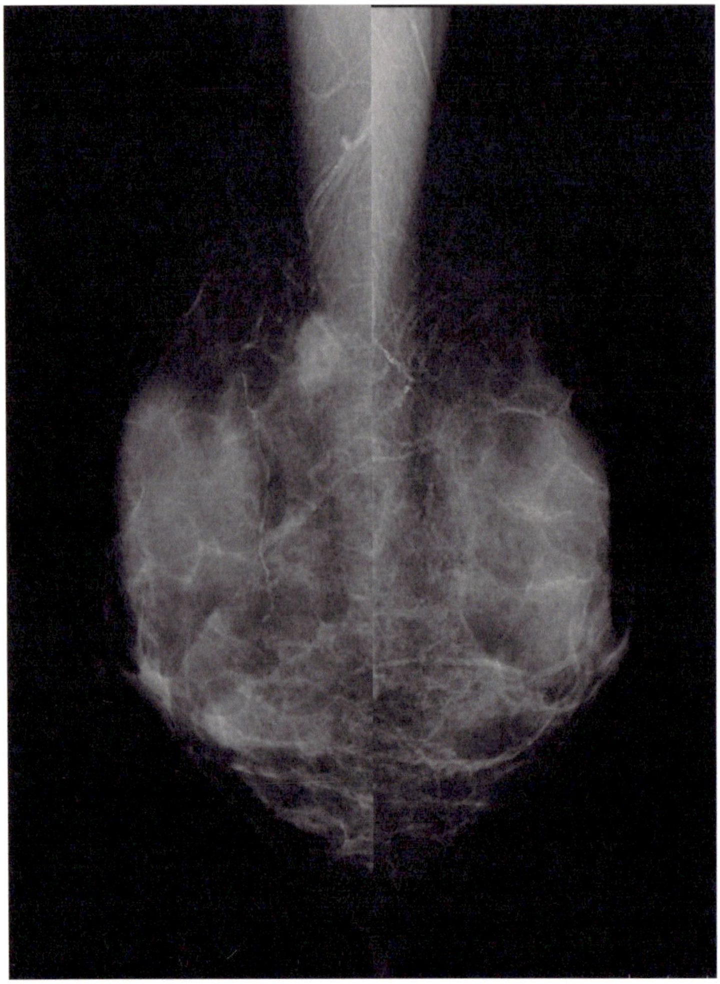

Fig. 4.1. A second representative case of IDC, mammography.

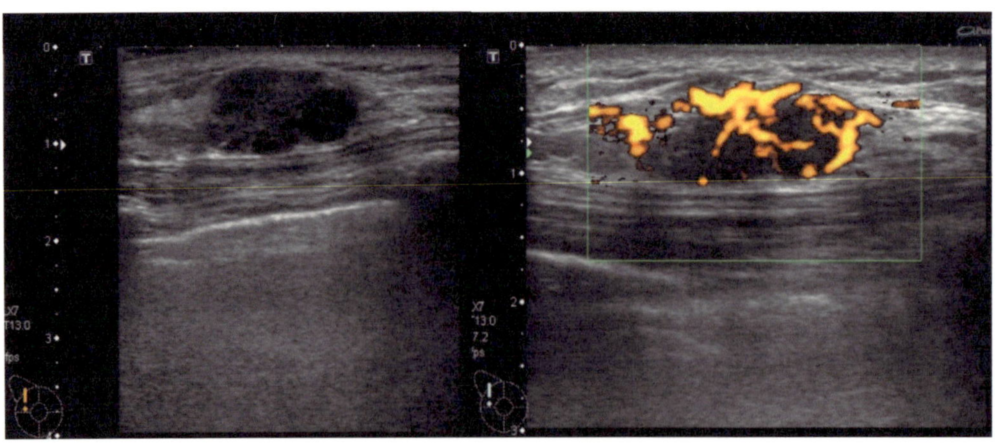

Fig. 4.2. A second representative case of IDC, Ultrasound; B-mode and power Doppler view.

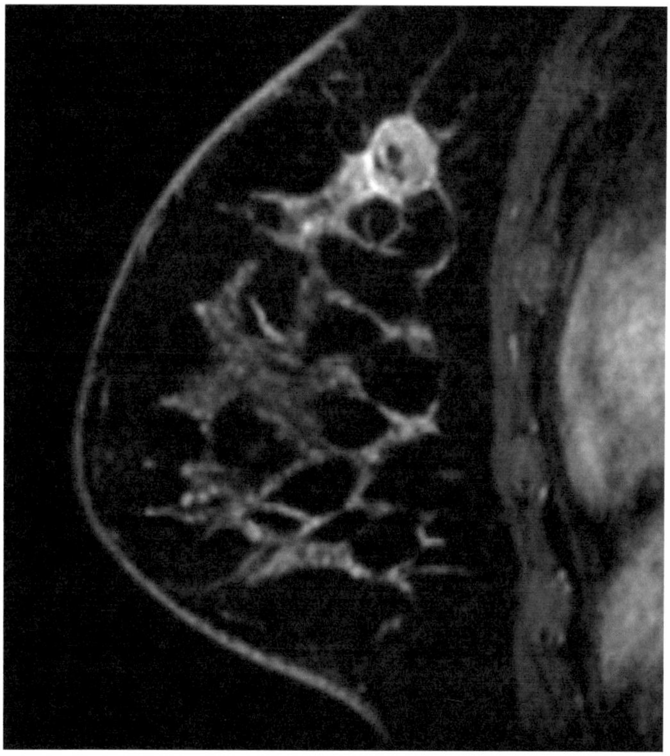

Fig. 4.3. A second representative case of IDC, MRI.

4. Discussion

There are a few reports describing mammography and ultrasound findings of triple-negative breast cancers (Ko ES et al., 2010; Wang Y et al., 2008; Yang WT et al., 2008). In those studies, comparisons were made between the mammography and ultrasound findings of hormone receptor negative, HER2-negative cancers with hormone receptor positive, HER2-negative cancers and hormone receptors negative, HER2-positive cancers. The radiological features of TN breast cancers included in our study were similar to the features described above. According to the Japanese data, hormone receptor positive breast cancer, such as luminal A or B, less likely to be found as a mass with pushing border compared to triple negative type cancers (Iwase H et al., 2010). Additionally, a few researchers have stated that triple-negative cancer is less frequently associated with calcifications, compared to the other subtypes. Collett et al. (Collett K et al., 2005) evaluated interval cancers diagnosed in a screening program between 1996 and 2001 and found that TN breast cancers were more likely than non-TN breast cancers to present in the interval between regular mammograms. The radiological features of TN breast cancer would give an answer to this.

Wang et al. showed that triple–negative cancers are less likely to be associated with spiculated margins on mammography than estrogen receptor–negative human epidermal growth factor receptor–positive cancers are. In their series of 23 TN breast cancers, 9% were mammographically occult and only 23% had associated calcifications. (Wang Y et al., 2008).

Dent et al determined that patients with TN breast cancers had a much lower proportion of breast cancers first detected by mammography or ultrasound than patients with other breast cancers (19.6% versus 36.0%) (Dent R et al., 2007).

Dogan et al reported that TN breast cancer features include; triple negative cancers were mammographically occult in 9% and sonographically occult in 7% of the patients (Dogan BE et al, 2010). When they could be visualized, the TN breast cancers had benign or indeterminate mammographic and sonographic findings, such as focal asymmetry (21%) and circumscribed round or oval masses (15.8%), despite their large size. Only three cases (6.8%) were identified as calcifications alone on mammography. Triple negative breast cancer is less likely to be detected in the routine screening using mammography alone. In contrast, all the cancers were visualized on MRI and showed characteristic findings associated with malignancy, as defined by the BI-RADS criteria. The most frequent MRI finding was a round or oval contrast-enhanced mass with irregular or spiculated margins and rim enhancements, (Schnall MD et al., 2006) and the characteristic shape is a common mammographic and ultrasound finding. Jinguji et al., who previously suggested an association of poor prognostic factors, such as nodal status, blood vessel invasion, and hormone receptor negativity, with rim enhancement on MRI, which are also some of the clinicopathological features of TN breast cancer. (Jinguji M et al., 2006)

Uematsu et al. suggested frequent association of rim enhancements and smooth mass margins on their series of TN breast cancers. (Uematsu T et al., 2009)

There are many reports describing the characteristic findings of MRI, although there are few describing those findings of mammogram or ultrasound.

In our study, we determined the radiological characteristics, which were often observed as a mass (65%) on mammography. In the ultrasound findings, we noted that TN breast cancers were more likely to be seen as mass lesions (71%), with oval or lobulated shapes, and hypo-echoic masses. Posterior echoes were less likely to attenuate, and vascularity was identified to some extent. From a previous report (Itoh A et al., 2006), the sensitivity, specificity, and accuracy of elastography were 83.3, 86.7, and 85.2%, respectively, with a cutoff score of between 3 and 4. Among the patients who were able to have elastography, TN breast cancer appeared as hard masses, with elasticity scores of 4 or 5. These findings represent TN tumor characteristics including high cellularity, less fibrous mass, and an elasticity score as high as ordinary invasive ductal carcinoma.

Our study showed that only 20% (4/20) of TN DCIS were detected because of mammographic abnormal calcifications. To gain a better understanding of the character of this rare type of DCIS, we retrospectively reviewed the charts and reports of each case.

Ordinarily, DCIS was first described a century ago by Dr. Joseph Bloodgood, but its natural history is poorly understood. In a large population-based surveillance, epidemiology, and end results series, Ernster et al. (Ernster VL et al., 2000) reported a 10-year mortality risk of DCIS of only 1.9%. Therefore, early detection is essential for improving the prognosis of breast cancer. The prognosis of TN invasive cancer is considered to be poor. If TN DCIS is a precursor of TN invasive carcinoma, detection of TN DCIS is attributed to appropriate treatment of the cases that may become TN invasive carcinoma.

DCIS was detected because of breast lumps or an abnormal discharge from the nipple. Through wider usage of MMG, and the development of radiological detection technologies capable of identifying breast abnormalities long before they become palpable, the frequency of DCIS detection has increased (Frykberg ER, 1997; Schnitt SJ et al., 1988; Dershaw DD, 1989; Stomper PC, 1989; Ikeda DM & Anderson I, 1989). Historically, most cases of DCIS (72–80%) have been diagnosed by MMG. This is mainly because of abnormal calcifications, such as necrotic calcifications representing dead tumor cells or secretory calcifications in tumor nests. Only 10–12% of DCIS cases have been discovered because of masses without calcifications revealed by MMG.

Abnormal calcifications are seen in approximately 62% (Ikeda DM & Andersson I, 1989) to 72% of common DCIS cases (Kopans DB, 1998). The percentage in TN DCIS cases of abnormal calcifications is considerably lower than in common DCIS cases.

In our cohort, the percentage of TN DCIS was only 3.0% of all DCIS. This percentage is much less than that of TN cancer rate in IDC cases.

When we investigated the reason why TN DCIS is so rare, we were able to identify a few possibilities. TN DCIS may grow rapidly in a short time span, which makes it difficult to detect during its noninvasive term. This is one possibility that TN cancers were reported more likely to present in the interval between regular mammograms. TN invasive carcinoma is known to have rapid growth characteristics and has a poor prognosis. On the basis of pathology and molecular studies, some DCIS represents a precursor to invasive breast cancer; however, the proportion of untreated DCIS that will progress to invasive breast cancer is uncertain (Bradley BB et al., 2006; Livasy CA, 2007; Flora Z, 2007). Ko et al. suggest that triple-negative breast cancer may develope rapidly to an invasive stage with no major in situ components or to a precancerous stage; hence, such tumors lack calcifications on mammography (Ko ES et al., 2010). Moriya et al. reported the incidence of TN DCIS among DCIS as being less than 5% (Moriya T et al., 2010). They also think it is possible that TN DCIS transforms to invasive cancer in its early stage, not remaining preinvasive DCIS. However, the presence of precursor lesions of TN breast cancer has not been clarified, and its origin and development remain to be investigated.

In our study, we identified a small number of patients (according to their mammograms) who were diagnosed as being without any abnormalities. If this were to happen in a normal screening process, such patients might slip through undiagnosed. We noted that ultrasound did indeed pick up all abnormalities. As a result, we can conclude that ultrasound used in combination with mammography is advantageous in detecting TN breast cancer.

Among DCIS, subtypes of DCIS correlate to the progression to invasive carcinoma; comedo type DCIS progresses to invasive carcinoma, both more often and more rapidly than low-grade DCIS (Pinder SE & Ellis IO, 2003; Ketcham AS & Moffat FL, 1990). From our findings, comedo components were frequently seen among lesions, and these comedo components are thought to be one reason for the rarity of TN DCIS. These results do not adequately explain the rarity of TN DCIS with its growth speed. The expression of ER, PgR, or HER2 is different between intraductal and invasive components within a patient in fewer cases, and its significance (whether it can be explained by dedifferentiation) has attracted a lot of interest recently. TN DCIS is thought to be a complex of several phenotypes. Not all TN DCIS cases progress rapidly to invasive cancer.

In lesions consistent with noninvasive and invasive components, the expression of HER2 differs between these two components, positive in the noninvasive part, and negative in the invasive part. ER positivity between these two components is almost the same (50–75%), however, HER2 positivity in DCIS is much higher than in invasive cancer, 32–55 and 20–25%, respectively. It is thought that a high proportion of DCIS lesions that progress to invasive lesions do lose overexpression of HER2 (Wiechmann L & Kuerer HM, 2008). Therefore, when hormone-negative and HER2-positive DCIS progresses to an invasive carcinoma, it becomes a TN invasive carcinoma, which might be another reason for the rarity of TN DCIS.

Our findings suggest that TN DCIS cases are less likely to have calcifications in comparison with non-TN DCIS. TN DCIS are also detected mainly as masses or asymmetry. US and MRI findings of TN DCIS are almost the same as those of DCIS as seen in previous studies. From our data, almost all TN DCIS were observed as low echoic masses by US, which leads us to believe that US is a more important diagnostic tool than MMG in detecting TN DCIS. By using US more frequently, the detection rate of TN DCIS should be elevated.

5. Conclusion

We diagnosed TN DCIS in 3.0% of all DCIS cases. There were fewer incidences of mammographic abnormal calcifications with TN DCIS than with non-TN DCIS. Mammography and ultrasound imaging together revealed that the morphological features of TN breast cancer include a lobulated mass, with less attenuating posterior echoes, some vascularity, and low elasticity.

6. References

Betsill, WLJ, Rosen, PP., Lieberman, PH. & Robbins, GF. (1987). Intraductal carcinoma. Long-term follow-up after treatment by biopsy alone. *JAMA*, Vol. 239, No.18, (May 1978), pp. 1863–7, ISSN 1538- 3598

Bradley, BB., Stuart, JS. & Laura, CC. (2006). Ductal carcinoma in situ with basal-like phenotype: a possible precursor to invasive basal-like breast cancer. *Mod Pathol.*, Vol.19, No.5, (May 2006), pp. 617–21, ISSN 1530-0285

Collett, K., Stefansson, IM., Eide, J., Braaten, A., Wang, H., Eide, GE., Thoresen, SØ., Foulkes, WD. & Akslen, LA. (2005). A basal epithelial phenotype is more frequent in interval breast cancers compared with screen detected tumors. *Cancer Epidemiol Biomarkers Prev.* Vol.14 No.5, (May 2005), pp. 1108-12, ISSN 1538-7755

Dent, R., Trudeau, M., Pritchard, KI., Hanna, WM., Kahn, HK., Sawka, CA., Lickley, LA., Rawlinson, E., Sun, P. & Narod, SA. (2007). Triple-negative breast cancer: clinical features and patterns of recurrence. *Clin Cancer Res.*, Vol.13, No,15, (Aug 2007), pp. 4429-4434, ISSN 1557-3265

Dershaw, DD., Abramson, A., Kinne, DW. (1989), Ductal carcinoma in situ: mammographic finings and clinical implications. *Radiology*, Vol. 170, No. 2, (Feb 1989), pp. 411–5, ISSN 1527-1315.

Dogan, BE., Gonzalez-Angulo, AM., Gilcrease, M., Dryden, MJ., Yang, WT. (2010). Multimodality imaging of triple receptor-negative tumors with mammography, ultrasound, and MRI. *Am J Roentgenol.* Vol.194, No.4, (Apr 2010), pp. 1160-6, ISSN 1546-3141

Ernster, VL., Barclay, J., Kerlikowske, K., Wilkie, H. & Ballard-Barbash, R. (2000). Mortality among women with ductal carcinoma in situ of the breast in the population-based surveillance, epidemiology and end results program. *Arch Intern Med.*, Vol.160, No.7, (Apr 2000), pp. 953–8, ISSN 1538-3679

Flora, Z., Theodoros, NS. & George, CZ. (2007). Precursors and preinvasive lesions of the breast: the role of molecular prognostic markers in the diagnostic and therapeutic dilemma. *World J Surg Oncol.*, Vol.5, (May 2007), pp. 57–68.

Frykberg, ER. (1997). An overview of the history and epidemiology of ductal carcinoma in situ of the breast. *Breast J.*, Vol.3, No.5, (Sep 1997), pp. 227–31, ISSN 1524-4741

Ikeda, DM., Anderson, I. (1989). Ductal carcinoma in situ: atypical mammographic appearances. *Radiology*. Vol.172, (Sep 1989), pp. 661–6, ISSN 1527-1315.

Itoh, A., Ueno, E., Tohno, E., Kamma, H., Takahashi, H., Shiina, T., Yamakawa, M., Matsumura, T. (2006). Breast disease: clinical application of US elastography for diagnosis. *Radiology*, Vol.239, No.2, (May 2006), pp. 341–50, ISSN 1527-1315

Iwase, H., Kurabayashi, J.,Tsuda, H., Ohta, T., Kurosumi, M., Miyamoto, K., Yamamoto, Y., Iwase, T. (2010). Clinicopathological analyses of triple negative breast cancer using surveillance data from the Registration Committee of the Japanese Breast Cancer Society. *Breast Cancer*, Vol.17, No.2, (Nov 2010), pp.118-24, ISSN 1880-4233

Jinguji, M., Kajiya, Y., Kamimura, K., Nakajo, M., Sagara, Y., Takahama, T., Ando, M., Rai, Y., Sagara, Y., Ohi, Y. & Yoshida, H. (2006). Rim enhancement of breast cancers on contrast-enhanced MR imaging: relationship with prognostic factors. *Breast Cancer*, Vol.13, No.1, (Jan 2006), pp. 64–73, ISSN 1880-4233

Ketcham, AS. & Moffat, FL. (1990). Vexed surgeons, perplexed patients, and breast cancers which may not be cancer. *Cancer*. Vol.65, No.3, (Feb 1990), pp. 387–93, ISSN 1097-0142

Ko, ES., Lee BH., Kim HA., Noh, WC., Kim, MS. & Lee, SA. (2010). Triplenegative breast cancer: correlation between imaging and pathological findings. *Eur Radiol*, Vol.20, No.5, (May 2010), pp. 1111–7, ISSN 0938-7994

Kopans, DB. (1998), *Breast imaging*, (2nd ed.), Lippincott-Raven, ISBN 0-397-51302-X, Philadelphia

Livasy, CA., Perou, CM., Karaca, G., Cowan, DW., Maia, D., Jackson, S., Tse, CK., Nyante, S. & Millikan, RC. (2007). Identification of a basal-like subtype of breast ductal carcinoma in situ. *Hum Pathol.*, Vol.38, No.2, (Feb 2007), pp. 197–204, ISSN 1532-8392

Moriya T, Kanomata N, Kozuka Y, Hirakawa H, Kimijima I, Kimura M, Watanabe M, Sasano H, Ishida T, Ohuchi N, Kurebayashi J. & Sonoo, H. (2010). Molecular morphological approach to the pathological study of development and advancement of human breast cancer, *Med Mol Morphol.*, Vol.43, No.2, (Jun 2010), pp. 67–73, ISSN 1860-1499

Page, DL., Dupont, WD., Rogers, LW. & Landenberger, M. (1982). Intraductal carcinoma of the breast: follow up after biopsy alone. *Cancer*, Vol.49, No. 4, (1982), pp. 751–8, ISSN 1097-0142

Page, DL., Dupont, WD., Rogers, LW., Jensen, RA. & Schuyler, PA. (1995). Continued local recurrence of carcinoma 15–25 years after a diagnosis of low grade ductal carcinoma in situ of the breast treated only by biopsy. *Cancer*, Vol.76, N0.7, (Oct 1995), pp. 1197–200, ISSN 1097-0142

Pinder, SE. & Ellis, IO. (2005). The diagnosis and management of preinvasive breast disease: ductal carcinoma in situ (DCIS) and atypical ductal hyperplasia (ADH)—current definitions and classification. *Breast Cancer Res.*, Vol.5, No. 5, (Jul 2003), pp. 254–7, ISSN 1465-5411

Schnall, MD., Blume, J., Bluemke, DA., DeAngelis, GA., DeBruhl, N., Harms, S., Heywang-Köbrunner, SH., Hylton, N., Kuhl, CK., Pisano, ED., Causer, P., Schnitt, SJ., Thickman, D., Stelling, CB., Weatherall, PT., Lehman, C. & Gatsonis, CA. (2006). Diagnostic architectural and dynamic features at breast MR imaging: multicenter study. *Radiology*, Vol.238, No.1, (Jan 2006), pp. 42–53, ISSN 1527-1315

Schnitt, SJ., Silen, W., Sadowsky, NL., Connolly, JL. & Harris JR. (1988). Ductal carcinoma in situ (intraductal carcinoma) of the breast. *N Engl J Med.*, Vol.318, No.14, (Apr 1988), pp. 898–903, ISSN 1533-4406

Simpson, JF. (2009). Update on atypical epithelial hyperplasia and ductal carcinoma in situ. *Pathology*, Vol.41, No.1, (Jan 2009), pp. 36–9, ISSN 1465-3931

Stomper, PC. (1989). Clinically occult ductal carcinoma in situ detected with mammography: analysis of 100 cases with radiologicpathologic correlation. *Radiology*, Vol.172, No.1, (Jul 1989), pp. 235–41, ISSN 1527-1315

The Committee of Mammography Guideline (Japan Radiological Society, Japanese Society of Radiological Technology). (December 2010). *Mammography guidelines* (3rd ed.), Igaku Syoin, ISBN978-4-260-01204-1, Tokyo, Japan

Uematsu, T., Kasami, M., Yuen, S. (2007). Triple-negative breast cancer: correlation between MR imaging and pathologic findings. *Radiology*, Vol.250, No.3, (Mar 2009), pp. 638–647, ISSN 1527-1315

Wang, Y., Ikeda, DM., Narasimhan, B., Longacre, TA., Bleicher, RJ., Pal, S., Jackman, RJ. & Jeffrey, SS. (2008) Estrogen receptor-negative invasive breast cancer: imaging features of tumors with and without human epidermal growth factor receptor type 2 overexpression. *Radiology*, Vol.246, No.2, (Feb 2008), pp. 367–75, ISSN 1527-1315

Wiechmann, L. & Kuerer, HM. (2008). The molecular journey from ductal carcinoma in situ to invasive breast cancer. *Cancer*. Vol.112, No.10, (May 2008), pp. 2130–42, ISSN 1097-0142

Yang, WT., Dryden, M., Broglio, K., Gilcrease, M., Dawood, S., Dempsey, PJ., Valero, V., Hortobagyi, G., Atchley, D. & Arun, B. (2008). Mammographic features of triple receptor negative primary breast cancers in young premenopausal women. *Breast Cancer Res Treat*, Vol.111, No.3, (Oct 2008), pp. 405–10, ISSN 0167-6806